Online Resources & Audiobook

Included with your purchase are multiple online resources. This includes the practice tests in an interactive format and this book in audiobook format. There is also a convenient study timer to help you manage your time.

Instructions for accessing these resources can be found on the last page of this book.

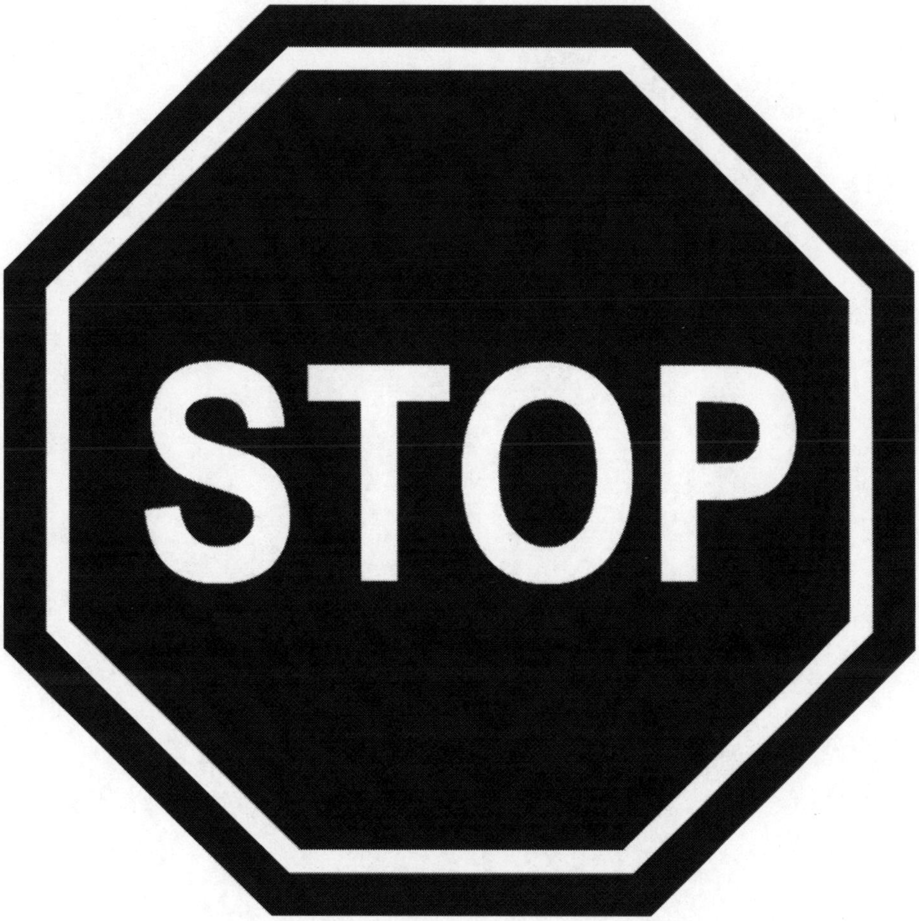

Nursing Professional Development Exam Study Guide

3 Practice Tests and NPD-BC Certification Prep Book [Includes Detailed Answer Explanations]

Lydia Morrison

Written and edited by TPB Publishing.

ISBN 13: 9781637758397

Table of Contents

Welcome

Dear Reader,

Welcome to your new Test Prep Books study guide! We are pleased that you chose us to help you prepare for your exam. There are many study options to choose from, and we appreciate you choosing us. Studying can be a daunting task, but we have designed a smart, effective study guide to help prepare you for what lies ahead.

Whether you're a parent helping your child learn and grow, a high school student working hard to get into your dream college, or a nursing student studying for a complex exam, we want to help give you the tools you need to succeed. We hope this study guide gives you the skills and the confidence to thrive, and we can't thank you enough for allowing us to be part of your journey.

In an effort to continue to improve our products, we welcome feedback from our customers. We look forward to hearing from you. Suggestions, success stories, and criticisms can all be communicated by emailing us at support@testprepbooks.com.

Sincerely,

Test Prep Books Team

Quick Overview

As you draw closer to taking your exam, effective preparation becomes more and more important. Thankfully, you have this study guide to help you get ready. Use this guide to help keep your studying on track and refer to it often.

This study guide contains several key sections that will help you be successful on your exam. The guide contains tips for what you should do the night before and the day of the test. Also included are test-taking tips. Knowing the right information is not always enough. Many well-prepared test takers struggle with exams. These tips will help equip you to accurately read, assess, and answer test questions.

A large part of the guide is devoted to showing you what content to expect on the exam and to helping you better understand that content. In this guide are practice test questions so that you can see how well you have grasped the content. Then, answer explanations are provided so that you can understand why you missed certain questions.

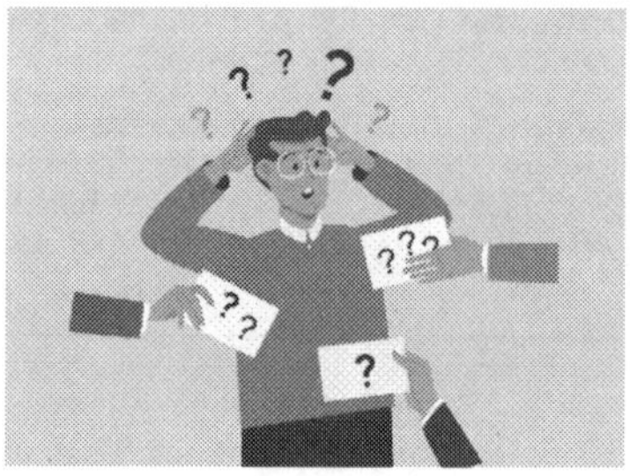

Don't try to cram the night before you take your exam. This is not a wise strategy for a few reasons. First, your retention of the information will be low. Your time would be better used by reviewing information you already know rather than trying to learn a lot of new information. Second, you will likely become stressed as you try to gain a large amount of knowledge in a short amount of time. Third, you will be depriving yourself of sleep. So be sure to go to bed at a reasonable time the night before. Being well-rested helps you focus and remain calm.

Be sure to eat a substantial breakfast the morning of the exam. If you are taking the exam in the afternoon, be sure to have a good lunch as well. Being hungry is distracting and can make it difficult to focus. You have hopefully spent lots of time preparing for the exam. Don't let an empty stomach get in the way of success!

When travelling to the testing center, leave earlier than needed. That way, you have a buffer in case you experience any delays. This will help you remain calm and will keep you from missing your appointment time at the testing center.

Be sure to pace yourself during the exam. Don't try to rush through the exam. There is no need to risk performing poorly on the exam just so you can leave the testing center early. Allow yourself to use all of the allotted time if needed.

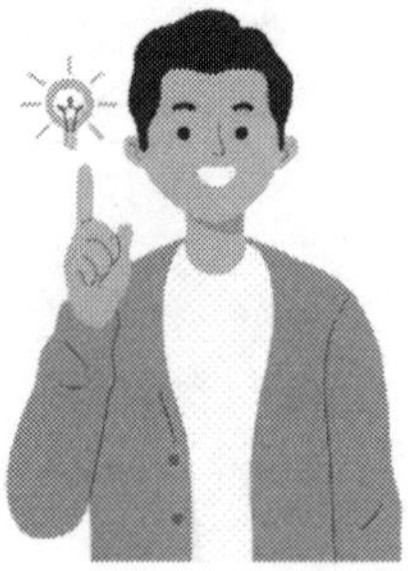

Remain positive while taking the exam even if you feel like you are performing poorly. Thinking about the content you should have mastered will not help you perform better on the exam.

Once the exam is complete, take some time to relax. Even if you feel that you need to take the exam again, you will be well served by some down time before you begin studying again. It's often easier to convince yourself to study if you know that it will come with a reward!

Test-Taking Strategies

1. Predicting the Answer

When you feel confident in your preparation for a multiple-choice test, try predicting the answer before reading the answer choices. This is especially useful on questions that test objective factual knowledge. By predicting the answer before reading the available choices, you eliminate the possibility that you will be distracted or led astray by an incorrect answer choice. You will feel more confident in your selection if you read the question, predict the answer, and then find your prediction among the answer choices. After using this strategy, be sure to still read all of the answer choices carefully and completely. If you feel unprepared, you should not attempt to predict the answers. This would be a waste of time and an opportunity for your mind to wander in the wrong direction.

2. Reading the Whole Question

Too often, test takers scan a multiple-choice question, recognize a few familiar words, and immediately jump to the answer choices. Test authors are aware of this common impatience, and they will sometimes prey upon it. For instance, a test author might subtly turn the question into a negative, or he or she might redirect the focus of the question right at the end. The only way to avoid falling into these traps is to read the entirety of the question carefully before reading the answer choices.

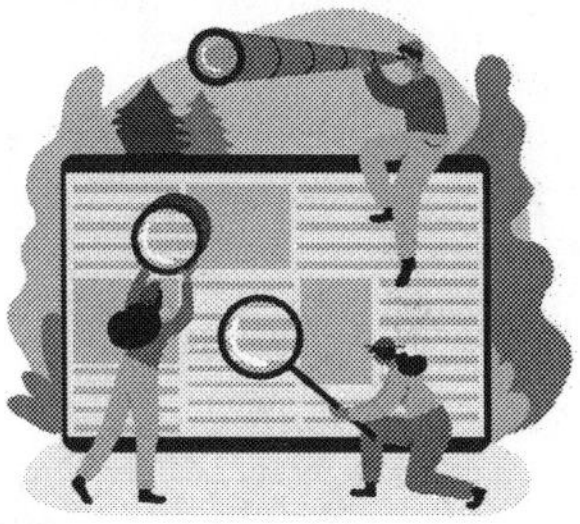

3. Looking for Wrong Answers

Long and complicated multiple-choice questions can be intimidating. One way to simplify a difficult multiple-choice question is to eliminate all of the answer choices that are clearly wrong. In most sets of answers, there will be at least one selection that can be dismissed right away. If the test is administered on paper, the test taker could draw a line through it to indicate that it may be ignored; otherwise, the test taker will have to perform this operation mentally or on scratch paper. In either case, once the obviously incorrect answers have been eliminated, the remaining choices may be considered. Sometimes identifying the clearly wrong answers will give the test taker some information about the correct answer. For instance, if one of the remaining answer choices is a direct opposite of one of the eliminated answer choices, it may well be the correct answer. The opposite of obviously wrong is obviously right! Of course, this is not always the case. Some answers are obviously incorrect simply because they are irrelevant to the question being asked. Still, identifying and eliminating some incorrect answer choices is a good way to simplify a multiple-choice question.

4. Don't Overanalyze

Anxious test takers often overanalyze questions. When you are nervous, your brain will often run wild, causing you to make associations and discover clues that don't actually exist. If you feel that this may be a problem for you, do whatever you can to slow down during the test. Try taking a deep breath or counting to ten. As you read and consider the question, restrict yourself to the particular words used by the author. Avoid thought tangents about what the author *really* meant, or what he or she was *trying* to say. The only things that matter on a multiple-choice test are the words that are actually in the question. You must avoid reading too much into a multiple-choice question, or supposing that the writer meant something other than what he or she wrote.

5. No Need for Panic

It is wise to learn as many strategies as possible before taking a multiple-choice test, but it is likely that you will come across a few questions for which you simply don't know the answer. In this situation, avoid panicking. Because most multiple-choice tests include dozens of questions, the relative value of a single wrong answer is small. As much as possible, you should compartmentalize each question on a multiple-choice test. In other words, you should not allow your feelings about one question to affect your success on the others. When you find a question that you either don't understand or don't know how to answer, just take a deep breath and do your best. Read the entire question slowly and carefully. Try rephrasing the question a couple of different ways. Then, read all of the answer choices carefully. After eliminating obviously wrong answers, make a selection and move on to the next question.

6. Confusing Answer Choices

When working on a difficult multiple-choice question, there may be a tendency to focus on the answer choices that are the easiest to understand. Many people, whether consciously or not, gravitate to the answer choices that require the least concentration, knowledge, and memory. This is a mistake. When you come across an answer choice that is confusing, you should give it extra attention. A question might be confusing because you do not know the subject matter to which it refers. If this is the case, don't eliminate the answer before you have affirmatively settled on another. When you come across an answer choice of this type, set it aside as you look at the remaining choices. If you can confidently assert that one of the other choices is correct, you can leave the confusing answer aside. Otherwise, you will need to take a moment to try to better understand the confusing answer choice. Rephrasing is one way to tease out the sense of a confusing answer choice.

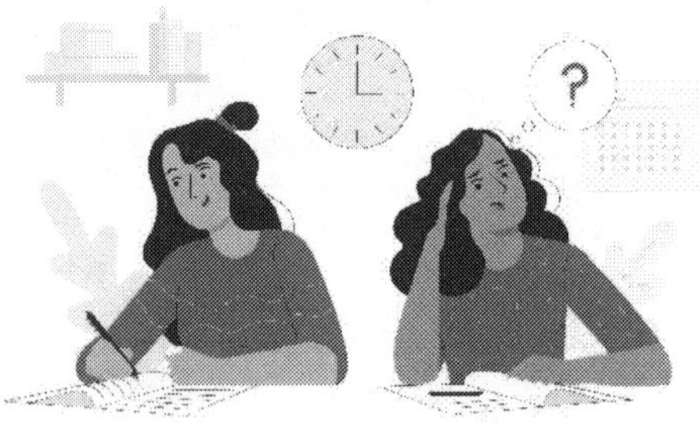

7. Your First Instinct

Many people struggle with multiple-choice tests because they overthink the questions. If you have studied sufficiently for the test, you should be prepared to trust your first instinct once you have carefully and completely read the question and all of the answer choices. There is a great deal of research suggesting that the mind can come to the correct conclusion very quickly once it has obtained all of the relevant information. At times, it may seem to you as if your intuition is working faster even than your reasoning mind. This may in fact be true. The knowledge you obtain while studying may be retrieved from your subconscious before you have a chance to work out the associations that support it. Verify your instinct by working out the reasons that it should be trusted.

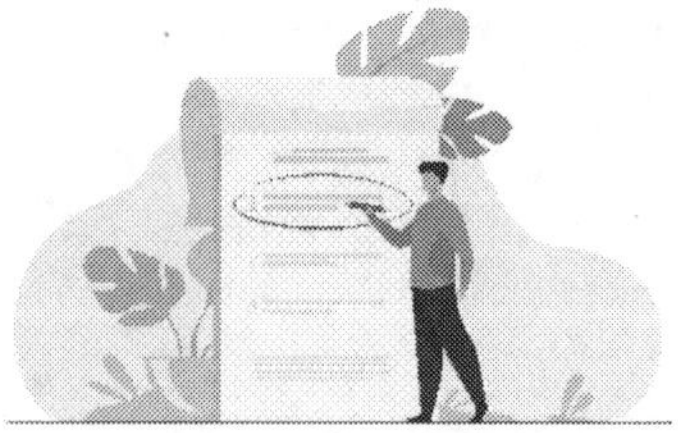

8. Key Words

Many test takers struggle with multiple-choice questions because they have poor reading comprehension skills. Quickly reading and understanding a multiple-choice question requires a mixture of skill and experience. To help with this, try jotting down a few key words and phrases on a piece of scrap paper. Doing this concentrates the process of reading and forces the mind to weigh the relative importance of the question's parts. In selecting words and phrases to write down, the test taker thinks about the question more deeply and carefully. This is especially true for multiple-choice questions that are preceded by a long prompt.

9. Subtle Negatives

One of the oldest tricks in the multiple-choice test writer's book is to subtly reverse the meaning of a question with a word like *not* or *except*. If you are not paying attention to each word in the question, you can easily be led astray by this trick. For instance, a common question format is, "Which of the following is...?" Obviously, if the question instead is, "Which of the following is not...?," then the answer will be quite different. Even worse, the test makers are aware of the potential for this mistake and will include one answer choice that would be correct if the question were not negated or reversed. A test taker who misses the reversal will find what he or she believes to be a correct answer and will be so confident that he or she will fail to reread the question and discover the original error. The only way to avoid this is to practice a wide variety of multiple-choice questions and to pay close attention to each and every word.

10. Reading Every Answer Choice

It may seem obvious, but you should always read every one of the answer choices! Too many test takers fall into the habit of scanning the question and assuming that they understand the question because they recognize a few key words. From there, they pick the first answer choice that answers the question they believe they have read. Test takers who read all of the answer choices might discover that one of the latter answer choices is actually *more* correct. Moreover, reading all of the answer choices can remind you of facts related to the question that can help you arrive at the correct answer. Sometimes, a misstatement or incorrect detail in one of the latter answer choices will trigger your memory of the subject and will enable you to find the right answer. Failing to read all of the answer choices is like not reading all of the items on a restaurant menu: you might miss out on the perfect choice.

11. Spot the Hedges

One of the keys to success on multiple-choice tests is paying close attention to every word. This is never truer than with words like *almost*, *most*, *some*, and *sometimes*. These words are called "hedges" because they

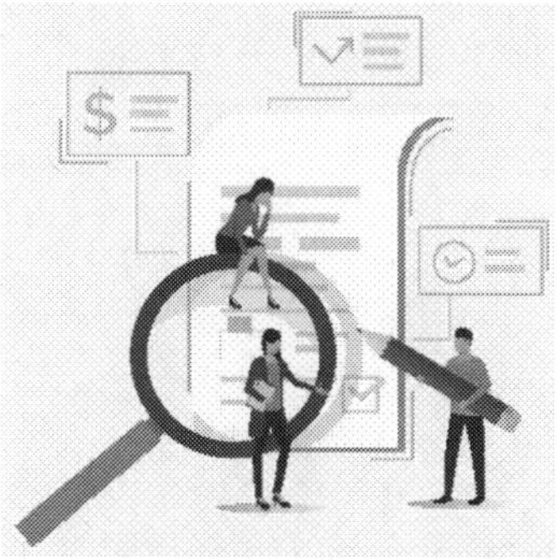

indicate that a statement is not totally true or not true in every place and time. An absolute statement will contain no hedges, but in many subjects, the answers are not always straightforward or absolute. There are always exceptions to the rules in these subjects. For this reason, you should favor those multiple-choice questions that contain hedging language. The presence of qualifying words indicates that the author is taking special care with his or her words, which is certainly important when composing the right answer. After all, there are many ways to be wrong, but there is only one way to be right! For this reason, it is wise to avoid answers that are absolute when taking a multiple-choice test. An absolute answer is one that says things are either all one way or all another. They often include words like *every*, *always*, *best*, and *never*. If you are taking a multiple-choice test in a subject that doesn't lend itself to absolute answers, be on your guard if you see any of these words.

12. Long Answers

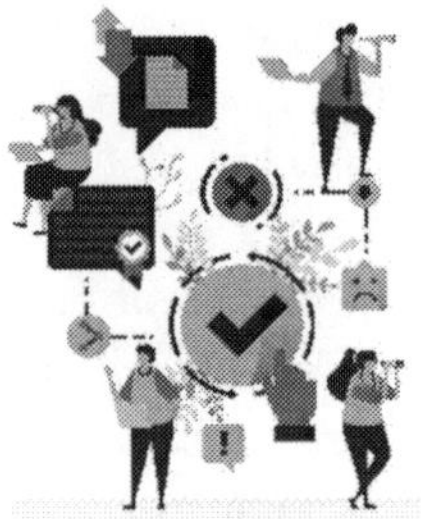

In many subject areas, the answers are not simple. As already mentioned, the right answer often requires hedges. Another common feature of the answers to a complex or subjective question are qualifying clauses, which are groups of words that subtly modify the meaning of the sentence. If the question or answer choice describes a rule to which there are exceptions or the subject matter is complicated, ambiguous, or confusing, the correct answer will require many words in order to be expressed clearly and accurately. In essence, you should not be deterred by answer choices that seem excessively long. Oftentimes, the author of the text will not be able to write the correct answer without offering some qualifications and modifications. Your job is to read the answer choices thoroughly and completely and to select the one that most accurately and precisely answers the question.

13. Restating to Understand

Sometimes, a question on a multiple-choice test is difficult not because of what it asks but because of how it is written. If this is the case, restate the question or answer choice in different words. This process serves a couple of important purposes. First, it forces you to concentrate on the core of the question. In order to rephrase the question accurately, you have to understand it well. Rephrasing the question will concentrate your mind on the key words and ideas. Second, it will present the information to your mind in a fresh way. This process may trigger your memory and render some useful scrap of information picked up while studying.

14. True Statements

Sometimes an answer choice will be true in itself, but it does not answer the question. This is one of the main reasons why it is essential to read the question carefully and completely before proceeding to the answer choices. Too often, test takers skip ahead to the answer choices and look for true statements. Having found one of these, they are content to select it without reference to the question above. The savvy test taker will always read the entire question before turning to the answer choices. Then, having settled on a correct answer choice, he or she will refer to the original question and ensure that the selected answer is relevant. The mistake of choosing a correct-but-irrelevant answer choice is especially common on questions related to specific pieces of objective knowledge.

15. No Patterns

One of the more dangerous ideas that circulates about multiple-choice tests is that the correct answers tend to fall into patterns. These erroneous ideas range from a belief that B and C are the most common right answers, to the idea that an unprepared test-taker should answer "A-B-A-C-A-D-A-B-A." It cannot be emphasized enough that pattern-seeking of this type is exactly the WRONG way to approach a multiple-choice test. To begin with, it is highly unlikely that the test maker will plot the correct answers according to some predetermined pattern. The questions are scrambled and delivered in a random order. Furthermore, even if the test maker was following a pattern in the assignation of correct answers, there is no reason why the test taker would know which pattern he or she was using. Any attempt to discern a pattern in the answer choices is a waste of time and a distraction from the real work of taking the test. A test taker would be much better served by extra preparation before the test than by reliance on a pattern in the answers.

Study Prep Plan

1. **Schedule** - Use one of our study schedules below or come up with one of your own.

2. **Relax** - Test anxiety can hurt even the best students. There are many ways to reduce stress. Find the one that works best for you.

3. **Execute** - Once you have a good plan in place, be sure to stick to it.

One Week Study Schedule

Day 1	Educational Process Standards
Day 2	Leadership
Day 3	Ethical, Legal, and Regulatory Standards
Day 4	Evidence-Based Practice and Research
Day 5	Program/Project Management and Process...
Day 6	Practice Test #1
Day 7	Take Your Exam!

Two Week Study Schedule

Day 1	Educational Process Standards	Day 8	Technology
Day 2	Leadership	Day 9	Program/Project Management and...
Day 3	Diversity, Equity, and Inclusion Advocacy	Day 10	Project Management
Day 4	Ethical, Legal, and Regulatory Standards	Day 11	Practice Test #1
Day 5	Analysis of Gaps in Practice that...	Day 12	Practice Test #2
Day 6	Legal and Compliance	Day 13	Practice Test #3
Day 7	Evidence-Based Practice and Research	Day 14	Take Your Exam!

One Month Study Schedule

Day 1	Educational Process Standards	Day 11	Ethical, Legal, and Regulatory Standards	Day 21	Organizational Performance Indicators...
Day 2	Learner Characteristics	Day 12	Risk Management	Day 22	Project Management
Day 3	Educational Design and Delivery	Day 13	Analysis of Gaps in Practice that...	Day 23	Performance Improvement
Day 4	Continuing Education and Accreditation	Day 14	Legal and Compliance	Day 24	Practice Test #1
Day 5	Leadership	Day 15	Integration of Legal and Regulatory...	Day 25	Answer Explanations #1
Day 6	Change Management	Day 16	Evidence-Based Practice and Research	Day 26	Practice Test #2
Day 7	Promotion of a Healthy Work...	Day 17	Processes, Translation, and Dissemination of...	Day 27	Answer Explanations #2
Day 8	Diversity, Equity, and Inclusion Advocacy	Day 18	Technology	Day 28	Practice Test #3
Day 9	Group Facilitation	Day 19	Technology Tools and Strategies	Day 29	Answer Explanations #3
Day 10	Mentoring Processes	Day 20	Program/Project Management and...	Day 30	Take Your Exam!

Build your own prep plan by visiting the Online Resources page.

Instructions and a QR code can be found on the last page of this guide.

As you study for your test, we'd like to take the opportunity to remind you that you are capable of great things! With the right tools and dedication, you truly can do anything you set your mind to. The fact that you are holding this book right now shows how committed you are. In case no one has told you lately, you've got this! Our intention behind including this coloring page is to give you the chance to take some time to engage your creative side when you need a little brain-break from studying. As a company, we want to encourage people like you to achieve their dreams by providing good quality study materials for the tests and certifications that improve careers and change lives. As individuals, many of us have taken such tests in our careers, and we know how challenging this process can be. While we can't come alongside you and cheer you on personally, we can offer you the space to recall your purpose, reconnect with your passion, and refresh your brain through an artistic practice. We wish you every success, and happy studying!

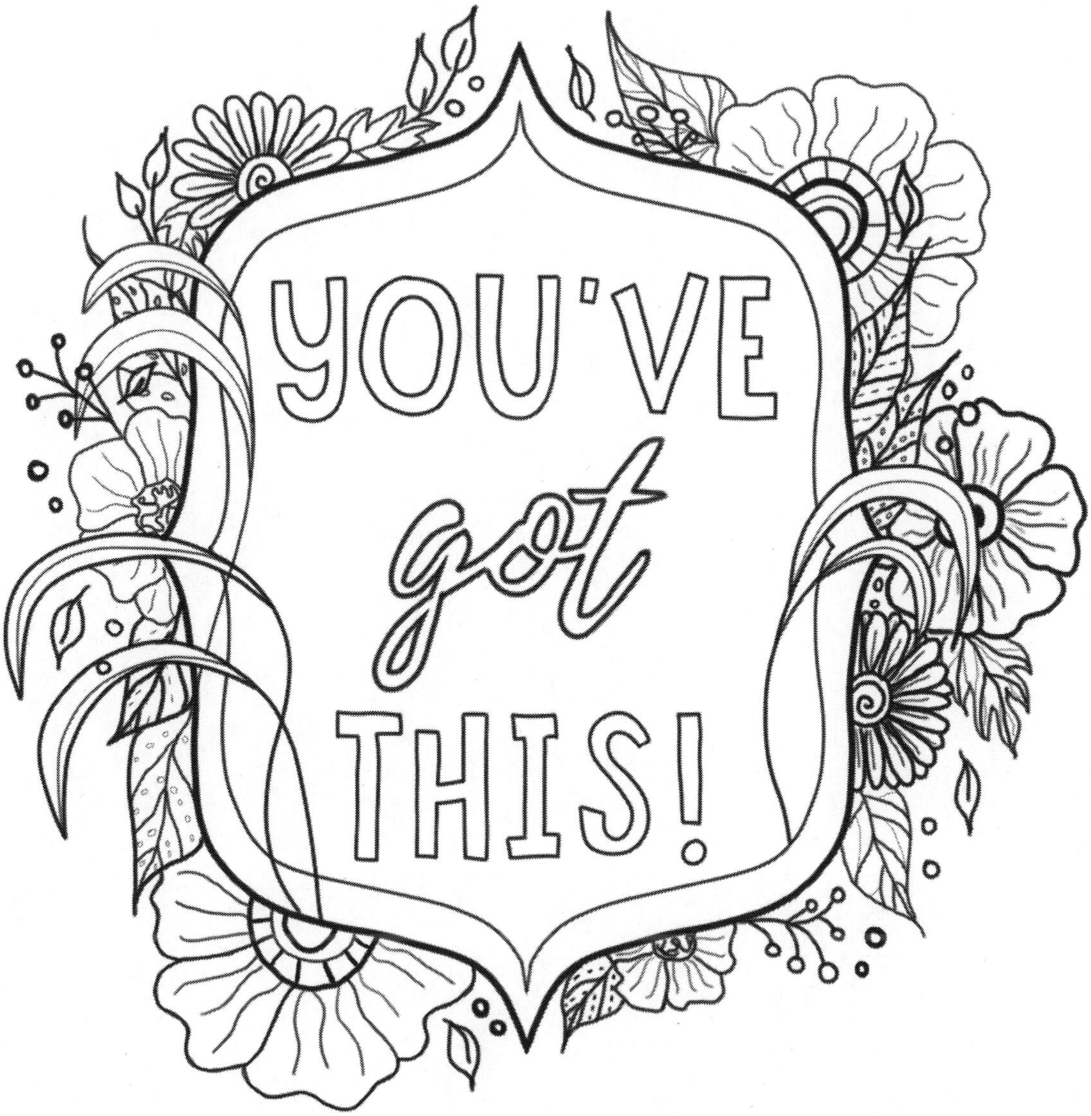

Introduction

Function of the Test

The Nursing Professional Development Board Certification Examination (NPD-BC) is one of many specialty certification exams administered by the American Nurses Credentialing Center (ANCC). This exam is designed for registered nurses working in the nursing professional development realm who seek to demonstrate competency in and commitment to their field. The exam is accredited by The Accreditation Board for Specialty Nursing Certification (ABSNC) and the National Commission for Certifying Agencies (NCCA). After receiving a passing score, the nurse will be awarded the NPD-BC credential, which is valid for five years.

The first step in taking the Nursing Professional Development Board Certification Examination begins with an online application. Eligibility requirements for the exam include the following:

- Active Registered Nurse (RN) licensure
- Bachelor's degree or higher in Nursing
- Minimum of two years of full-time RN practice
- Minimum of 2,000 hours of nursing professional development practice within the last three years
- Minimum of 30 hours of continuing education in nursing professional development within the last three years

The content of the exam is developed by a panel of experts and certified nurses in the specialty area. Based on the results of a role delineation study, the exam focuses on six areas of competency: Educational Process Standards; Leadership; Ethical, Legal, and Regulatory Standards; Evidence-Based Practice and Research; Technology; and Program/Project Management and Process Improvement. This supports the goal of accurately validating the candidate's knowledge and skillset in the field of nursing professional development.

Test Administration

Candidates who meet eligibility requirements will receive approval to schedule their exam within a 120-day testing window. The exam is delivered in a computer-based format at Prometric testing centers. For special testing accommodations, a signed document from the candidate's physician or healthcare professional must be submitted prior to scheduling the exam. Appointments may be rescheduled or canceled at least two days prior to the testing date to avoid loss of exam fees. If needed, a one-time extension to the 120-day testing window may be requested for an additional cost. To provide proof of identity on the day of the exam, candidates must bring at least one form of identification (e.g., driver's license or passport). Prohibited items in the testing area include items such as cell phones, books, study notes, and food/drink. Candidates should plan to arrive at least fifteen minutes prior to their appointment time to allow adequate time for check-in and preparation for the exam.

Test Format

The Nursing Professional Development Board Certification Examination (NPD-BC) consists of 150 questions. Of these questions, 125 are scored and the remaining 25 are unscored pretest questions. While the pretest questions do not affect the candidate's results, all test questions must be answered since the difference between the two is not distinguished on the exam. Candidates will have three hours in which to complete the exam. The following table represents a breakdown of exam topics by number of questions and percentage:

Competency Area	Questions	Percentage
Educational Process Standards	32	26%
Leadership	34	27%
Ethical, Legal, and Regulatory Standards	19	15%
Evidence-Based Practice and Research	7	6%
Technology	19	15%
Program/Project Management and Process Improvement	14	11%
Total	**125**	**100%**

Scoring

Test results are determined based on the established minimum passing score for the exam. Upon completion of the exam, candidates will receive a score of pass or fail. For those who do not pass the exam, a detailed report of performance in each content area will be provided to aid in studying for a future attempt. Following a 60-day time period and submission of a new application, retesting can be scheduled. Candidates can retest a maximum of three times within a 12-month time period.

Educational Process Standards

Theories, Models, and Principles

Nursing Philosophy

Nursing philosophy refers to a definition of what is considered to be the most important aspect or aspects of nursing practice and its foundation. Many great nursing scholars have established changing ideas of what the philosophy of nursing is meant to be. Florence Nightingale's philosophy of nursing focused on the improvement of environmental factors to improve patient health. Jean Watson, on the other hand, focused more on the belief that the most important aspect of nursing is caring for patients. Similarly, Ernestine Wiedenbach encouraged providing for the individualized needs of each patient, and Virginia Henderson believed in helping patients achieve their highest level of independence and self-care. Modern nursing philosophy and practice may include all or most of these sentiments depending on the patient, the situation, and even the specific nurse. It is important for nurses to determine which philosophy or philosophies best fit their practice to provide the best outcomes for their patients. It is also important to be aware that nurses from different backgrounds with different values and experiences may have slightly different beliefs on which nursing philosophy is best for their practice. These differences working together can benefit the nursing profession as a whole, providing different perspectives that may better meet patient needs.

Standards of Nursing Professional Development Practice

Established to provide guidance and direction to the nursing body, nursing professional development standards are ever evolving and adapting to nursing science. The standards are developed by the American Nurses Association (ANA) for all registered nurses, including advanced roles. These standards set precedence for building competencies that encourage nurses to meet and exceed the skills, knowledge, and abilities needed to successfully perform duties.

The nursing professional development practice model comprises several functions that support and engage nurses to promote a high level of competency in nursing practice. These roles include serving as a mentor, learning facilitator, leader, and champion of scientific inquiry, and advocating for advancing nursing autonomy. Working at the highest level of the nursing scope of practice is an expectation encouraged through higher education, professional nursing practice enrichment, and professional development plans to meet individualized career goals.

There are six primary standards of nursing professional development advocated for by ANA. The first is Assessment, which includes data collection, analysis, and presenting the facts and figures in a meaningful way to enhance understanding and sharing. Data is obtained from sources based on the query and must be thoroughly checked for accuracy and non-bias.

Diagnosis is the next standard; this consists of interpreting and applying data to develop an action plan that addresses gaps in practice and vulnerabilities to patient care outcomes. This information is important to the goal of differentiating between performance issues versus failures in systems. Instituting a culture of safety begins here with conducting non-punitive investigations to mitigate risk. Emphasis is placed on finding solutions to process problems rather than assigning blame.

The third standard is outcomes identification; this focuses on developing goals that are evidence-based, measurable, and that distinguish the objective. After the goal is established, the process moves into planning, the fourth standard. Planning incorporates the application of a systems outlook to develop initiatives, improve cultural norms, and create content aimed at achieving the identified goals.

The final standards, implementation and evaluation, are the confirmed execution of action from the work completed through the previous standards. Implementation requires buy-in from all healthcare services affected, alignment with organizational goals, and support for learning and sustainment of new practices. Evaluating the activities requires assessment through the change process, which involves gathering feedback and analyzing outcome measures to determine the efficacy and adoption of change.

Nursing professional development standards may be fulfilled on micro and macro levels to enhance nursing care and elevate the status of the collective as a fully contributing member within the multidisciplinary health team. Individuals can focus on this merit by increasing knowledge in their specialty, seeking certification, and employing evidence-based practices at the bedside to drive patient care. Mentoring is another way that nurses can engage with other nurses, healthcare staff, or students to share expertise and cultivate professionalism. Self-directed education and continuous learning can be achieved through reading current nursing publications and journal articles or by taking on projects within the workplace to improve patient care and safety. Healthcare organizations can strive to support nursing professionalism by achieving recognition as a facility that promotes nursing practice, provides quality outcomes, and reduces attrition rates. Organizational elements that align with established best practices in nursing foster these standards and frameworks.

Teaching/Learning Theories, Models, and Principles

When a new nurse joins a unit or when further education may be required, the nurse can refer to different coaching and learning theories in order to best assess the needs of the learner and where they are in their learning process. Within nursing, most learning theories relate to how the learner acts and how they express their thoughts and understanding. Examples of different theories that can be used include behaviorism, cognitive learning, constructivism, educational neuroscience, humanism, and connectivism. These may be used independently or interconnectedly depending on the learner and the learning situation, but when applied effectively, they can promote successful coaching and learning.

Behaviorism

Behaviorism refers to the observable aspects of learning or the actions of the learner. This is most strongly applicable to teaching new skills. For example, the coach may demonstrate the skill to the learner and then observe the learner repeat the skill. Corrections may be made until the skill is demonstrated accurately. Nurse educators may use this method when new equipment is being introduced to ensure that all staff know how to use them properly. While this theory of learning is helpful for specific tasks, it does not go any deeper to show that the learner knows when to or why they should perform this skill.

Cognitive Learning

Cognitive learning refers to more brain-based learning. This can be in the form of providing written resources or even classroom learning to better understand the fundamentals of something. Cognitive learning is generally demonstrated verbally or through testing to ensure that the learner has retained the new knowledge. However, this is mainly a demonstration of knowledge on a more surface level, such as regurgitation of facts or new policies. For example, the learner may be able to say that it is procedure to keep the head-bleed patient's head of the bed elevated but may not necessarily know why or be able to come to that conclusion on their own.

Social Constructivism

Constructivism is a theory that combines knowledge from behaviorism and cognitive learning and adds critical thinking and creativity to the mix. The learner may apply what they have learned to new situations or even create hypothetical situations to show understanding. This learning may be demonstrated through both verbalization and action. The learner may find a unique way to perform a skill that is more appropriate for a specific situation or may better advocate for a patient given their overall presentation rather than just hospital policy. In order to coach the learner through constructivism, it is important to ask the questions "why?" and "how would you act if…?"

Educational Neuroscience

Within the past decade, the application of neuroscience to enhance learning has been explored within academia. Learning comprises various aspects involving sensory input, information processing, and storage. Students use each of their sensory inputs to learn, including touch, sight, feel, hearing, and taste. Research has shown that in order to learn and retain information more effectively, there must be a knowledge base to build upon when processing data that is being received. The stronger the knowledge base, the more likely the information will be retained. Retention occurs through an immediate process, where information is used immediately. This is also referred to as the working memory. For long-term storage, the information must be memorized. This is developed through repetition and applying the information to a previous context. Repetition comes from repeated exposure to a concept while relating this memory to an event. By using a multimodal system of learning, including senses, repetition, and building upon knowledge, learning experiences become beneficial and engaging to the student. Educational neuroscience draws upon and aligns with other learning theories, including social learning theory, constructivism, behaviorism, and cognitivism.

Humanism and Connectivism

The final two theories, humanism and connectivism, focus more on how the coach interacts with the learner than how to assess the learner's retention of knowledge. Humanism refers to the need to focus on the learner and find out what their goals and needs are. When the coach works to help the learner meet their goals, it increases the learner's sense of autonomy and pride in their work and accomplishments. This theory may not apply, however, if the learner's goals do not align with the needs or goals of the unit. Connectivism refers to identifying holes in the learner's knowledge and providing them with the resources to independently find answers. Examples of this could be showing the learner how to access the hospital or unit's policy and procedure databases, how to find medication references, and how to contact someone if they need help. This is especially important so that the learner feels they have the resources they need and know where to look if they don't know the answer once they no longer have a coach by their side.

Learning Styles

Patient education is a critical part of empowering patients to make informed decisions and be actively involved in their health care. Additionally, patient health education after they have received a serious diagnosis may be the most intensive health education that the patient has ever received. Therefore, it is important that nurses have a comprehensive understanding of the different styles in which people learn and barriers they may face. People primarily learn best through auditory, visual, or kinetic learning techniques; often, an integrated approach provides the best educational value. **Auditory education** techniques may include having a conversation with the patient, providing a relevant podcast for the patient to listen to, or holding an open lecture on a specific health topic. **Visual education** techniques may involve the use of charts, 3-D models, printed materials, pictures, or a presentation. **Kinetic education** techniques allow the patient to apply the material in a hands-on way, such as by practicing injecting a medication into a mannequin before trying to do so at home. Barriers to patient learning may include a lack of interest or the inability to take their health status seriously, poor literacy or comprehension skills, or an inability to attend educational sessions (e.g., due to lack of transportation or childcare). Other barriers may involve the healthcare provider. For example, the healthcare provider must ensure that they are communicating in a way that is easily understandable to the patient rather than using complex medical lingo. They also must ensure that they create a warm environment and build a relationship with the patient, so that the patient feels comfortable discussing topics he or she doesn't understand. Patient discomfort or unwillingness to discuss topics with the healthcare provider, due to embarrassment or shame, is a barrier that can be easily prevented.

Teaching Methods

Patient teaching takes place in different settings and formats. The method of choice can be determined by a variety of factors, including learner preference, educator preference, the topic, the setting, and the availability of time and resources. Learning can occur with the help of audio, visual, written, or activity-based methods, and learners tend to fall on a wide spectrum of preference. Typically, individuals require several exposures to new information before it is retained. Additionally, factors such as age, level of education, language barriers, emotional state, desire to learn, pain level, disability, and many others can significantly impact the ability of an individual to take in and retain new information. Therefore, patient teaching requires individual consideration and benefits from the use of a variety of teaching methods over a span of time.

The following are some of the common methods used to facilitate teaching:

- **Written materials:** Written handouts, brochures, or pamphlets include information about various topics (e.g., disease, procedure, treatment, or medication). These are often accompanied by visual tools to support written information and are often more affordable and convenient for teachers. They can be reviewed repeatedly over time and taken from the care site to the patient's home.
- **Visual tools:** Charts, graphs, pictures, posters, and drawings can provide a visual way to convey a significant amount of information at once and can organize complex ideas. They can be reviewed repeatedly over time and are cost-effective resources. Some visual materials, like brochures, can be taken from the care site, while other materials, like posters, remain at the care site.
- **Audio and audiovisual materials:** Video clips, video programs, recorded interviews, podcasts, or recorded demonstrations can provide learners with opportunities to review information as often as needed and can also be a more interesting method of facilitating patient learning. This can be more costly for organizations to create and is also somewhat limited to individuals who possess the technology required to view the materials; it is also limited by a patient's comfort and desire to use the given media.
- **Discussion:** In-person, virtual, telephonic, email, support group, workshop, or classes provide an opportunity for two-way dialogue between learner and teacher. Discussions can be individual or group-based and can occur in a variety of settings. Teachers have an opportunity to provide learners with a variety of teaching methods to facilitate learning.
- **Demonstration:** Models and training equipment can be utilized in live or recorded sessions to supplement learning through visual representation of a process or procedure. This method is often accompanied by verbal discussion. Live demonstration can provide opportunities for repetition or focus on a specific portion of the demonstration. Patients can also sometimes have the opportunity to handle and practice with training equipment or models in order to increase comfort and decrease anxiety.

Teach Back Method

The "Teach Back" method is an interactive educational technique that fosters rapport, communication, and information sharing between healthcare providers and patients. It encourages the healthcare providers to explain medical diagnoses, prognoses, and plans of care to patients in clear, non-medical terms. Then, patients are asked to explain the medical situation and plan of care to the healthcare professional, utilizing their own understanding. This empowers patients to actively engage in their care plans and understand their health in a new way. It also allows the healthcare provider to determine whether or not the patient has an appropriate understanding of their health situation and how to manage care once they are out of the medical setting. Providers should remain calm, compassionate, and responsive during this process, even if the patient is unable to correctly teach back right away.

Adult Learning Principles

Facilitation of Learning

Facilitation of learning refers to the process of assessing the learning needs of the patient and family, the nursing staff, and caregivers in the community, and creating, implementing, and evaluating formal and informal educational programs to address those needs. Novice nurses often view patient care and patient education as separate entities;

however, experienced nurses are able to integrate the patient's educational needs into the plan of care. Nurses are aware that the patient often requires continued reinforcement of the educational plan after discharge, which necessitates coordination with home care services.

As facilitators of learning, nurses may be involved in a large-scale effort to educate all patients over 65 admitted to the nursing unit about the need for both Prevnar 13 and Pneumovax 23 to prevent pneumonia. In contrast, nurses may provide one-on-one instruction for a patient recently diagnosed with diabetes. The first step of any teaching-learning initiative is the assessment of the learning needs of the participants. Specific needs that influence the design and content of the educational offering include the language preference and reading level of the participants. Nurses must also consider the effect of certain characteristics, identified in the Synergy Model, on the patient's capacity to process information. Diminished resiliency or stability, as well as extreme complexity, are examples of characteristics that must be considered in the development of the educational plan. Nurses are also responsible for creating a bridge between teaching and learning in the acute care setting and the home environment. A detailed discharge plan, close coordination with outpatient providers, and follow-up phone calls to the patient may be used to reinforce the patient's knowledge of the plan of care.

Successful learning plans for staff members and colleagues also consider the motivation of the participants to engage in the process. Successful facilitators include a variety of teaching strategies to develop the content and evaluate learning, in order to address adult learning needs and preferences, such as preferred language and reading level. Research indicates that when adults do not have a vested interest in the outcomes of the teaching/learning process, they may not participate as active learners.

The remaining element of successful facilitation of learning is the availability and quality of learning resources. There is evidence that individuals with different learning styles respond differently to various learning devices. The minimum requirements for successful facilitation of learning include the skilled staff to develop the educational materials, paper, a copy machine, and staff to interact with the patient in the learning session.

Barriers to the facilitation of learning must be anticipated and accommodated. Changes in the patient's condition commonly require reduction in the time spent in each learning session due to fatigue. Cognitive impairment can impede comprehension and retention of the information and will require appropriate teaching aids. The learning abilities of the patient's family members must also be assessed. Adequate instruction time might be the greatest barrier. Learning needs are assessed and discharge planning is begun on the day of admission; however, shortened inpatient stays require evaluation of the patient's comprehension of the plan of care.

Encouraging Critical Thinking

Critical thinking is a skill that comes from experience (both successes and failures). The nurse-to-be can be the smartest person in the classroom, making perfect scores on every test, but will not be able to provide quality care without using critical thinking. Common practices for using critical thinking in nursing include the following:

- Using self-regulation
- Practicing problem-solving
- Analyzing and interpreting information
- Making appropriate inferences
- Using the nursing process

Self-Regulation

Self-regulation is a responsibility of every nurse. To self-regulate, the nurse must first fully understand their individual scope of practice (federal, state, and agency regulations). Practicing within the established scope of practice, the nurse's goal is to provide effective, safe, and ethical care practices.

Problem Solving

Problem-solving skills are essential in the practice of critical thinking. Using critical thinking to recognize the problem is important, but the nurse must also cultivate the mindset of finding potential solutions. Problem solving can be seen formally in care plans, but the nurse will need to understand the importance of putting this into practice.

For example, say a patient is prescribed digoxin, and the nurse is due to administer the medication. The nurse with critical thinking skills will check the heart rate prior to administering the medication. Upon further assessment, the heart rate is 40 bpm. The nurse with problem-solving skills will recognize that this medication should not be administered, and the medical provider should be contacted for further orders.

Analysis, Interpretation, and Making Inferences

Additional key practices in critical thinking include analyzing data, interpreting results, and making inferences based on that interpretation. Why is the patient's heart rate 40 bpm? That would be the question the nurse needs to analyze, and they could find that information by looking through past vital sign trends, medications, comorbidities, and procedures. It is important for the healthcare team not to stop at just recognizing the problem and solving it, as that does not likely prevent the problem from happening again. Analyzing the data gives the nurse the information to interpret and then allows them to make clinical inferences based on the results.

For example, if the previously mentioned patient was also taking ivabradine, an HCN channel blocker for progressing heart failure, the nurse could infer that the combination of ivabradine and digoxin is the culprit of the patient's bradycardia. The following is a breakdown of the critical-thinking process in this scenario:

- **Analyzing** the medication administration record
- Interpreting the results
- **Inferring** that the synergistic effect of the medications can cause the problem

This process of critical thinking allows the medical team to either closely monitor the patient on both medications or make a medication change to acknowledge the problem.

Therapeutic Communication

Overcoming barriers to communication requires practicing therapeutic communication. Therapeutic communication is a type of communication that assists the patient in the healing process rather than hindering it. There are a number of useful communication techniques the nurse can employ to aid in therapeutic communication.

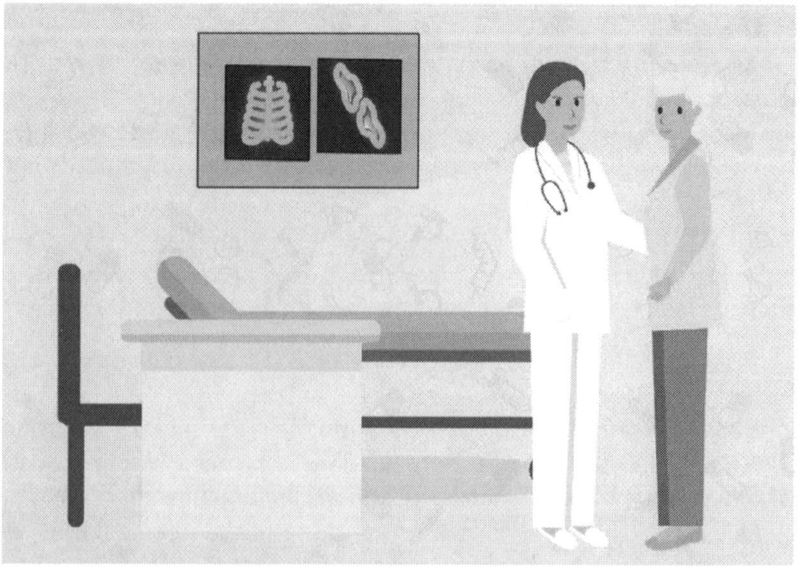

Sometimes, silence is the best way to get clarification from a patient, or simply asking them to clarify when one does not understand. Nurses may offer themselves to support the patient without providing personal details, by sympathizing and saying, "Yes, I have been through something similar." The nurse may ask the patient to summarize their thoughts or identify a theme when stories go on at length. This helps redirect communication in a positive direction.

Asking the patient how certain events made them feel is a way to investigate the patient's emotional status. The nurse may give information about their role and make observations, such as "I noticed you seem tense," to open the door to more fluent conversation. Giving the patient praise and recognition without overt flattery is a way to show support, such as complimenting a noticeable effort during a physical therapy session. The nurse may want to determine the chronological order of events, which can be helpful for reporting information.

Employing therapeutic communication aids smooth collaboration and cooperation between members of the healthcare team. Incorporating smart, simple, therapeutic communication techniques and overcoming barriers to communication are important parts of achieving this goal.

Motivational Interviewing

Motivational interviewing (MI) is a communication technique that focuses on altering the patient's behavior. It is often used as a counseling tool for patients with substance use disorders, behavioral alterations, smoking, and obesity. There is a subset of skills used in MI that facilitate the progress in each of the MI phases. The **OARS** skills are a set of verbal and non-verbal interview techniques, which can be tailored to the specific needs of the MI process. The acronym OARS stands for **open-ended questions**, **affirmations**, **reflections**, and **summaries**.

Open-ended questions encourage two-way conversation because they are not generally answerable with a simple "yes" or "no." Questions beginning with the word "why" can potentially elicit a defensive patient response and should be avoided. **Affirmations** acknowledge the patient and convey a message of empathetic understanding. These statements can also build a patient's self-efficacy which positively affects motivation. **Reflections**, or reflective listening, improve the interviewer's understanding of the patient's narrative. Periods of reflection after the patient speaks slow the pace of the conversation so that it is not simply a series of questions and answers. **Summaries** provide a review of the substance of the conversation and an opportunity for closure by the interviewer and the patient.

The OARS skills are used with each process of MI to maximize the outcomes. If the work of the MI process is slowed down or is unsuccessful at any point, the provider returns to the initial process and reestablishes it. MI is not a linear process; it is responsive to the flow of the conversation, which depends on the skill of the interviewer and the use of the OARS techniques. The four processes of MI include engaging, focusing, evoking, and planning. **Engaging** is the process of establishing a rapport, assessing and reducing any defensive behavior, and creating a collaborative environment for the discussion of change. The interviewer is able to assess the focus of the patient's conversation; in other words, is the patient actually engaged in the work of MI. If the patient is resistant to participating in the process of MI, the interviewer often finds that empathy is effective in re-establishing the interviewer-patient relationship.

The second process of MI is **focusing**. Communication experts advise that it may take several sessions before the interviewer can direct the conversation to the issue at hand. The potential for success at this stage is enhanced when the patient has already reached a state of contemplation for the desired change. The process of **evoking** focuses on the discussion or "**change talk**" for two behaviors: identification of the specific steps necessary for the desired change and the steps required for an ongoing commitment to the changed behavior. There are two forms of change talk: **preparatory** refers to the desire to change, and **mobilizing** addresses commitment and action. The **planning** process may be optional, but when it is included in MI, it identifies the "how" for the planned change.

Shared Decision-Making

Shared decision-making is a patient care model that focuses on the patients' involvement in care decisions for every aspect of their own care, in partnership with the primary care providers. Although patients currently have access to vast amounts of information in many forms, the average patient continues to voice frustration with the perceived amount of personal input into the plan of care. The **SHARE approach** is a five-step program that was developed by the Agency for Healthcare Research and Quality (AHRQ) to give primary care providers the necessary tools to improve patient satisfaction through increased participation in decision-making. One of the key elements of this model is enhanced communication between the provider and the patient. Researchers found that providers wait an average of 17 seconds after their first question before asking their second question. Clearly, this does not provide the patient with sufficient time to participate in the care planning process. Providers are reminded to provide the patient with appropriate information sources and to then use "teach back" to verify the patient's understanding. In addition, providers should avoid the use of medical jargon, use skilled interpreters as necessary, and actively listen to the patient and family.

The initial step of the SHARE program is to engage the patients and encourage their participation in the process of shared decision-making. The patients should understand that their participation is voluntary, their families are welcome to participate as well, and their decisions will be based on their understanding of their care options. Many providers first enroll patients in the electronic patient portals that can then be used as a recruitment delivery system for the SHARE program.

The second step of the SHARE program is to present the patient with all available evidence-based treatment options while recognizing that the choice of no treatment is also a viable option. The AHRQ provides extensive patient education resources for a wide range of clinical conditions. The provider is encouraged to present the information in several different forms to be sure to match the patient's learning style. The third step of the SHARE program asks the provider to identify the patient's values by using empathetic open-ended questions. This step also involves considering the potential differences between patient-centered outcomes and clinical outcomes. Providers must recognize that the patients' priorities are often not the same as the provider's priorities. The fourth step is to assist the patient in making the final choice of the available options.

Once the treatment decisions have been made, the provider will schedule follow-up visits to complete the treatment and to monitor the treatment outcomes. The final step is ongoing evaluation of the patient's treatment decisions with appropriate modifications as the patient's condition changes. There have been modest decreases in emergency room visits for patients who participated in shared decision-making and received information about acute coronary syndrome. Although shared decision-making is appropriate for all patients, in most cases, only the treatment outcomes and patient satisfaction have been measured.

Learner Characteristics

Assessing and Adapting to Level of Understanding (Sender-Receiver-Feedback)

An understanding of the basics of communication, involving the **communication cycle**, is important for the nurse to know how to communicate effectively with their patients. The communication cycle starts with a **sender**. The sender sends the message to the receiver and looks for feedback. This goes on and on through a circular cycle until transmission is ended, such as the end of a conversation.

Educational Needs Assessment

An educational needs assessment is a goal-oriented assessment meant to better understand a person's level of knowledge, what they need to know, and how best to help them learn. Educational needs assessments are a useful tool in all levels of nursing practice and can be used between the nurse educator or preceptor and staff nurse as well as between the nurse and the patient.

In the mentor/mentee role, an educational needs assessment is meant to establish a baseline of the mentee's current knowledge and how best to help the mentee improve their knowledge and skills to meet unit expectations. This involves establishing the best learning styles and communication methods. This assessment often takes place during the orientation stage of a nurse's career or when a mistake is made to ensure that just culture is practiced.

In the nurse/patient role, an educational needs assessment is also necessary to establish a baseline understanding of the patient's knowledge and goals for their health. Not everyone enters the hospital with the same level of education or medical experience. This assessment is important to give the patient autonomy and to allow them to make informed decisions about their health.

Health Literacy

Health literacy refers to how capable patients are of understanding their diagnosis, treatment plans, prognosis, and follow-up health instructions. A high degree of health literacy is associated with the ability to make personal health decisions, higher confidence in personal health decisions, and higher compliance with medical instructions.

Barriers to Communication

Internal Distractions

- Pain: If a patient is in pain, their ability to communicate will break down. Treating the pain first will facilitate communication between the patient and the healthcare team.
- Hunger: A patient who is hungry will have difficulty concentrating on sending and receiving messages effectively. In some instances, it is impossible to avoid a hungry patient, as many must fast for tests and procedures. Alleviating hunger, where possible, will ensure better communication.
- Anger: If there is something angering a patient, this could pose a potential blockade to effective communication. Identifying the inflammatory stimulus and working toward a resolution will improve future communications with the patient.

External/Environmental Distractions

- Temperature: A patient who is distracted by feeling too hot or too cold will have difficulty maintaining a normal conversation with the nurse. Warm blankets for a cold patient and fans/open windows/air conditioning for a hot patient are helpful for fixing this problem.
- Noise: The nurse would be wise to eliminate unnecessary noise when communicating with a patient. This may entail closing the door of the patient's room to block hallway chatter and/or turning a TV's volume down.

Age-Specific Therapeutic/Adaptive Responses

There are considerations to be made regarding the age of the person the nurse is communicating with.

Geriatric

Geriatric refers to an older adult, a population of patients the nurse may work with quite frequently. The nurse should remember that active listening is as important as, if not more important than, speaking as far as communication goes. The nurse should ask questions but listen intently to the answers to ascertain if the patient understands. The nurse needs to remember that interrupting is rude and can compromise trust and good communication. The nurse should take their time when giving instructions, ensuring understanding. It is not wise to use jargon, slang, or other language that the geriatric patient may not understand. If the patient needs to use new technology such as an online patient account, an assessment of Internet usage and proficiency would be useful.

Pediatric

There are a few tricks a nurse should have up their sleeve when addressing a **pediatric** patient to make them feel comfortable and safe in a medical environment. The nurse should address the child by name to create a tone of familiarity. Getting down to the child's level physically—in other words, squatting down to eye level—will help the child feel they are on the same level as their caregiver, rather than the nurse towering over them. Smiling and exuding a positive attitude will create the right environment for the nurse to care for the child. Making medical tools and equipment into toys when appropriate, such as gloves or tongue depressors, can help the child feel at ease. The nurse should enlist the parents as team members in the child's care.

Adolescent

Communicating with teenagers can present its own unique challenges for the nurse. No longer a child and not quite an adult, the **adolescent** must feel they are part of the care team and that they have a say in decision-making. It may be useful to conduct interviews with adolescents without their parents being present, if possible. This will help when trying to conduct a frank discussion on the patient's sexual activity as well as potential drug/alcohol usage. The assessment of an adolescent should include questions about mental health issues, such as depression and anxiety. The teen may feel more comfortable discussing these issues without their parent present, though the parent should be made a member of the team when addressing any issues that are discovered. Another important topic to approach with teens is stress, its causes, and coping mechanisms. In some cases, it is important to inform the adolescent which topics will remain confidential. This may encourage them to share more with the nurse.

Approach to Communication Barriers

Death and Dying

Not only will each individual respond differently to grief based on personality and relationship with the deceased, but also the response will differ based on their own spiritual beliefs and cultural influences. These beliefs and influences affect how a person thinks they should act during the mourning period, what to wear, what rituals need to be performed, and what happens after a person dies.

Each individual culture will not be discussed since there are many variations of how different people handle this process. It is not necessary for the nurse to know each and every one, but rather have a general knowledge of differences and be respectful towards them.

Some cultures believe an outward show of emotion is appropriate and necessary. Sometimes, this entails an outward expression of weeping and wailing. Other cultures may be more conservative and think it is appropriate to be stoic, serious, and somber, without crying and losing one's composure. Some have specific rituals before and after the death, involving holy men, priests, or other clergy who prepare the person and/or the body for an afterlife. Some may not have any religious affiliation and may not believe in a life after this one.

Regardless of what cultural and spiritual beliefs are present, the role of the healthcare team is to respect those wishes as much as possible. It is imperative that the team explore the resident and family's wishes in this respect, rather than overlooking or refusing to allow them. It is always appropriate to politely ask how best to respect the resident and family's wishes when performing tasks for the dying or deceased resident. For example, some family members may prefer to clean the body themselves after death, an important ritual to express grief and ensure proper care in their view.

Each member of the healthcare team, including the nurse, needs to assess their own beliefs about death and dying. Self-knowledge on the subject is valuable as it may not be something one has consciously acknowledged. This self-assessment also helps reveal any unfair biases and prejudices towards cultures and people whose worldview is different than one's own. Discovering what one's own beliefs and others' beliefs are leads to a better understanding between groups. These groups can then begin to find ways to work together during the difficult end-of-life period.

Terminal Illness

Navigating the tricky area of communicating with a patient who is diagnosed with a **terminal illness** can present a real challenge to the nurse. It is important to be honest with the patient. The nurse should be an active listener, looking for opportunities to connect the patient with valuable resources and support. The nurse should offer compassion but not false hope. The nurse may want to say something meaningful or helpful, but this is not always the best option. Sometimes simply being present, offering a hug, or holding a patient's hand is better than any words. The nurse should also look for opportunities to communicate with and support the family of the terminally ill patient. After the patient passes, they will need guidance to bereavement, loss, and grief resources.

Visually Impaired

A patient with a **visual impairment** will require adaptations to the nurse's communications techniques to ensure a clear message is sent and received. The nurse should identify themselves clearly when beginning their assessment. The nurse should never treat the patient who has a visual impairment as if they have a deficit in intellect or as if they are deaf. The nurse should check the environment to make sure there are no distractions, such as a loud TV, that may make it difficult to be heard. The nurse should ask questions to ensure the message has been received and understood by the patient. Assessing the level of visual impairment will assist in knowing how much assistance the patient will need. Someone who is legally blind versus someone with complete vision loss from birth will have different needs for assistance.

Deaf and Hard of Hearing

When communicating with persons who are **deaf** or **hard of hearing**, an important first step is to assess the level of hearing loss. This will guide further communication. Depending on the amount of hearing loss, lip reading, visual tools, hearing aids, an increased volume of the nurse's voice, or the hiring of a sign language interpreter may or may not be useful. The nurse should directly face the person with a hearing impairment when addressing them so that understanding can be better assessed. The nurse should not be in another room, have their back to the patient, or compete with a loud TV or other distraction while trying to communicate. The nurse may ask the patient questions to ensure understanding of the message.

Non-English Speaking/English as a Second Language/Interpreter

In the case of a **non-English-speaking** patient, the nurse should seek out translation services. This can come from a family member who accompanies the patient or possibly be provided by the facility where the nurse works. Seeking educational materials in the patient's native tongue will be helpful in clearly communicating with the patient after they leave the facility.

Americans with Disabilities Act Amendments Act (ADAAA) Compliance

Passed in 2008, the **ADAAA** amends a previous act, the ADA, to better define what "disability" means for certain Americans as well as protecting and upholding the rights of those with **disabilities** in the United States. The ADAAA was a response to several Supreme Court decisions that were thought to have limited the rights of those with disabilities.

Illiterate

A person who is **illiterate** cannot read and/or write. It is not always apparent to a nurse which patients may have this problem. There is a type of illiteracy called **health illiteracy** in which a patient is highly unfamiliar with medical information and is, therefore, unable to apply it to their own health and healthcare management. In illiteracy and health illiteracy, asking questions and listening for comprehension are both tools the nurse can use to determine how well the patient understands their individual healthcare plan. If a patient cannot read or write, the nurse can offer their health information to them in a different format. The nurse can read through instructions for home care and ensure that a literate caregiver is accessible to the patient to assist them with written materials. Patients with low healthcare literacy tend to make their healthcare decisions based on emotions and practical considerations such as if they will be able to get a ride to the doctor. An example of emotional decision-making would be a patient who doesn't go to the doctor because he "doesn't like needles"; this is irrational, since not every doctor visit implies needles, yet it creates a barrier to successful healthcare. Identifying these barriers is the first step to overcoming illiteracy.

Intellectually Challenged

A patient who is **intellectually challenged** may need additional help communicating with the healthcare team. The nurse will need to practice patience and allow extra time for communicating messages with and receiving messages from a person with an intellectual disability. The nurse should work with caregivers to get helpful tips for working with a patient. Every patient is different, and a full-time caregiver or loved one will know what works best when trying to communicate with the patient. The nurse should try to explain care in the simplest terms possible, avoiding complicated medical jargon. The nurse should focus on the patient's strengths rather than pointing out and focusing on weaknesses. As with all communication, the nurse should concentrate on being an active listener, open to receiving the patient's concerns and giving them time to voice them.

Professional Development Models

Models of Caring

There are several models that were created to define the art and science of nursing. This is different from the practice of medicine, although nurses also expertly use assessment, diagnosing, planning, intervention, and evaluation to provide holistic care for all patients. Caring is the most commonly identified characteristic of nursing care, and it is the central concept of most nursing models. One such framework is the **6 C's of Caring** model that was proposed to define the unique characteristics of nursing practice that distinguish nursing from the remaining patient care disciplines. These personal attributes shape the skilled nursing practice of nurses.

In the 6 C's of Caring model, **compassion** is defined as being in a state of empathy with another individual, especially with regard to pain and suffering. **Competence** requires the active pursuit of knowledge, and it is demonstrated by nurses' performance in each domain of learning, including the psychomotor, cognitive, and affective domains. The **conscience** directs nurses' moral and ethical decisions and prompts a response to instances of injustice. **Confidence** is a direct reflection of nurses' trust in their own ability to provide appropriate care for all assigned patients. Confidence is gained through formal and informal education, clinical experience, and life experience. It is evident in all aspects of the nurses' professional practice, including the clinical environment and the community. **Commitment** is the pursuit of excellence in all areas of professional nursing practice, including direct patient care, promotion of the profession, personal enrichment through education, mentoring of novice nurses, and support of public health initiatives at all levels of government. **Comportment** refers to all aspects of nurses' professional behavior in the clinical setting and the community.

While the 6 C's model is used to define nursing as a caring profession, the **Synergy Model** proposes a novel paradigm for nursing that considers patients' specific needs as the driving force in healthcare. Nursing is viewed as a coordinated, competence-based response to such needs rather than as a series of tasks that may or may not satisfy them. The model is based on the following assumptions: the patient is viewed holistically with attention to the mind, body, and spirit dimensions; the patient, the family, and the community all contribute context to the nurse-patient relationship; characteristics of either the patient or the nurse cannot be viewed in isolation because they are interrelated; and the goal of nursing is the return of the patient to the optimal level of wellness as defined by the patient. Death is considered an acceptable outcome of care to all nurses, but to different degrees according to their experience level. Novice, or level 1 nurses, understand that the patient's death is a possibility, yet they do not comprehend that the death is inevitable or acceptable. Experienced, or level 2 nurses, know from interacting with the patient and family, and from expert assessment of the patient's progress, that death may be an acceptable outcome. Expert, or level 3 nurses, recognize death as an acceptable outcome, and demonstrate skills in managing end-of-life care. They create care plans to manage patient death in the best way possible, to the benefit of the patient and the family.

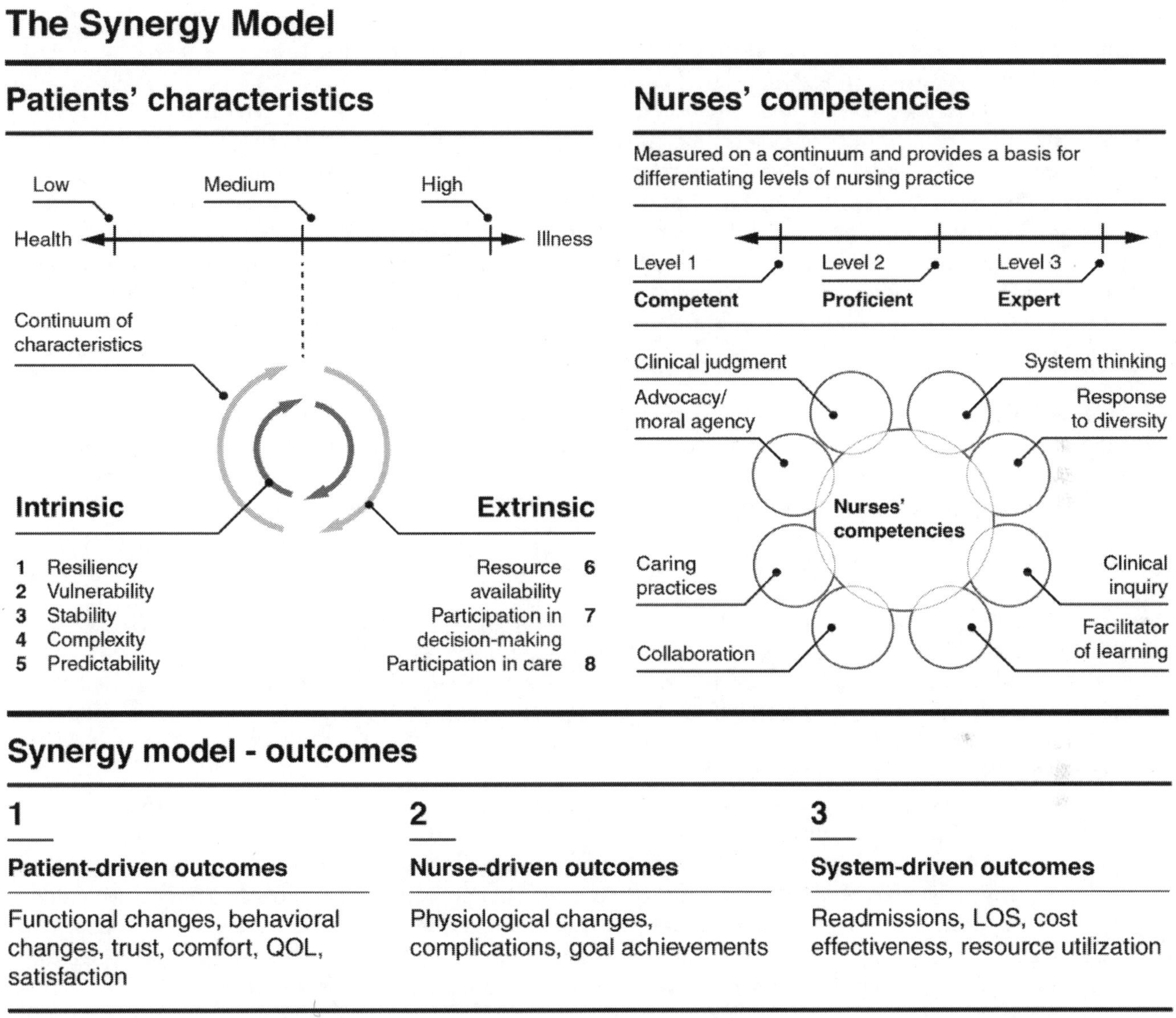

Caring practices are identified as one of the eight nursing competencies in the Synergy Model. Nurses establish and maintain a therapeutic patient-care environment, based on consideration of the needs of the patient and the family, that promotes healing and minimizes discomfort and stress. The model identifies vigilance and engagement as essential elements of the caring practices. **Vigilance** as a caring skill is viewed on a continuum according to the ability of nurses to recognize and respond to patient needs. Novice nurses are capable of responding to usual and predictable changes in the patient's condition; however, responding to more subtle cues requires an increased level of clinical competence, and preventing any potential hazards requires even greater nursing skill. **Engagement** refers to the degree to which nurses commit to the nurse-patient relationship. Researchers note that favorable patient outcomes are associated with the degree of caregiver engagement; however, there is also evidence that the incidence of burnout in experienced nurses is related to the degree of their engagement in patient care. The third attribute of the caring practices is **responsiveness**, which means that the reaction of the patient's family, the healthcare institution, and the nursing staff will all have an effect on the patient's progress.

Novice-to-Expert

Nurses acquire clinical inquiry skills on a continuum that is based on education and clinical experience. As is the case with the other nursing competencies included in the Synergy Model, this progressive development is consistent with Benner's novice to expert model that views the development of nursing expertise as a progressive process that requires ongoing education and clinical experience. Novice nurses are able to implement clinical innovations developed by others, to identify their own learning needs, and to enlist the aid of other nurses to identify critical needs of the patient. Experienced nurses are able to question the adequacy of interventions and to begin to challenge the "we have always done it this way" philosophy that is the most common rationale for many nursing interventions. They are also able to assess the utility of alternative interventions. The Synergy Model views the practice of expert nurses as the point at which clinical inquiry and clinical reasoning become inseparable elements of clinical practice. Expert nurses are able to predict changes in the patient's condition that require revision of the plan of care, and they are also able to develop and implement alternative approaches to address those changes.

Transition to Practice

Also referred to as a nurse residency, the Transition to Practice model assists in guiding newly graduated nurses through their first year as a registered nurse. Attrition rates among first-year nursing graduates are high—approximately 25 percent. Beginning any new career can be stressful; however, when faced with accountability for increasingly complex and chronic conditions coupled with high acuity levels, becoming familiarized with the healthcare culture can prove overwhelming. Providing support to first-year nurses through the journey from didactic learning to clinical practice can ease this adjustment.

The Transition to Practice model is an essential framework that often comprises a preceptorship that extends beyond the typical nurse role onboarding. This is paired with additional training that may include hands-on simulation or clinical application at the bedside. Utilizing a novice to expert approach, new nurses are guided through the skills and knowledge required to provide care that enhances outcomes.

Performance-Based Competencies

There are several ways that professional development nurses can assess the staff. The nurses can perform **self-assessments**, in which the nurse considers specific questions about their own performance and abilities. These assessments may ask the nurse to list their best attributes or strongest skills, along with areas where they feel they could improve. They might be asked to describe situations in which they feel like they excelled as well as situations that they found difficult to manage. Self-assessments can also include information about career goals, feedback about their current job description, and execution of the required duties. Formatting of the assessments can include both open-ended questions and checklists for nurses to rank the information (e.g., on an agree-disagree scale).

Professional development nurses can also assess staff through observation, by accompanying them on their rounds, for example, and having the nurse explain what they are doing and why. The professional development nurse can pose questions to the staff member to get a fuller picture of the nurse's knowledge and thought process when dealing with patient care. Additionally, professional development nurses can perform audits of the nursing staff's notes, review patient files, and conduct peer reviews to get a full picture of a nurse's performance. If the professional development nurse finds areas that may be weak, having the nurse review information or complete practice simulations can help assess whether the weakness is due to knowledge, skills, lack of attention to detail, or a poor attitude about the job.

Periodically, a full appraisal of each nurse and staff member should be completed. An **employee appraisal** generally consists of ratings as well as written notes and observations. For example, the nurse may be given a score of one to five on a particular aspect of the job, and then the appraiser may include notes supporting or explaining that score.

Employee appraisals often include information about the employee's schedule, attendance record, interactions with management and peers, and patient feedback. Ideally, the appraisal should also include direct information from the nurse, including any concerns they may have, their career goals, and their feedback about their work and their position within the organization. These appraisals are usually completed by the nurse's immediate supervisor or manager, reviewed by upper management, and placed into the nurse's permanent employment record.

Regardless of the type of evaluation, professional development nurses should ensure that the information and analysis align with the organization's mission and values. It would be unfair to evaluate a nurse based on criteria that they were unaware were part of their job requirements. Similarly, nurses should be given frequent feedback, both positive and critical, so that they can make adjustments on an ongoing basis. It would not be fair or effective management to withhold information or observations just so they can be included in an evaluation or appraisal at a later time. Nurses and staff want to be good at their jobs and want to know both what they are doing well as well as how they can improve.

Additionally, evaluation feedback should be clear and well-documented to avoid any type of "he said, she said" situation. If a nurse is given critical feedback and instructed on techniques for making improvements in that area, that feedback should be documented and acknowledged by both parties. By doing this, misunderstanding can be avoided if the nurse fails to make the necessary improvements or if the nurse makes changes that the professional development nurse says were unnecessary and/or incorrect.

Finally, evaluations and feedback should focus on employee retention and growth. Overly critical analysis without any acknowledgment of successes only serves to make the employee less satisfied with their job. It creates feelings of inadequacy and adds unnecessary stress to the employee. Instead, feedback should be growth-focused. While it is important to let staff know when an area needs improvement, this must be done in a way that allows the employee to learn and grow rather than making them feel as though they are incompetent or unvalued.

Similarly, when an employee is doing well and receives a good evaluation, the assessment should include specific details and explanations about what they are doing well and how that can translate to career growth and future potential. This way, the employee knows what they should continue doing and can take pride and ownership of a job well done.

Clinical Ladder

The clinical ladder is a method of nurse promotion based on experience and performance. This option for nurse advancement was first introduced in the 1980s by Patricia Benner and has gained popularity since. Based on Benner's model of clinical competence, there are five levels of proficiency in nursing care that make up the clinical ladder: novice, advanced beginner, competent, proficient, and expert.

Promotions and career advancements are based on the nurse's competencies, skills, and leadership abilities, which are graded through proposed activities. Healthcare organizations may elect to institute a professional nursing committee that develops a framework of a series of steps to achieve each ranking within a reward system. The rewards may include one-time monetary bonuses, granted time off, or pay raises. This type of reward system encourages nurse engagement through completion of quality improvement projects and involvement in nursing professional development activities. Examples of these activities include shared governance, committee work, and empowerment to assume leadership roles.

Educational Design and Delivery

Education Design Process

The nurse will need to understand the cycles of the nursing and educational design process. Below is a visual to demonstrate the steps of the nursing process.

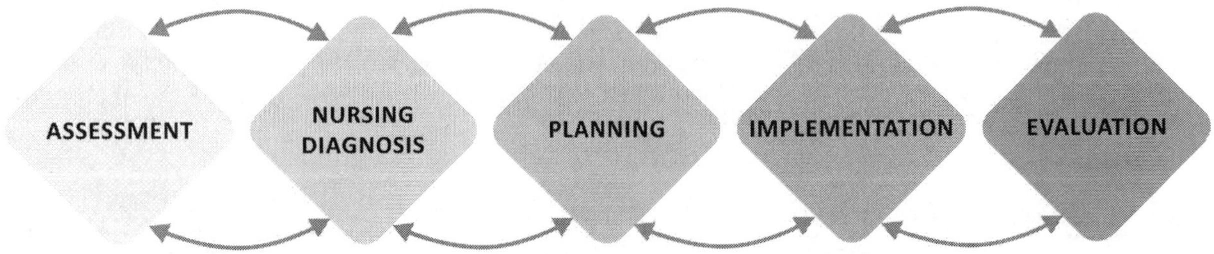

It is important to note that the cycle of the nursing process does not just move in one direction, and it may take multiple steps back to get to the solution. If the nursing diagnosis is no longer applicable, the nurse will need to go back to the assessment phase. Using this method of critical thinking gives the nurse an overview of the procedural process while also allowing for the flexibility needed in healthcare.

Assessment Domain

The assessment aspect of the education design process refers to the active gathering of information regarding the current knowledge, abilities, skills, and experiences of the target audience. First, the educator must decide on the expected learning objective to provide validity of the assessment. This may also be referred to as a needs assessment. When developing assessments, emphasis should be placed on the progression of cognitive skills. Bloom's taxonomy is a helpful tool to measure levels of thinking, from rote memorization to analytical and critical thinking.

Measuring these characteristics requires a clear definition of the purpose of the assessment. Establishing strong learning objectives that align with the curriculum will guide the focus of the types of knowledge, skills, and abilities being appraised. From the perspective of improving nursing professionalism, examples of targeted outcomes may include a gap in the standard of care, practice deviation or drift from best practice, and improvement of current practices. Assessing the baseline is required to determine the current state, establish hypotheses, and identify and plan for barriers before moving into the planning phase to address the needs or changes that will provide improvement.

Planning Domain

Once the baseline of knowledge is determined and the gap or deficit is identified through the assessment, the education design process moves into the planning domain. Individuals that can assist with planning of the educational activity must be selected based on their status as a subject matter expert, influence on the members being taught, and ability to provide unbiased opinions and input on the root cause of the problem. There should be at least two individuals involved in this phase, a nurse planner and a subject matter expert, though it may be beneficial to have additional insight and contribution from a collaborative committee.

Once this is discovered, the planning committee will determine the instructional plan and learning activities required for acquiring the necessary skills and knowledge needed to address the problem. There are several frameworks that can be used to design instructional plans. These include backward design, integrated course design, the 5E model, and the accelerated learning cycle.

Implementation Domain

Once the education has been planned, the implementation phase involves development and delivery to the intended audience. As determined by the goal, materials may be acquired from outside sources or produced internally. Education should be reviewed to ensure that it meets the needs of the learners and revised when necessary. This can include updating any changes in best practice or content that is not meeting the learning goals.

The characteristics of the target audience will drive the type of education to be delivered. Some aspects to consider when presenting the information are the work schedules of the audience, time required for learning, and delivery format (in-person versus online lecture). Methodologies that can enhance learning include simulation, role-play, case studies, story sharing, game playing, and concept mapping.

The team delivering the education, which may include trainers, subject matter experts, instructors, and facilitators, must be adequately knowledgeable on the subject matter. The training may be provided in a live format or need to be developed within a learning management system. Training and education may be delivered via any one of these methods or as a hybrid approach, depending on which would be the most effective for the target audience.

Evaluation Domain

While the evaluation domain follows the assessment, implementation, and planning phases of the educational design process, it must be incorporated at each step for the purpose of testing applicability and progression towards goals. This may be evaluated through testing, facilitator observations, assessments such as surveys, and tracking the targeted outcome of the education. For example, if the education is aimed at reducing catheter-associated urinary tract infections (CAUTI), data can be gathered for a set period following education delivery and analyzed for improvement.

Tracers can be completed with staff at the point of care or where the learning will be used by utilizing the teach-back method. The learners may be assessed through direct observation of the skill or through demonstration of knowledge. Any deviation or drift that signals that the teaching goal was not met or partially met can be mitigated by revising the material and providing follow-up education. The baseline and post-implementation metrics should be shared widely with leadership and staff through huddles and related committees for transparency and awareness of initiative progress.

Learning Domain

The learning domain plays a vital role in shaping professional nursing development through education and comprises three integrated domains: cognitive, affective, and psychomotor. Cognitive skills, from basic to advanced using Bloom's taxonomy, include remembering, understanding, applying, analyzing, evaluating, and creating. In nursing education, this framework encourages learners to not only memorize facts but also comprehend concepts, apply knowledge in clinical settings, analyze complex patient situations, and develop innovative solutions. The affective domain incorporates the feelings, opinions, interests, attitudes, and values of the receiver. Through reflection, the learner gains insight into the order in which they apply these factors to their environment. This provides understanding of influential external factors in relationship development. Finally, the psychomotor domain is focused on motor skill development, which can include clinical performance skills through hands-on practice. Development of this domain through experiential learning fosters competence, promotes confidence, and prepares learners for real-world clinical challenges.

By progressing through these levels, critical thinking, decision making, and problem-solving abilities are enhanced to promote evidence-driven patient care and improved outcomes. Incorporating Bloom's taxonomy into nursing curricula fosters a structured approach to learning, ensuring that educational activities promote deep understanding and practical competence. This progression supports continuous professional development by empowering nurses to adapt to evolving healthcare environments, improve patient outcomes, and contribute to healthcare innovation. Incorporating these domains into educational plans facilitates a comprehensive learning experience, which is essential to produce competent and confident nursing professionals.

Types of Educational Activities

Orientation

Orientation Planning

Orientation planning refers to the necessary preliminary step of preparing to orient new staff. Depending on available resources, this phase of precepting may be started by nurse educators and preceptors before new staff starts working or it may take place the first time the new hire and preceptor meet. The main point of orientation planning is to establish an idea of what the teaching goals and desired outcomes will be for the nurse entering a new role. Orientation planning should also establish an expected or desired timeline of how long precepting should take and when progress evaluations should take place.

Preceptor Best Practices

Following the orientation-planning phase, preceptors should apply ongoing best practices in order to ensure the success of the new hire or preceptee. This begins with assessing the preceptee's current knowledge and learning style, as well as assessing how best to meet the goals established in the orientation plan. This may be a continuous assessment throughout the orientation phase or as the preceptee encounters new hurdles. Any feedback provided should be given in a respectful and timely manner. If there is not an immediate safety issue that needs to be corrected, offering feedback is generally best done when not in front of a patient or other staff that might make the preceptee feel humiliated or criticized. However, feedback should also be given soon enough that corrections can be made in the moment rather than after orientation is expected to be completed. It is also important to encourage the preceptee by showing them where their strengths lie and how they can contribute to the unit as a whole. Finally, preceptor best practices do not end when the preceptee has completed orientation. Providing continued support and mentorship throughout the nurse's career establishes an environment of support and growth.

On-Boarding

On-boarding, also known as organizational socialization, is the process by which new hires obtain the knowledge, skills, and behaviors they need in order to become valued, productive contributors to the company. The success of on-boarding programs is crucial because new employees decide if they will stay with an organization during their first six months of work. Therefore, it is important for companies to ensure that new employees feel supported and adjust to the social and performance aspects of their new roles quickly.

On-boarding can begin by having an employee's new managers and teammates reach out to them via email to welcome them even prior to their formal start date with the company. On the first day at work, the manager can introduce the new hire to the team member who will serve as their "buddy," to whom they can feel free to go to with any questions or concerns. Taking the new hire out of the office for a welcome lunch on the first day with a couple of staff members is always a nice gesture, as well as ensuring they have lunch partners for the first couple of weeks on the job.

Other aspects of successful on-boarding programs involve the new hire's manager scheduling meet-and-greet appointments to learn more about the roles that each teammate in the department plays and how the new hire will interact with them. These types of meetings can also be scheduled with individuals throughout the company who have key relationships with the department, such as members of IT, Marketing, Human Resources, etc. Additionally, providing the new hire with an on-boarding schedule that involves a variety of team members who will train on various processes and applications can be helpful. It is also important for the manager to provide clear expectations by meeting with the new hire to discuss their performance and development plans for the first three months. Finally, to help a new hire build contacts throughout the company, it is imperative to get them involved in a cross-functional project.

There is no set time limit for on-boarding programs, but at some companies, these programs can last throughout an employee's first year.

In-service

In-service nursing education plays a vital role in the ongoing professional development of nurses. Structured training sessions, workshops, and seminars are conducted within healthcare facilities to enhance nurses' knowledge, skills, and competencies. This form of education ensures that nurses stay current with mandatory specialty skills, technological advancements, and regulatory requirements. In-service education promotes continuous learning, which is essential for maintaining high standards of patient care and safety.

Organizational support and encouragement of lifelong learning and professional growth among nursing staff is essential to foster nursing professional development. Through regular in-service programs, nurses can update their clinical skills, learn new procedures, and deepen their understanding of disease management. Additionally, these programs promote teamwork, improve communication, and boost morale. Ultimately, in-service nursing education contributes to improved patient outcomes, increased job satisfaction, and the higher quality of healthcare delivery.

Continuing Education

Since the medical and healthcare fields are always rapidly changing due to technological advances, new research, organizational and governmental regulations, and through continuous process improvements in healthcare delivery, nurses can expect to continue their education throughout the course of their careers. Consequently, the ability to learn new topics will be a necessary skill in order to remain a competent practitioner. Lifelong learning and **continuing education** are associated with improved patient outcomes, job satisfaction, personal validation and achievement, and obtaining skills that were not taught or available at the time that the nurse was enrolled in a formal education program. The most crucial association with lifelong learning activities is the improvement in quality of care. Incompetent or unaware nursing staff means a great deal of risk for the patient. By constantly striving to improve their knowledge and practical skills, nurses decrease the chance that they will be held liable for negligence or malpractice, and they are taking tangible actions to adhere to the ethical tenets of the healthcare profession.

While avenues to continue professional development in the nursing field may be formal (e.g., obtaining extra relevant degrees or certifications, publishing research, or enrolling in trainings offered by the nurse's workplace), many opportunities require intrinsic motivation (e.g., taking personal initiative to keep abreast of current relevant literature, consulting with mentors, or experiencing different responsibilities within the field). However, even with these varied opportunities and the multitude of personal and professional benefits associated with lifelong learning activities, there are still some barriers for nurses. These include obstacles like disinterest, lack of time on the job or outside of the job to participate in activities, an inability to balance work and life needs with job demands, and lack of financial resources (to pay for educational activities and/or to take the time off to participate in them). In this regard, it is helpful for leadership and subordinate employees to work together to overcome these barriers.

Nurses who are in positions of leadership can promote a culture of lifelong learning by pushing for organizational support for development activities. In the event that development activities are free or hosted by the nurse's workplace, the nurse should recognize the valuable opportunity and take the time to attend and fully engage in the experience. This shows that such activities are in demand and valued and is likely to make affordable and accessible professional development activities part of the workplace culture.

Interprofessional Education

Interprofessional educational activities are vital in nursing education and professional development, fostering collaboration among a multidisciplinary team. These activities promote understanding of different roles, responsibilities, and perspectives within the healthcare team, enhancing communication and teamwork. Engaging professionals from a wide range of disciplines develops the necessary skills to achieve coordinated patient care, leading to improved safety and outcomes. Examples of such activities include simulations, case discussions, workshops, and collaborative projects that are reflective of actual clinical settings. Interprofessional education encourages mutual respect and understanding, reducing siloed practices and fostering a culture of shared responsibility. This engagement also prepares nurses to work effectively with physicians, pharmacists, social workers, and other healthcare professionals. Incorporating these activities into nursing curricula and ongoing professional development ensures that nurses are equipped with the competencies needed to provide comprehensive, patient-centered care. Ultimately, interprofessional education enhances healthcare quality, efficiency, and safety, benefiting both practitioners and patients.

Competency Management Process

When management and staff have good communication, it becomes easier for managers to convey important information, such as employee evaluations and performance assessments. **Nursing competency** involves several aspects, including general knowledge, job skills, attitudes, and behaviors. The nurse must have sufficient knowledge to do the job effectively. They must also have the necessary skills to apply that knowledge to patient care, and they must be able to do the job with an appropriate attitude and behavior. A nurse who is knowledgeable and skilled may not do well if the patients feel uncomfortable with them or do not trust them. Similarly, a nurse can have the best personal rapport with their patients, but without the proper knowledge or skills, they could do more harm than good. It is the responsibility of the manager, therefore, to ensure that each staff member has a suitable mix of knowledge, skills, and attitudes to do their jobs effectively.

Individual Competencies

Professional nursing practice includes behaviors and norms that are expected to be demonstrated by the successful nurse. These behaviors include demonstrating effective communication and teamwork, placing the patient first, and having an attitude of growth and positivity. This growth mentality is exemplified by improving and advancing individual competencies.

Effective communication may look different depending on the situation and the other participants the nurse is interacting with. For example, when communicating with peers, the nurse may be respectful but will likely be able to use technical terminology that is understood amongst peers. Communication with those in a leadership position may be slightly different—less relaxed than with peers and with an increased level of professionalism. Communication with patients may also be different, as the nurse will need to assess the patients' healthcare knowledge and show a level of care while providing education. Finally, situations may change how the nurse communicates effectively. Communication in an emergency situation may be more concise and require more of a closed loop than day-to-day problem solving with a team.

Effective teamwork is essential to a functioning healthcare facility and nursing unit. Care of a single patient may involve multiple nurses, ancillary staff, and doctors. The professional nurse understands these roles and works within the team effectively to promote positive patient outcomes.

Finally, a nurse shows professional behaviors through putting the patients first and exemplifying a positive, growth-oriented attitude. Nurses must act as advocates for their patients, prioritizing their needs and safety within their role. Negative attitudes do not encourage a safe environment for nurses or patients. As the patient may be in a frightening and unfamiliar world on the unit, positivity can provide the patient with a feeling that they are in capable hands. Additionally, nurses who advance in their skills and competencies are more likely to have greater satisfaction within the profession and are able to provide more skilled care to patients. It is generally expected that as a nurse advances in their career, they become more competent, moving from novice to expert and potentially taking on new roles as their individual competency improves.

Clinical Judgment

Clinical judgment is the art of assessing and understanding what is happening in a particular medical situation and what actions should be taken based on this assessment. Clinical judgment develops with time, experience, and furthering education. The novice nurse may struggle to identify a disease process within a patient and need to ask more questions before acting, while a seasoned nurse may identify signs and symptoms quickly and take appropriate action. This advancement in clinical judgment comes from continued application of the nursing process and having more experience opportunities throughout one's career.

In its most fundamental and basic form, the nursing process generally refers to ADPIE (assess, diagnose, planning, implementation, and evaluation). Within this structure, the nurse will first assess the patient's presentation and then come up with an applicable nursing diagnosis. From there the nurse will create a plan of care, implement the plan, and then evaluate if the intervention was successful or not. As the nurse gains more experience, this process can become more efficient and effective with improved application of critical-thinking skills. In fact, the more experienced nurse may be able to jump more quickly from assessment to implementation and evaluation as they better understand a disease process or patient presentation within their clinical judgment.

While clinical judgment does come with time and experience, nurses must be proactive in working to improve it. Some nurses may be tempted to embrace comfort in their career, following doctors' orders with few questions and avoiding difficult situations whenever possible. These nurses may advance their clinical judgment for certain situations, but it is possible they will have difficulty thinking outside of the box when they are outside of their comfort zone. Nurses who push outside of their comfort zone, say "yes" to a more challenging patient assignment, continually ask questions of more clinically experienced individuals, and advocate for themselves to have further opportunities and educational experiences will be more successful improving their clinical judgment.

Peer Review Methods

Peer review methods refer to the processes of assessing the validity and use of clinical articles, journals, studies, or nursing practices. The intent behind peer review is to ensure the integrity of the science behind the article or study and to ensure that practice is evidence based. The hope is to minimize harm from inaccurate or deceptive information. Peer review can be used in the academic setting and within the professional setting using several different methods.

Two forms of peer review within the academic setting are meant to emphasize anonymity. One is "single anonymized," where the author does not know who will be reviewing their article or study. This prevents the author from leaning the article's bias in favor of the reviewer and allows the reviewer to feel more comfortable providing negative feedback. The other is "double anonymized," where both the author and reviewer are anonymous in the review process to prevent bias in either direction. While these methods can be useful in reviewing academic articles and studies, it is important for nurses to be aware that the American Nurses Association does not consider anonymized peer review to be the standard of practice within the professional setting as it does not allow for accountability for either party.

Peer review methods that provide more transparency are open peer review and transparent peer review. Within open peer review, all parties are known to one another and accountability from all parties is encouraged. However, this method may discourage some reviewers from providing negative feedback. In order to encourage unbiased feedback, transparent peer review may be employed, in which the reviewer may choose whether or not to have their identity known. These methods can be applied both in the academic setting and within professional practice. A mentor may use open peer review with a mentee to provide feedback to ensure that their practice is evidence-based. On the other hand, a nurse may use transparent peer review when submitting a quality improvement form regarding an incident that had a negative outcome when it might not be appropriate or possible to provide negative feedback to a specific individual.

Continuing Education and Accreditation

Process for Providing Continuing Education

Contact Hours

Providing nursing continuing education (CE) contact hours is a requirement for maintaining nursing licensure and ensuring that nurses stay current with best practices. To offer CE contact hours, organizations must be accredited and comply with the standards set by the relevant accrediting bodies, such as the American Nurses Credentialing Center (ANCC) or state nursing boards. The curriculum must be evidence-based, relevant, and must meet the needs of the learners. CE contact hours are based on an algorithm of difficulty, word count, and learner assessment. A tool available for assessing appropriate content adherence is the Mergener formula. Once the curriculum is prepared, the program is submitted for approval to the accrediting organization, which reviews the content for quality and compliance.

Delivery methods of continuing education may vary, often including live seminars, webinars, online courses, or workshops. It's important to accurately record attendance, participation, and assessment scores to verify completion. After completion, participants should receive a certificate that specifies the number of contact hours earned, along with the accreditation statement and expiration date, if applicable. Thorough documentation and record-keeping must be accurate to meet compliance regulations and potential audits. Providing post-education evaluations can assess the effectiveness of the program and identify areas for improvement. By adhering to these steps, organizations can ensure that nursing continuing education offerings are credible, compliant, and valuable for professional development.

Continuing Education Requirements

Each state and/or board of nursing requires a specified number of continuing education (CE) content hours per year or period for licensure renewal. This is to ensure that licensed nurses stay current with evolving healthcare practices, maintain licensure, and provide high-quality patient care. The number of mandated hours typically ranges from 20 to 30 hours every two years. These hours cover areas such as patient safety, infection control, ethics, pharmacology, pain control, and critical updates in clinical practice.

To fulfill CE requirements, nurses can attend accredited courses, workshops, seminars, or online programs approved by recognized bodies. Some states may specify that a certain number of CE hours are dedicated to topics such as cultural competency or human trafficking. CE content hours may also be required for advanced practice licensure or specialty certifications renewal. Failure to complete required CE hours can result in licensure suspension and monetary penalties.

Managing Process for Continuing Education Credits

The process of managing continuing education (CE) credits requires a systematic approach to ensure compliance, accuracy, and participation tracking. This begins with establishing clear accreditation standards that align with industry requirements. CE content providers must offer courses approved by accrediting bodies, including training and activities that align with CE regulations. A database that displays eligible CE content offerings should be easily accessible for learners and include systems that record attendance, course completion, and number of credits earned. Utilizing learning management systems (LMS) can streamline this process, providing automated tracking and reporting features. Registration tracking must be able to verify participant identities and attendance to ensure credits are awarded appropriately.

After course completion, CE content providers issue certificates that specify the number of credits earned, course details, and completion dates. Records must be securely stored and accessible by the CE content provider as well as the participants for future verification and audit purposes. Regularly updating course content and accreditation status ensures ongoing compliance and relevance. Organizations that utilize LMS benefit from the ease of sending reminders about upcoming courses and deadlines for credit submission. Evaluating participant feedback and maintaining accurate documentation helps improve the process continually.

Practice Quiz

1. The Synergy Model views the practice of expert nurses as which of the following?
    a. Being able to anticipate the patient needs
    b. Being able to address change
    c. The point where clinical reasoning and clinical inquiry are inseparable
    d. Being able to incorporate research findings

2. A nurse is caring for a patient who had a colectomy two days ago. While assisting the patient back to bed, the nurse notes that the patient's heart rate and respiratory rate are slightly elevated, and the patient states, "I can feel my pulse." The nurse assesses the patient for additional signs of heart failure. This intervention is an example of which of the following caring practices according to the Synergy Model?
    a. Engagement by a novice nurse
    b. Vigilance by an experienced nurse
    c. An expected response to predictable changes by the novice nurse
    d. Collaboration by an experienced nurse

3. The clinical practice of expert nurses reflects all of the nursing competencies identified in the Synergy Model. Which of the following ethical principles is the overall principle guiding nurses' actions?
    a. Beneficence
    b. Advocacy
    c. Autonomy
    d. Justice

4. Which of the following choices represents the learning sequence of a nurse, in the correct order from novice to expert, with regard to caring practices?
    a. The nurse anticipates the needs of the patient in the community; then, acknowledges death as a potential outcome; and finally, learns to respond to subtle changes in the patient's condition.
    b. The nurse facilitates solutions to patient and family concerns related to death and dying; then, modifies caring practices to the individual patient; and finally, learns to maintain a safe physical environment.
    c. The nurse bases care on standards and protocols; then, views death as an acceptable outcome; and finally, learns to anticipate and avoid patient problems.
    d. The nurse recognizes the patient as a unique being; then, facilitates the care of the patient across the caring continuum; and finally, learns to focus on the patient's customary needs.

5. Which of the following is a common barrier to successful patient education?
    a. Poor literacy
    b. Lack of disease prevalence
    c. Lack of safe places to hold patient education sessions
    d. Patient ego

See answers on the next page.

Answer Explanations

1. C: Expert nurses are those who reach the point in their clinical practice where clinical reasoning and inquiry are intertwined, allowing the nurse to make clinical judgements quickly and appropriately, according to best practice standards.

2. B: Vigilance refers to the ability of the nurse to recognize and respond to changes in the patient's condition. According to the Synergy Model, vigilance as a caring practice is a learned behavior that evolves with clinical experience, which means that the novice nurse will identify predictable alterations in the patient's condition, while the experienced nurse will identify and respond to more subtle changes. The most experienced nurse is capable of intervening to prevent some adverse events. Engagement refers to committing to the patient care relationship, rather than responding to changes in the patient's condition. The changes noted in the patient's condition are early, subtle indications of heart failure. The novice nurse would initially associate the changes with the surgical procedure, while the experienced nurse would assess the patient for heart failure. Although collaboration with other providers may have been an outcome of the nurse's assessment, the initial care was an independent action.

3. A: Beneficence is defined as doing good for another individual, which would include acting as an advocate, supporting the individual's autonomy, and working to ensure justice. While advocacy, autonomy, and justice (Choices *B*, *C*, and *D*) are relevant considerations in nursing practice, they are not the overall principle guiding nursing actions.

4. C: Novice nurses base their care on standards and protocols, experienced nurses view death as an acceptable outcome, and expert nurses anticipate and avoid patient problems. Choices *A*, *B*, and *D* identify the progression of novice to expert caring practices in random order. Choice *A*: Expert nurses anticipate the needs of the patient in the community, novice nurses acknowledge death as a potential outcome, and experienced nurses respond to subtle changes in the patient's condition. Choice *B*: Expert nurses facilitate solutions to patient and family concerns related to death and dying, experienced nurses modify caring practices for the individual patient, and novice nurses maintain a safe physical environment. Choice *D*: Experienced nurses recognize the patient as a unique being, expert nurses facilitate the care of the patient across the caring continuum, and novice nurses focus on the patient's customary needs.

5. A: Patient literacy plays a major role in understanding educational material, especially written handouts. Many healthcare providers rely on written materials, such as pamphlets and discharge papers, to provide patient education. When the patient struggles with literacy, these items may not be useful. If the patient fails to fully understand their diagnosis, treatment, and follow up instructions, they are more likely to be readmitted to the hospital. Therefore, healthcare providers should also offer to talk through the material with the patient in simple language. They can also ask if the patient prefers other forms of media, such as online videos. This can be done in an objective way, framed as asking for the patient's personal preference, in order to not potentially embarrass the patient. The other options are not accepted as common barriers to education.

Leadership

Leadership Principles, Concepts, and Structures

Leadership Principles

Authority

Authority refers to who oversees each task and individual person in an organization. There are three basic types of authority: line authority, staff authority, and team authority. **Line authority** refers to the direct line of supervision from supervisors to staff. Line authority usually involves a chain of command, with staff reporting concerns to their immediate supervisor and information continuing up the "chain" as needed until it reaches the person who has the ability and authority to resolve the issue. For example, a question about how to complete a task can likely be resolved by the employee's immediate supervisor, but a request for a raise in pay would likely need to be moved up the "chain" to someone with a higher authority who can make that determination. By establishing a clear chain of command, resolution of potential problems becomes a clear and straightforward process.

Staff authority refers to a management system based on experience, where supervisors have authority over their area of expertise. Employees report to the appropriate supervisor, depending on what type of issue or concern they are having. For example, if an employee has a concern about a patient, they would see the person designated as the nursing supervisor. If the concern is a janitorial issue, the employee would need to talk to the supervisor of the janitorial department. While this type of authority organization can lead to more immediate resolutions to issues, it can become confusing if the staff is not entirely clear about who is actually in charge of a given situation.

The third type of authority structure is **team authority**. This can be a temporary organizational structure established to manage specific tasks, committees, or work groups. Someone may be designated as the supervisor for their particular team or work group, though they may not hold any authority or supervisory duties outside of that group.

Delegation

Nursing staff take on many responsibilities that can be delegated to other clinical and non-clinical colleagues. However, learning how to safely delegate tasks, while still making patients feel cared for, is a skill that can take time to develop. It requires knowing not only what the needs of the patient are, but also the strengths and weaknesses of assistive personnel and how to best communicate professional needs with them. It also requires personal development in becoming comfortable with outsourcing responsibilities, as the nurse who delegates still remains accountable for the patient.

There are different types of assistive personnel that may be supervised by nurses. **Clinical assistive staff** can provide basic medical assistance, such as taking patients' vital signs, assisting with caretaking duties, monitoring any abnormalities or changes in the patient, maintaining a sterile and safe environment, and any other request made directly by nursing staff. **Non-clinical assistive personnel**, such as front desk staff, can assist with patient communication (such as wait times), managing paperwork and ensuring it is complete, and performing any other administrative task that may support the nursing staff's cases.

When nursing staff choose to delegate tasks, they may feel worried about risking their own accountability or work ethic. However, communicating with assistive personnel, understanding their strengths and weaknesses, and remaining transparent about the needs that are present in the department can ensure that delegated tasks are a good fit for the person who is taking the responsibility. In this regard, nursing staff take on a leadership and managerial role that requires developing their problem-solving, time management, and interpersonal skills. Some effective tools for delegation include standardized checklists that cover the procedure that is being delegated, meetings with assistive personnel to assess their comfort levels in performing certain tasks, and matching professional needs with individual qualifications. When **delegation** is effective, it can help the entire department work in a more efficient manner. Additionally, both nursing staff and assistive personnel are more likely to feel like part of a cohesive team and less likely to feel overworked or undervalued.

Supervision

After the nurse has successfully and effectively delegated a task, the nurse then takes on the role of supervisor of the person to whom they delegated the task. Delegation requires supervision to ensure the task is done appropriately and protect the nurse's own licensure.

The key to supervision is the follow-up. After the task is delegated, the nurse must then make a note to investigate whether the task was completed correctly and in a timely manner. Asking the person who was supposed to perform the task to report back is appropriate. All conversations and interactions must be performed professionally and with respect for both the inferior and superior party.

Many nurses were once **certified nursing assistants** (**CNAs**) and understand the role and responsibility of the person they now delegate to. If the two nurses were former co-workers and one has risen to the role of nurse from CNA, tensions may arise. Tensions that arise between nursing staff and those they delegate to may be resolved through careful interactions. Each party must be respectful and recognize they are working together with the best interest of the patient at the forefront of their minds.

At times, it may be necessary for the nurse to coach and support the staff member, giving tips for better performance where appropriate. Again, this interaction must be done with professionalism and respect. It is important as an employee in any field to be receptive to constructive criticism, as well as being able to offer it when appropriate and allowing plenty of discussion on the point.

The nurse must ensure that the task delegated, such as taking vital signs or cleaning up an incontinent patient, has been appropriately documented. Documentation is necessary for legal reasons, to show that proper care was given to the patient. If the person to whom the task was delegated did not document the task, it is necessary for the nurse to confront them directly and confirm that it was done.

Leadership Styles

The most effective and efficient way for those in leadership positions in healthcare to utilize the resources at their disposal is for them to carefully consider how they interact with those they lead. Regardless of how perfect a provider's understanding of a disease may be, they will still need to rely on other individuals (e.g., emergency medical technicians [EMTs], nurses, and laboratory personnel) to treat patients with that disease effectively and efficiently. They must understand how to communicate with others, utilize their staff members, and balance each person's unique assets and potential liabilities. Each of these diverse tasks, and how best to navigate them as a leader, form the basis for discussions around leadership styles—specifically, which styles of leadership work best in healthcare settings.

Discussions on the best traits for those seeking to be leaders have existed for as long as humans have lived in organized society. One dominant theory for much of recorded history is called the **"Great Man Theory of Leadership"**. According to the theory, great leaders are born, not made. Implicit in such a theory is the idea that leadership cannot be taught—either one has the ability to lead, and will, or one does not, and will not. The Great Man Theory of Leadership is largely dismissed today. Increasing psychological and scientific evidence has sufficiently attested to the idea that characteristics associated with effective and efficient leadership are not only given to a select few; instead, they are patterns of behavior that can be understood, taught, and replicated.

Autocratic, Democratic, and Laissez-Faire Leadership

Almost all other theories on leadership styles promote the idea that being a great leader is a learnable and practicable skill. In the mid-20th century, psychologist Kurt Lewin was credited with popularizing three basic styles of leadership: Autocratic, Democratic, and Laissez-Faire. Lewin had formulated these three distinct styles of leadership while watching schoolchildren complete a project together, although intending his theory to be applied directly to the business world. According to his theory, an **autocratic leadership** style (also sometimes referred to as an authoritarian leadership style) occurs when only the leader is involved in the decision-making process, and input from other team members is not expected or invited. On the other end of the scale, a **democratic leadership** style involves the active gathering of input from team members by the leader, with the goal of incorporating feedback into the final decision-making process. A leader can still be democratic even if they make the decision alone; what makes a leader democratic is how they go about their decision-making process. Finally, a **laissez-faire leadership** style occurs when a leader is largely not involved in the decision-making process. Even if a laissez-faire leader does ultimately decide on a course of action at the end of a process, they are still considered laissez-faire, as they were hands-off in the majority of the work process.

Transactional and Transformational Leadership

In the time since Lewin's theories on leadership first became popular, there has been much further research done on the various techniques and strategies individuals employ in leadership positions. One distinction that has been highlighted is the difference between transformational leadership and transactional leadership. Central to both styles is the concept that a leader is most effective when those they lead are most satisfied in their work, because satisfied workers will have more natural motivation to work hard. With the **transactional leadership** style, the belief is that team members are most satisfied when their objectives and rewards are clear. In other words, the transactional aspect of the relationship, in which the team members put in effort with the expectation of an appropriate reward, is what defines the leadership style. In a **transformational leadership** style, there is the same focus on motivating employees to perform, but the type of motivation is different. Instead of trying to transactionally motivate their employees, a transformational leader is one who motivates their employees by establishing an environment in which the employees feel the most personal growth and connection to their work. Whereas a transactional leader may look to entice an employee into better performance by offering a bonus for a certain quality of performance, a transformational leader will look to improve employee performance by ensuring there is a workplace culture of caring for and nurturing employees.

In order to better understand the kind of mindset and behaviors that underlie transformational leadership style, consider the style's four main components, typically called the "four I's." First, *intellectual stimulation* refers to the quality among transformational leaders to inspire and support innovative ways of thinking in the workplace. Instead of working under the assumption that past policy should dictate present and future action, transformational leaders encourage new ways of thinking and problem solving. Second, *individual consideration* refers to transformational leaders' ability to serve as mentors to their employees. Rather than simply behaving as a boss to their subordinates, a transformational leader seeks to engage with their employees and encourage them to improve both themselves and the organization. Third, *inspirational motivation* is embodied by leaders who can motivate their employees to commit to the organization's vision. Such leaders can convince their employees to internalize the goals and objectives of the organization, resulting in better alignment with their own goals and objectives. Finally, idealized influence refers to leaders who serve as **role models** to their employees. In this way, a transformational leader might inspire their employees simply by leading by example, displaying the behaviors they wish to see more of in their employees. Unlike the other leadership styles, the more ephemeral nature of transformational change and leadership makes it more difficult to discuss the exact actions and behaviors one may want to exhibit. Therefore, the "four I's" provide a multifaceted, if not comprehensive, view of how a transformational leader may act.

Situational Leadership

One leadership style that has gained popularity in recent years is called **situational leadership**. As the name suggests, situational leadership maintains that the most important quality for a leader to have is the ability to adapt to a specific situation. Implicit in such a theory is the idea that no single disposition or mentality for a leader will result in the best outcome every time. For example, a democratic leadership style, although potentially advantageous when considering treatment options for a patient, may not be acceptable in an emergency in which discussion needs to be quick and to the point. Situational leadership style, like transformational leadership style, can be practiced in many ways; however, it is the philosophy supporting the actions that matters.

The main reason situational leadership has gained prominence in recent years, especially in discussions around healthcare leadership, is a growing acknowledgment that for certain workplaces, there is no single style of leadership that will always garner the best outcomes. This is particularly true in a healthcare setting where different patients and scenarios will require leaders to act and plan in different ways. For example, a patient who arrives to the emergency room in some stage of cardiac arrest will clearly require a more direct and autocratic leadership style than a patient who arrives at the hospital stable but with chronic pain of unknown origin. There are also certain types of healthcare environments, such as the operating room, that can better support a democratic leadership style due to the team-based nature of the unit. A situational leadership perspective best prepares healthcare professionals and leaders for any circumstance that may arise by acknowledging that the best way to lead will vary depending on the patient, the team members, and the resources at hand.

For a healthcare leader to best engage with and practice a situational leadership style, it is necessary for them to have a complete and thorough understanding of their team members' strengths and weaknesses. Having an in-depth knowledge of other leadership styles will improve a leader's ability to lead situationally, since they will be better equipped to properly handle a wide variety of circumstances. As a result, such leaders will be capable of preparing and organizing not only themselves, but also the distinct members of their team. Such adaptability can be helpful in both managing the day-to-day activities of a healthcare facility as well as preparing for the often difficult process of securing proper public health accreditation. When the leaders of a healthcare organization are adaptable and cognizant of the varying abilities of their team members, they are best prepared to handle whatever challenges may come their way, whether they involve caring for a patient or caring for the financial health of the entire organization.

Organizational Structures, Principles, and Concepts

Organizational Structure

Organizational structure refers to the framework an organization uses to allot power and responsibilities to its employees and those in leadership positions. While this structure may differ, an example of an organizational structure would be the Chief Nursing Officer (CNO) as top nursing leader making overall organizational decisions for nursing staff, nurse managers running individual departments or units, house supervisors acting as resources for the entire hospital, charge nurses acting as resource and leadership for individual shifts on a unit, and then staff nurses generally following the leadership of the previously listed individuals. Each role has different expectations of responsibility, and facilities will often provide a guide to employees on the hierarchy of the organization's structure and what to expect from each role. This guide can also act as a way to understand what resources are available and to know which person to ask for help. For example, it might be more appropriate to ask the unit nurse manager about scheduling and days off than to ask the CNO. However, the CNO may be the person to go to when a practice council wants to recommend a facility-wide change. It is important for nurses to understand the organizational structure of their facility in order to best advocate for themselves and their patients and to best understand expectations of their own roles.

Shared Governance

Shared governance is a theoretical model used in the nursing profession to promote high quality care and a healthy work environment. Shared governance combines the inputs and skills of both superiors and subordinate staff to hold nursing professionals accountable for their work. This model also aims to nurture collaborative efforts to provide care that is safe, effective, and considered valuable by the patients. It promotes high levels of cooperation and aims to foster respect between all employees in a hierarchical structure, believing that this leads to improved worker productivity and satisfaction, and consequently, better service delivery. Ways to implement shared governance in a medical setting include defining collaborative efforts and boundaries between different professional roles, soliciting input from all staff members, regular in-person meetings where all members feel comfortable sharing opinions, ideas, and concerns, and reliable modes of communication outside of meetings. Shared governance is associated with stronger feelings of responsibility, group collaboration, and professional support in the work setting.

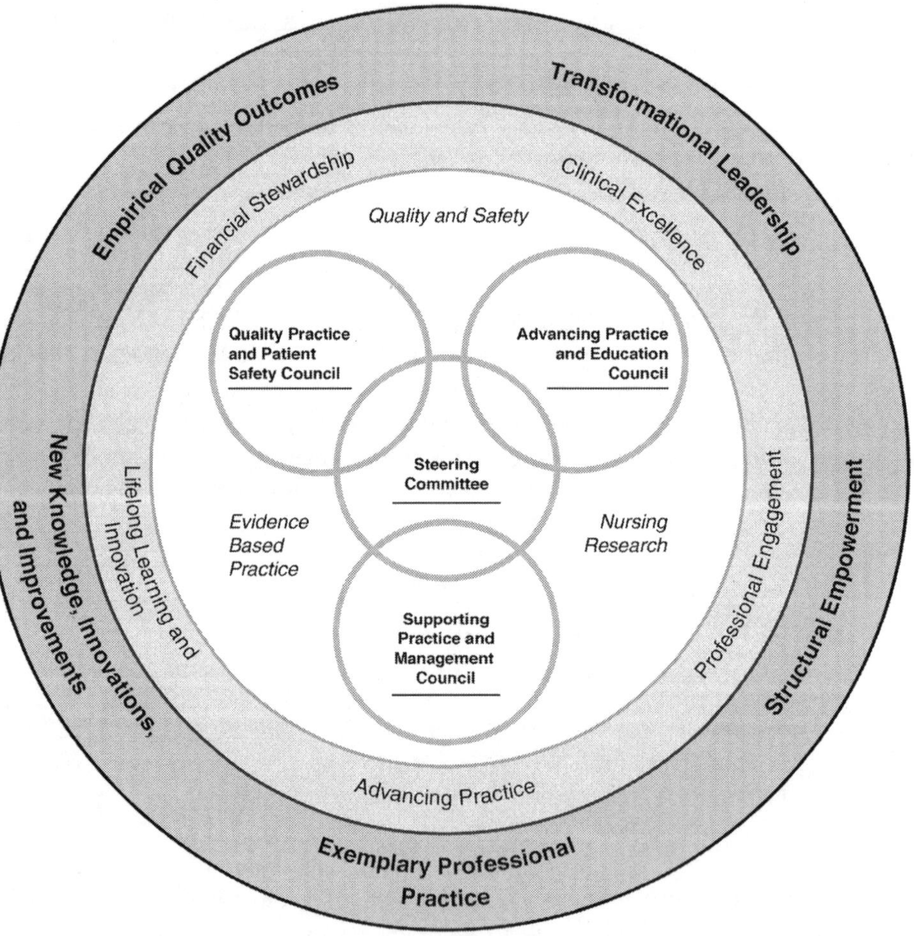

Nursing Care Delivery Systems

Nursing care delivery systems refer to the different methods or structures used to decide roles and responsibilities in the care provided to patients. Some of the different care delivery systems include functional nursing, team nursing, primary nursing, and total patient care or individual nursing. These different systems depend on resources available in an organization, staff abilities, and the goals of specific patient care. Each hospital system may use a combination of these nursing care delivery systems to provide the best care possible.

Functional nursing is a very task-oriented nursing care delivery system. There is generally one primary or leading nurse who then delegates tasks to other nurses. For example, one nurse may administer medications, one may perform wound care, and one may focus on dietary needs. This care delivery system may be less common certain settings, but it is possible that hospitals will have staffed nurses to focus on certain specialized tasks, such as wound care, to ensure increased quality of those specific tasks. However, if this method is applied for all care of the patient, care may become disjointed, as each nurse is task-focused rather than understanding the whole patient care continuum.

The team nursing method of nursing care delivery involves a team leader—someone who is responsible for all patients—assigning a group of nurses to a group of patients. The assigned nurses are then responsible for ensuring that all patient care is completed, and they may delegate tasks to ancillary staff as needed. This method is helpful in environments that encourage flexibility. For example, if one nurse is needed with a particularly acute patient for an extended period of time, the other nurses in the group can take on the care of the other patients. This delivery method can be more common in emergency departments but can also be applied to other areas of nursing when there is a need. Care in this method is more individualized than in functional nursing, but the nurses may have less contact with specific patients and patients may struggle to know who is responsible for their care.

Total patient care (or individual) nursing is likely the care delivery system most commonly seen in nursing. Within this system, there is a head nurse in charge of a unit of patients, who then assigns each nurse on the unit a group of patients who will be the focus of their care for that specific shift. The assigned nurse is responsible for the planning and delivery of care to these patients, delegating tasks as needed.

Finally, in a primary nursing structure of care delivery, one specific nurse is assigned to a specific patient from admission to discharge. The nurse may delegate the care of the patient when the primary nurse is not available at the hospital, but all care responsibilities fall to the primary nurse. This nursing care delivery system allows for a much stronger relationship between nurse and patient, as well as improved continuity of care. However, this method is rare, as there are generally not enough nurses available to make this system possible at most hospitals.

Organizational Climate and Culture

How employees think and feel about a company is critical to an employer. If members of an organization have negative associations with their workplace, it can be difficult to motivate them. The overall "mood" of an organization is known as its **climate**, and organizational climate cannot be directly controlled. However, climate is closely affected by work environment, company standards, interactions, and a general sense of "how things are done around here." Together, these factors add up to what is called organizational culture. So, if an employer wants to improve the company's climate, they need to make changes to the company culture.

Encouraging Communication and Involvement

Encouraging communication and involvement is often a step in the right direction toward changing company culture. And much like climate and culture, communication and involvement are closely related, but not necessarily identical. For example, if John's boss gives him increased responsibility over an aspect of his work, then John has become more involved. However, if John does not have input from his boss on the decision process or a formal way to share his ideas with management, then the boss has not encouraged communication. Conversely, if John's boss starts sending regular memos detailing company activities and the strategies behind them, this is an increase in communication. However, if John and other employees do not have a way to contribute to this knowledge, then the boss has not encouraged involvement. To make meaningful changes to company culture, both communication and involvement should be addressed.

Involvement Strategies

There are numerous involvement strategies that companies can use. For example, the act of delegating authority allows an employee to make more decisions. By granting a staff member more responsibility, an employer can encourage them to take a greater sense of ownership over a company's successes. An employee survey can be used to ask employees how they feel about the company. Surveys can be formal (written or online) or informal (casual conversation), and can address topics such as concerns, suggestions for improvement, and priorities. It should be noted that, even in an anonymous survey, employees may feel hesitant to share their true feelings if the workplace culture is viewed as unfriendly.

In addition to surveys, a **suggestion program**, via an idea box or an online submission form, allows employees to recommend ways to address company problems. Unlike a survey, a suggestion program is an ongoing part of company involvement. Employees can also work together in a formal capacity as part of a committee to address company concerns. Committees may be temporary or ongoing, and employees' service on a committee may also be for a specific term or a permanent appointment.

Moreover, an **employee-management committee** is a specific kind of committee where employees work alongside management to address company concerns. Sometimes known as employee participation groups, these committees also can be temporary or ongoing, depending on the needs of the organization.

Finally, employees can also serve on a **task force**, which is similar to a committee but focused on a specific problem and is usually temporary in nature. Employees on a task force work to determine the cause of a problem and develop a solution.

Change Management

In order to remain competitive, adopt industry best practices, and adapt to changing markets, an organization will undergo change at many points. Change might be implemented to benefit company shareholders and increase the profitability of the company. Change can also occur to reduce costs and increase efficiency. However, especially from an HR perspective, it's important to keep in mind how change affects employees. The truth is that most people don't like change. Workforce changes, such as outsourcing or downsizing, are certain to be met with employee resistance. Even more minor changes like revised vacation policies may go through an unpopular adjustment period. Change management helps to smooth over these difficulties.

Change is inevitable for any organization, especially in fields affected by global markets and technological innovation. **Change management** seeks to aid organizations through significant transitions in resource allocation, operations, business processes, or any other large-scale changes. Careful change management helps the organization to function effectively even while undergoing a major evolution.

Implementing Change

How should an organization implement change? The classic 1961 text *The Planning of Change* tackles this question. The book outlines three strategies for managing change: the empirical-rational strategy, the normative-reductive strategy, and the power-coercive strategy.

The **empirical-rational strategy** assumes that people are rational and will naturally follow any course that's in their self-interest. Therefore, they are more likely to accept change when they think it will directly benefit them. To implement change in line with this strategy, an organization must either 1) demonstrate the benefit of the change or 2) demonstrate the harm of the status quo (or both). One way of accomplishing this is to incentivize change. For example, a growing company is gaining new employees, but it doesn't want to expand its available parking. The company decides to limit the number of parking spots and encourage public transportation use. Employees are reluctant to give up the freedom to drive, so the company holds an educational seminar about how to save money by using public transportation and offers monthly reimbursement for employees who use public transportation.

The next approach proposed in *The Planning of Change* is the **normative-reductive strategy**. This strategy assumes that people will closely follow social norms and expectations. In order to implement change, it's necessary to first change one's idea of what is socially acceptable. This is the strategy that harnesses the power of advertising. For example, think of anti-tobacco advertising campaigns over the past few decades. Throughout most of the twentieth century, smoking was socially acceptable just about anywhere. However, especially in the 1990s and 2000s, aggressive anti-smoking advertisements attacked the tobacco industry and started anti-smoking education programs for students. The social norm turned against smoking in most public places, and now there are more anti-smoking laws than ever before.

Finally, the **power-coercive strategy** assumes that people are followers who will listen to authority and do as they are told. This approach to change is basically, "My way or the highway!" Where the empirical-rational strategy seeks to demonstrate how change will benefit employees, the power-coercive strategy argues that not following change will be harmful to employees, who might be punished or even fired for failure to comply. For example, a factory undergoes an intense safety inspection and decides to completely renovate its safety standards. Employees now have new dress code requirements. If they don't follow the dress code, they aren't allowed to work that day; after the third dress code violation, they will be fired.

Deciding which strategy to employ depends on the overall character of the organization as well as the importance and sensitivity of the change. For example, an otherwise friendly and collegial office might respond negatively to usage of the power-coercive strategy. The power-coercive strategy would be useful for changes with clear legal or financial liabilities, such as when an organization must follow new government regulations.

ADKAR Model

One useful model for implementing and managing change is ADKAR (awareness, desire, knowledge, ability, reinforcement).

Within the ADKAR model, "awareness" refers to the need to ensure that staff are aware that change is coming. If a change is suddenly required of staff without warning, they have lost some autonomy within their role in the team. They are much more likely to oppose the change they did not know was coming and had no chance to prepare for. Because of this, leadership should provide staff with knowledge of the change before it is implemented, allowing staff time to feel prepared and to potentially contribute to its implementation.

"Desire" refers to the practice of convincing the staff that the change is both wanted and necessary. Staff will be more likely to participate in change implementation if they believe that the change is needed and will be beneficial to them. Staff that believe change is unnecessary or even a hindrance to their practice may be resistant and get in the way of progress made in implementing the change.

"Knowledge" refers to the need to provide staff with knowledge of how to make the change happen. Providing more information on what the change is, why it is necessary, and what is expected of them increases the staff's chances of accepting the change. This can be done through continuing education opportunities, meetings, fliers, and even in-service training as applicable.

"Ability" refers to making use of the staff's knowledge to implement the change. This may be from the new knowledge about the change discussed above or it may also include previous knowledge and experiences that may apply to making the change a success. For example, the nurse leader may encourage feedback from those within the staff on how to employ the change or even create a committee dedicated to ensuring success with the change. When staff feel they have contributed to the change, they are less likely to resist it, and the change is more likely to take place.

Finally, once the change has been implemented, "reinforcement" may be necessary to ensure that the change remains in place and continues to be successful. This may mean reminders if staff fail to follow through with the change, or it may mean further assessment to see how the change has affected the unit as a whole.

Resource Management

As managers of client care, nurses must decide which supplies, materials, and equipment are necessary to fulfill the patient's needs as part of the preliminary and ongoing client evaluation. They do this by assessing and determining the patient's condition, at time of primary contact. This involves measuring and recording a patient's vital signs using healthcare tools such as stethoscopes, blood pressure cuffs and thermometers, as well as other patient care equipment, medical technology, and devices. After this initial determination, the next step is ensuring that the patient is supplied with the proper resources, such as patient lifts, ventilators, compression devices, or catheters.

Each nursing team member has varying skills and duties according to the training and degrees he or she received. These skill sets are matched with the client care requirements in the healthcare setting. Depending on the training received, a nurse will be licensed to handle a specific range of materials and supplies. **Nursing assistive personnel (NAPs)** are responsible for providing support services such as assistance with daily living activities, basic hygiene, and comfort care. It is important for all team members to understand how to utilize these associated materials efficiently and effectively.

Nurses should review each function of patient care materials with the NAPs. A good knowledge check is to quiz or question staff members on the various medical devices under their care. This provides an extra level of patient safety, ensuring that all team members are aware of the required equipment and how to utilize it correctly.

The term **cost-effective** means that the cost of a product or service is not too high for what is being purchased. Therefore, a **cost-benefit ratio** refers to weighing the value or likely costs of a project or plan with its desired benefit. Both effective patient care and cost-benefit ratios must be weighed to determine care standards. For example, it has been shown that the length of time between some routine tests could be altered, such as a Pap smear screening, which has been determined to be just as effective to get checked once every three years instead of annually for most women. Regardless, patient care and services must be as cost-efficient as possible while still maintaining high quality standards and client needs requirements.

As a result, providing cost-effective healthcare is often a balancing act performed by all involved. Client care planning by nurses and other members of the healthcare team is determined according to what they deem suitable, economical, and cost beneficial without sacrificing optimal care quality and results. Therefore, the nursing team must carefully select therapies, interventions, and resources that are not only cost-effective, but also the most useful and applicable based on the patient's needs.

For instance, nurses could determine the costs of patient falls within their facility and show how nursing assistance could help prevent them. Another example would be to use cost-analysis data to determine the cost benefit and birth outcome (premature vs. full-term births) for pregnant teens who received prenatal care in a school setting compared those who received routine care. A third example would be to assess the rate of various community health issues, such as smoking, car accidents, elderly injuries, teen drinking, and drug usage, and determine how nursing intervention could improve these outcomes, ultimately decreasing the rate of admissions at their facility.

Accessibility

Healthcare accessibility means an individual can obtain timely attention for all their healthcare needs in order to realize optimal clinical and humanistic outcomes. There are three separate components to accessing healthcare:

- Entering the healthcare system, which generally requires some form of insurance coverage
- Having services available in the patient's geographic area
- Entering a caring relationship with a skilled provider

Each of these steps is a barrier to significant numbers of individuals, in spite of government plans like Medicare, Medicaid, veteran's health benefits, and the Affordable Care Act (ACA) plans.

As healthcare costs and insurance costs continue to escalate, fewer patients have insurance. Employers increase employee contributions to health insurance costs, elderly patients discontinue supplemental Medicare policies, and healthy young people pay fines that are less expensive than insurance coverage. As technology expands the available care options, more of the advanced procedures are provided only in large medical centers in major cities, making the therapies unavailable to large numbers of patients. In addition, acute care and even primary care services are not available in many rural areas. Individuals with insurance coverage may find that their choice of provider is dictated by the network restrictions of that policy, or they may find that their chosen provider does not accept their insurance coverage. Patients without insurance coverage have even greater difficulty accessing a primary care provider and may resort to using emergency services for routine healthcare needs. Accessibility for vulnerable populations such as the homeless who have a disproportionate incidence of mental illness is also a significant problem in the United States.

Efforts to address these disparities include incentive programs to provide primary care coverage for rural areas, expansion of outpatient primary care services for uninsured and under-insured patients, and increased preventive and health-promoting care for all patients. Lack of accessibility is associated with the increased costs of caring for patients with greater morbidity and more complications that require emergency services and hospitalization.

Allocation

Resource allocation in healthcare is a complex topic without a clear-cut solution. There are some key points for understanding the nurse's role in resource allocation, and the bulk of it revolves around being a patient advocate. Adequate staffing, reducing staff turnover, and ensuring equipment safety (both in availability of equipment and in proper usage and storage) are all important aspects of resource allocation. Adequate staffing and reducing staff turnover can go hand in hand. If the nurse feels comfortable with the patient caseload and that there are adequate resources available, there is a lower likelihood of turnover. Reduced staff turnover also results in effective cost management, improved patient satisfaction, and safer patient care.

Coordination

Resource coordination occurs at the federal and state levels, at the care organization level, and at the provider and patient level. The goal at each level is the same: for all patients, provide comprehensive, cost-effective, timely, and individualized care that results in positive patient outcomes. Poor resource management is associated with duplication of services, lengthy wait times for care delivery, and decreased patient satisfaction. The purpose of the patient-centered medical home (PCMH) is to provide access to primary care and specialty providers, timely completion of preventive, diagnostic, and therapeutic services, and the ongoing evaluation and revision of the plan of care.

Care coordination in this model also requires the expertise of certified medical assistants who might manage insurance claims and reimbursement, provide patient care, or manage the agency's calendar. Coordination of services in the primary care setting also addresses support for patients' self-care management for specific patient populations such as patients with chronic illnesses such as diabetes, modifiable risk factors such as obesity and smoking, and special needs such as pregnancy. Improved self-management skills are associated with improved outcomes. The patient portal can be used for patient-provider messaging, coaching, and e-visits to monitor the patient's progress when face to face visits are not required. The downside of the electronic patient interfaces is that the technology remains inaccessible to many patients, either because of the inability to negotiate the websites or the lack of internet access.

The use of the **electronic health record** (**EHR**) is an important element for the coordination of care at the agency level. The EHR is regulated by the **Office of the National Coordinator for Health Information** (**ONC**). Currently, most providers choose onsite architecture for the HER; however, cloud-based systems are increasingly available. There are several ONC-approved software providers for the onsite management of the EHR, such as Epic, Cerner, and MEDITECH. This expensive but necessary technology can be configured to meet all the coordination needs of the provider, including data that support reimbursement and regulatory requirements and enhanced patient interactions that can track the progress of clinical therapies such as hypertension or blood glucose management.

Financial Stewardship

Financial stewardship refers to taking on the responsibility of using another person's or organization's finances and resources and doing so in a responsible and wise manner. In nursing, this refers to not causing undue financial hardship to the patient. It is important to be mindful of how patient care can affect the patient financially and how finances may affect a patient's decisions about their care. On the most basic level, nurses should be careful not to be wasteful of things like medications or supplies that patients may be charged for. Additionally, nurses should advocate for patients when an unnecessary procedure or treatment is being encouraged. It is important to listen to the patient's concerns about cost and work within the interdisciplinary team to find ways to reduce costs when possible while still providing quality care. Nurse leaders can also improve financial stewardship by implementing programs to decrease costs in areas of efficiency, supplies used, and resource management.

Cost-Effectiveness

Cost-effectiveness related to resource management compares the effectiveness of the patient outcomes with the costs associated with the outcome. Consumer groups collaborated with physician's groups to establish the **Choosing Wisely** initiative which calls attention to the wide-spread use of low-value interventions in primary care. One of the initial targets of this initiative was the identification of low-value interventions used to treat patients that were covered by Medicare. Currently, the database contains more than six hundred recommendations from physician's groups that are updated as the guidelines as necessary. The Choosing Wisely website also includes a patient database that prepares patients to ask all the right questions when considering treatment options. A national study recently identified three common low-value treatments that should be reconsidered by providers. These treatments include spinal injections to treat lower back pain, imaging for non-specific lower back pain, and head imaging for non-specific headache complaints. Low-value interventions are more commonly prescribed for patients with insurance coverage, or by providers that are concerned about litigation, or by providers in agencies with reimbursement plans that support utilization.

Providers and patients should understand the process of **cost-effectiveness analysis** (**CEA**) that calculates the effectiveness of an intervention relative to the costs of the intervention. Additional cost versus effectiveness information is provided by **comparative effectiveness research** (**CER**), which generates outcome comparisons for two or more interventions for a specific disease. The information obtained from these analyses provides patients and providers with evidence-based options. CER can address, for example, hypertension, diabetes care for patients receiving chemotherapy, and myocardial infarction drug therapy. There are procedural questions surrounding the use of observational studies in CER; however, there is also agreement that **randomized controlled trials** (**RCT**) studies are expensive and unnecessary.

Utilization

For a more ground-level view of **resource utilization** practices, it can be helpful to consider how such efforts may play out on the scale of a single patient. When it comes to the care of an individual patient, the cornerstone of their treatment plan should always be the efficacy of the interventions selected. The cost of such interventions should not be a deciding factor, and cost should only be taken into consideration as it pertains to delivering the highest quality of care to the patient. As an example, consider a medical condition that has two common courses of treatment with similar levels of efficacy, but one treatment costs significantly less than the other. With such a condition, providing the highest quality care goes hand in hand with reducing costs—choosing the more expensive course of treatment would cost both the healthcare provider and the patient more. In addition, it would generate medical waste while exposing the patient to unnecessary treatments with potentially harmful side effects. Often, the most important way for healthcare professionals to practice proper resource utilization is to ensure that all individuals involved in a patient's treatment plan are fully aware of the exact specifications of that plan and their role in it. Whether a surgical team is reviewing the exact objectives and specifications of a patient's procedure, a nurse is ensuring that a particular medication is properly administered, or a doctor is providing a patient the appropriate outpatient service, any action taken to provide the most effective and efficient treatment options is a form of resource utilization.

The increasing cost of healthcare for both patients and providers has given rise to more in-depth discussion among providers and management about to how to accurately measure the effectiveness and efficiency of the treatment received by their patients. From an operational standpoint, one of the most commonly used metrics to assess efficiency of care is **hours per patient day (HPPD)**. As opposed to many of the metrics used to assess quality of care in healthcare, HPPD is an incredibly easy value to calculate and utilize. In order to calculate HPPD, only two pieces of data need to be gathered. First, one must know the total number of hours that have been worked by the care provider of interest in a 24-hour period. Second, one must know the number of patients at the medical facility of interest for the same 24-hour period. By dividing the number of hours worked by the number of patients, the HPPD value for that healthcare provider is found. As an example, a hospital that has 250 hours of work completed by their nursing staff and 100 patients under their care would have an HPPD value of 2.5.

A practical way to conceptualize HPPD is that it represents how many hours of care, on average, each patient received that day. On its own, an HPPD value can provide a healthcare provider with an image of both the effectiveness and efficiency of its care. Yet, it's important to note that there is no perfect or best HPPD value for a provider to have, and what that value means may be very different across providers. For example, the burn ward of a hospital may consider an HPPD value of 8 to be desirable because they have relatively few patients who require around-the-clock care. However, the emergency room at that same hospital may find it difficult and impractical to aim for an HPPD value of even 1 because they may see thousands of patients in a day. Although it is clearly preferable in most circumstances to have each patient attended to as much as possible, HPPD serves as a reminder of the cost of that care—both the cost to healthcare companies and to their patients. HPPD can therefore be understood as a metric that informs and reminds healthcare providers of this balance between quality of care and cost of the resources, rather than as a grade with a good or bad score.

Promotion of a Healthy Work Environment

Physical/Psychological Safety

Federal Workplace Safety Laws

Workplace policies should strictly follow federal laws in order to legally secure a workplace that satisfies minimum health, safety, security, and privacy standards. Failure to meet federal standards can result in fines or the loss of a license. Federal laws and regulations function as minimum standards that all workplace policies must meet. Employers are allowed to pursue policies that go beyond what is legally required if they believe such policies will benefit the organization. Many employers strive to understand the delicate balance between meeting federal guidelines and maintaining high profit margins. Therefore, organizations often find innovative ways to meet federal standards while using efficient business strategies.

Four examples of federal agencies and laws regarding workplace issues are the Occupational Safety and Health Administration (OSHA), the Drug-Free Work Place Act, the Health Insurance Portability and Accountability Act, and the Sarbanes-Oxley Act.

The **Occupational Safety and Health Act,** passed in 1970, established the Occupational Safety and Health Administration (OSHA) of the federal government in 1971. This agency creates and enforces workplace safety standards. Employers who are engaged in commerce and have one or more employees must observe the regulations established by OSHA. However, partial exemptions are allowed to employers with fewer than 10 employees. These employers do not need to keep OSHA injury and illness records unless requested, however, work-related fatalities, hospitalizations, and amputations must still be reported. Not only does OSHA set minimum standards, but the agency also ensures job training for workers in a language they can understand. Additionally,

OSHA protects employees who work in substandard conditions and informs them of their rights. A critical provision of OSHA is the protection of employees who file a complaint to open an investigation of their working conditions; these employees are protected by OSHA from employer retaliation. OSHA regulations empower employees to advocate for safety and security in their workplace.

OSHA regulations focus on employer and employee rights and responsibilities. Employers are required to meet all OSHA safety standards, attempt to reduce hazards to workers, and supply free protective equipment to workers. Additionally, they must provide safety training and prominently display OSHA posters that detail employee rights. Employers must keep accurate records of any injuries or illnesses that occur in the workplace and notify OSHA promptly of any injuries. Furthermore, employers may not retaliate if an employee uses their right to report an OSHA violation.

OSHA regulations provide specific rights to employees. Examples of these include the right to obtain information concerning work hazards, request a workplace inspection without fear of employer retaliation, and meet privately with a licensed OSHA inspector. Additionally, OSHA regulations allow employees to refuse work that may be abnormally dangerous or life-threatening.

The **Drug-Free Workplace Act of 1988** requires organizations to establish a drug-free workplace, provide a copy of this policy to their employees, and institute a drug awareness program. This law applies to federal contractors with contracts of $100,000 or more and all organizations that are federal grantees. Penalties exist for employers who do not comply with the act, including contract suspension or contract termination. Although an employer may discuss alcohol and tobacco use in its policies, the Drug-Free Workplace Act does not address the use of these substances.

The **Health Insurance Portability and Accountability Act** of 1996 (**HIPAA**) addresses issues of healthcare access and portability as well as aspects of healthcare administration. HIPAA provisions allow workers that change jobs or become unemployed to transfer and continue their healthcare coverage. Additionally, HIPAA regulations establish standards for healthcare administration in order to reduce waste, fraud, and abuse. HIPAA laws strengthen privacy standards and provide benchmarks for medical records in areas such as electronic billing.

HIPAA is applicable to health insurance plans issued by companies, HMOs, Medicare, and Medicaid. Moreover, these regulations apply to healthcare providers who conduct transactions electronically and healthcare clearinghouses that process certain information. HIPAA's Privacy Rule gives rights to the insured regarding the disclosure of medical information, such as the ability to view health records and request an edit of inaccurate information. Additionally, individuals may file a complaint if rights are denied or health information is not protected. Patient information with heightened protection is placed in the insurer's database and may include conversations about patients between medical professionals and billing information. Lastly, HIPAA creates strict rules regarding how healthcare information is disseminated and specifies who is given access.

The **Sarbanes-Oxley Act of 2002**, or **SOX**, is federal legislation that is designed to establish higher levels of accountability and standards for U.S. public institution boards and senior management. The act was passed in reaction to major global corporate and accounting scandals such as WorldCom and Enron, companies that were caught engaging in dubious financial practices. Sarbanes-Oxley specifically targets senior executives responsible for accounting misconduct and record manipulation. The law protects shareholders from any activity that conceals or misleads investors about the firm's finances. The firm has a mandate to report financial information transparently and accurately either to shareholders or the Securities and Exchange Commission (SEC). Moreover, SOX imposes more stringent penalties for white-collar crime and requires detailed reporting to the SEC if a company's finances significantly alter.

Ergonomic Principles

Ergonomics is the science of matching the physical requirements of a job to the physical abilities of the worker. Musculoskeletal injuries can occur if physical demands are greater than the employee's physical capabilities. **Body**

mechanics refers to how the body moves during activities of daily living. Understanding and practicing the use of proper body mechanics is imperative to preventing associate injury. The physical requirements of a job are explained during the interview process, and the physical capabilities of the associate are assessed during the pre-employment physical examination. Education on the use of proper body mechanics begins in nursing school and continues during employment. New associate orientation should include validation of proper body mechanics.

Principles of Body Mechanics

One way the nurse can take care of themselves is to employ proper body mechanics since the job is often highly physical in nature. Common physical tasks include turning patients in bed, transferring them to the chair or bedside commode, and assisting with ambulation to the bathroom or around the unit. Moving another person, especially one with limited ability to assist, can be extremely difficult and taxing on the body.

Depending on the facility in which the nurse works, different equipment will be available to assist with moving patients. Becoming acquainted with how and when to use this equipment will be part of the nurse's training in that facility. The nurse should use this equipment whenever possible, even if it takes a little more time to do so.

Basic **safe lifting techniques** include lifting with the legs, avoiding twisting and awkward positions, and keeping the back upright as much as possible to avoid straining. The individual should make sure to keep their feet as balanced as possible and not rush lifting or moving a patient. The nurse should ask for help from other nurses whenever needed to avoid injury.

The medical environment can present potential hazards that increase risk of injury to the nurse. Examples of these situations include transferring the patient from the stretcher to the operating room bed, positioning the patient, and standing for prolonged periods of time. Repetitive motions, such as turning the head to one side for visualization of monitoring equipment and holding a retractor for an extended time period, can also present ergonomic hazards. Proper body mechanics should be consistently followed to prevent injury. There are three foundational principles of proper body mechanics that should be followed by nurses. First, bending at the hips and knees, instead of at the waist, uses the large muscle groups of the legs to prevent back injury. Second, standing with feet at about shoulder-width apart helps to reduce risk of injury by providing foundational support. Finally, the nurse should keep the back, neck, pelvis, and feet aligned when turning or moving. Twisting and bending at the neck and waist can increase risk of associate injury.

As a standard of care, many healthcare institutions have mandated use of **safe patient mobilization** (**SPM**) equipment to reduce associate injuries and promote patient safety. SPM equipment in the medical environment can be used during patient transfers and positioning. For example, slide sheets are often used in patient transfers. These sheets are placed underneath the patient prior to lateral or vertical transfer. They decrease the surface tension, making transfers easier for the associates. However, since the slide sheets decrease surface tension, they must be removed after use to prevent the patient from sliding off the operating room bed.

Inflatable blankets can be placed under the patient to assist in lateral transfers as well. When engaged, the forced air blanket helps to support the weight of the patient, making lateral transfers easier. The mattress should be deflated after completion of transfer. Another type of SPM equipment is lift equipment. **Lift equipment** works by placing a sling under the patient's limb or underneath the entire patient, connecting the sling to the lift machine, and programming the machine to lift the body to the desired height. The weight limits of these machines vary, so the nurse must ensure the patient's weight does not exceed the weight limit set by the manufacturer.

Injury Prevention

Team members who are not careful to follow guidelines increase their potential for injury, which can result in physical harm, missed days of work, lost wages, and medical bills. Nurses are at high risk for injury due to the amount of lifting required during a shift. Using the appropriate lifting techniques can prevent back injuries and joint strains or sprains. The nurse should employ assistive devices, such as gait belts and mechanical lifting devices, whenever possible. It is important to ask for help whenever necessary to prevent injury. The following list details eight steps to use when lifting a heavy object:

1. Plan for lift and test the load
2. Ask someone for help
3. Get a firm footing
4. Bend knees
5. Tighten stomach muscles
6. Lift with legs
7. Keep the load close to the body
8. Keep back straight

Handling Hazardous and Infectious Materials

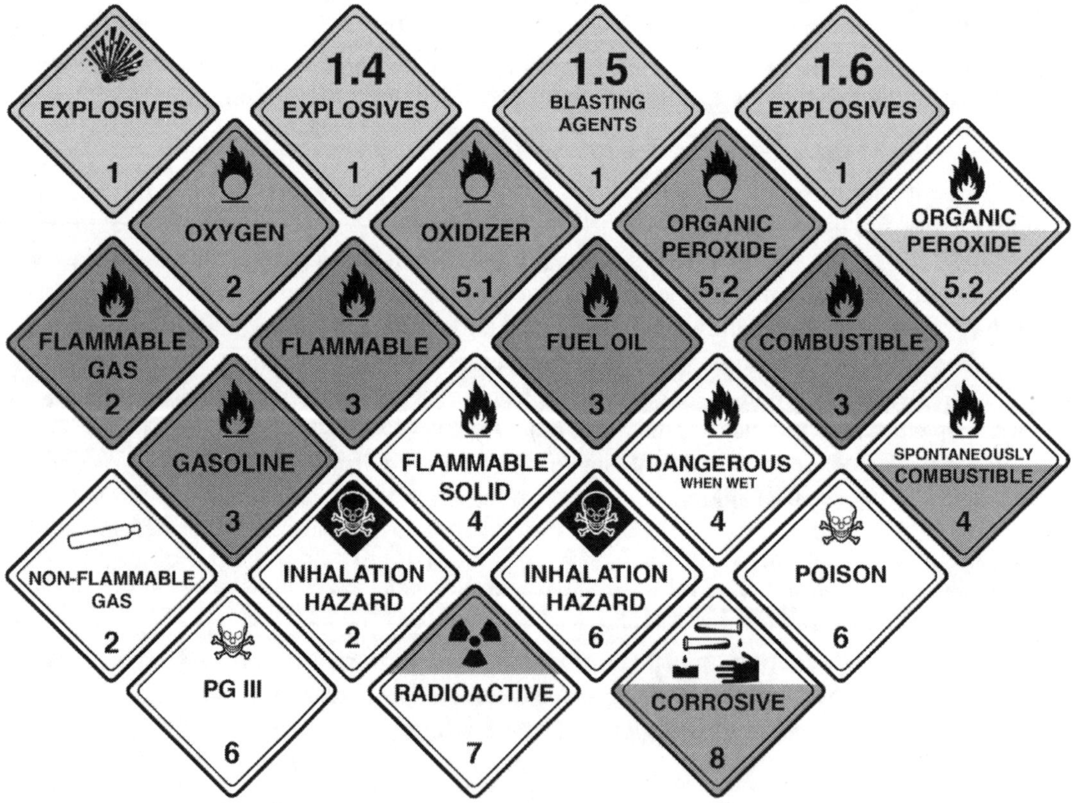

According to the **Institute of Hazardous Materials Management** (**IHMM**), a hazardous material is defined as "any item that has the potential to cause harm to humans, animals, or the environment, either by itself or through interaction with other factors." A hazardous item may be biological, chemical, radiological, and/or physical in nature. Agencies such as the United States **Environmental Protection Agency** (**EPA**) and the Occupational Safety and Health Administration (OSHA) provide regulation and guidelines as to how hazardous materials are handled.

Biological hazardous materials are commonly referred to as **biohazards**. These are materials that present a threat to the health of living things, primarily humans. Biohazards are typically introduced into the medical environment in the form of patient body fluids and excreta. Examples of biohazardous materials are blood, body fluids, viruses, and bacteria. Items in the medical environment that have been exposed to biohazardous materials are considered biohazardous as well, until the decontamination process is completed. For example, used surgical instruments are considered biohazardous until they have been cleaned of bioburden and sterilized.

Chemical hazardous materials in the medical environment include solid, liquid, or gas materials that pose a threat to health. Primarily, solid and liquid chemical hazards include materials used to clean, disinfect, and sanitize the medical environment. They may also include cytotoxic and chemotherapy medications. Gas chemical hazards are primarily anesthetic gases. Containers for chemical hazards are labeled with symbols representing the type of potential hazard, along with instructions for steps to take in the event of exposure.

Radiological hazards found in the medical environment are seen in the forms of thermal, radioactive isotopes, and electromagnetic radiation. The most common thermal radiological hazard is in the form of laser. The use of **lasers** exposes the patient and the healthcare team to risk of eye damage, as well as increasing the risk of fire in the operating room. Laser operators must be trained on the correct usage of the laser, along with indicated safety precautions. Radioactive isotopes are used in brachytherapy. Brachytherapy is a form of cancer treatment where radioactive beads are inserted near or inside a cancerous tumor, delivering a high dose of radiation to the tumor while sparing the surrounding healthy tissue. **Electromagnetic radiation** is seen in the form of X-ray and ultraviolet radiation. During a procedure where electromagnetic radiation is used, the patient is protected by shields and/or drapes specifically designed to minimize exposure to the radiation. The perioperative team utilizes shields, gowns, and eyewear to minimize radiation exposure.

Physical hazards also exist in the medical area. Autoclaves are used to steam sterilize surgical instruments, and this steam can potentially cause burns. Removing surgical instruments straight from the autoclave can cause burns to the hands if the proper gloves are not used. Liquid on the floor can cause someone to slip or fall, causing injury. Handling carbon dioxide tanks or cryogenic material can cause severe burns to the hands if gloves are not worn.

The types of hazards should be discussed at the beginning of employment in the medical environment. This should include identifying the potential hazards and known hazards, steps to minimize exposure to them, and discussing the necessary steps to take in case of exposure. Healthcare facilities are required to provide **Safety Data Sheets** (**SDS**) and keep them in a central area. For most healthcare facilities, education on hazardous materials management is done on an annual basis.

Fire Hazards

Recognizing **fire hazards** in the workplace is important in the prevention of fires and the promotion of safety for patients and employees. Staff will be trained on the fire policy and regular drills should be performed so that each staff person's role is known and practiced. Below are some potential workplace fire hazards:

- Candles may not be allowed in certain facilities. If they are allowed, make sure they are never left unattended, are not within reach of children or pets, and are not placed near windows or material that could burn.
- To mitigate electrical hazards, unplug appliances when not in use and keep them clean and in good working order. If there is concern about a piece of electrical equipment that is not working properly, report it and stop using it. Keep three feet of space around heaters. Do not overload outlets with too many cords, pinch cords behind devices or furniture, or use cords that are cracked or broken.
- Use of a stove and cooking appliances may not be allowed in certain facilities, but these guidelines are useful for anyone that may be cooking:
    - Never leave cooking unattended.
    - Don't cook if too sleepy or if taking medication that causes drowsiness.

- Use back burners on the stove to prevent spills and burns.
- Turn handles away from the front of the stove.
- Don't leave towels or potholders laying on the stovetop.
- Keep the oven and stove clean and wipe up spills.
- In case of a grease fire, do not use a fire extinguisher. Smother the fire in the pot or pan with a lid and turn off the burner.
- For an oven fire, turn off the oven and leave the door closed.
- For a microwave fire, leave the door closed, turn off the microwave, and unplug it.

- Healthcare facilities are smoke-free, but there may be designated smoking areas outside. Ensure that guests or employees use the appropriate area and extinguish the cigarette completely.
- Do not allow smoking near someone who is using oxygen because oxygen can increase the strength of a fire.

Each year, there are many structure fires in health care facilities. These fires happen in nursing homes, hospitals or hospice houses, mental health facilities, and doctors' offices or clinics. Cooking equipment is the primary cause of fires. Other causes of fires include clothes dryers or washers, intentional fires, smoking materials, heating equipment, electrical distribution or lighting equipment, and playing with a heat source.

Employees will be educated on the location of fire alarms, sprinklers, fire extinguishers, and any additional **alarm systems** that are in place. The danger of a fire is mainly from the smoke it creates. Smoke can travel quickly in a fire and affect areas in a building that are not close to the fire itself. With elderly and sick patients, lack of mobility inhibits a quick escape; therefore, proper evacuation and rescue planning is essential. When responding to a fire or an alarm, always treat it as a true emergency. Call 911, even if an alarm system is monitored and activated, to ensure that help is on the way. If it is a false alarm, the fire department may still search to make sure everything is safe.

Safe Use of Equipment

Nurses should ensure that all equipment that is to be used is safe and functioning properly. The use of medical devices is regulated by the United States **Food and Drug Administration** (**FDA**), **The Joint Commission** (**TJC**), and the **Centers for Medicare and Medicaid Services** (**CMS**). Both TJC and CMS require the presence of **manufacturer's instructions for use** (**IFU**) to be present in areas where the equipment is used. Prior to medical equipment being used on patients, the IFU are established by the device manufacturer. It is important for care providers to use the equipment only per manufacturer guidelines, since these guidelines are the ones tested and approved as safe for patient use by the FDA. If a safety concern regarding the equipment arises, the FDA recalls the product until the safety issue is resolved. For example, if a specific type of surgical guidewire breaks off at the tip and causes patient harm, the product may be recalled and pulled from circulation until further investigation.

The product manufacturer's IFU indicates if the equipment poses a fire, electrical, laser, or radiation hazard. If the product does pose one of these hazards, the IFU indicates the type of hazard and recommendations for protecting the patient and equipment users. For instance, if the product poses a fire hazard, the IFU contains information stating which type of fire extinguisher should be available. Also, the IFU advises if liquid, such as sterile water or sterile saline, should be available on the surgical field as a precautionary measure.

TJC and CMS observe **infection control** practices, such as chemical disinfection and sterilization of surgical instruments, during site visits to ensure healthcare facility compliance. If disinfection and sterilization are not performed according to manufacturer guidelines, the cleanliness and sterility of the surgical equipment cannot be verified. Manufacturer instructions for use should be available in each area where surgical equipment is used. Many healthcare facilities utilize **OneSource**, an online database of manufacturer instructions for use. Since OneSource is an electronic database, the contents are updated automatically, eliminating the need to update unit-based binders.

Standard Precautions/Transmission-Based Precautions

Infection prevention is an important focus in all patient care areas to protect patients and staff from transmission of infectious organisms. Standard precautions are practiced during direct contact with the patient and their environment. Followed universally by healthcare providers, **standard precautions** are the foundation for preventing disease transmission in all patient care settings. Included in standard precautions are hand hygiene, **personal protective equipment** (**PPE**), environmental control, and sharps safety. **Hand hygiene** is the gold standard for preventing disease transmission. In compliance with standard precautions, the nurse performs hand hygiene before and after patient contact, before and after applying exam gloves, after touching anything in the patient's environment, before eating, and after using the restroom. PPE protects the nurse from coming into contact with the patient's bodily fluids and other potentially infectious material.

Examples of PPE are gloves, masks, gowns, shoe covers, and eye shields. Surfaces in the patient environment are laden with bacteria and other infectious agents. Environmental contamination is directly linked to pathogen transmission and **hospital-acquired infections** (**HAIs**). Reusable laundry and textiles should be changed and laundered between each patient in a healthcare-accredited laundry facility. Syringes and needles should be limited to single-patient use in compliance with evidence-based care related to infection control. **Sharps** should include safety devices, when possible. Angiocaths (IV needles) and surgical blades are available with built-in safety features that cover the sharp when not in use, decreasing the chance of needle-stick exposure to patient body fluids. In addition to standard precautions, transmission-based precautions are to be used for patients with known or suspected infection of highly transmissible pathogens.

Transmission-based precautions are classified in three ways: contact, droplet, and airborne. **Contact precautions** are used with patients infected or colonized with microorganisms transmitted by direct or indirect contact. These include *Clostridium difficile (C. diff),* methicillin-resistant *Staphylococcus aureus* (MRSA), and vancomycin-resistant *Enterococcus* (VRE). When caring for these patients, the nurse dons a gown and gloves prior to entering the patient room. The PPE is discarded just prior to leaving the patient room, and hand hygiene is performed immediately. **Droplet precautions**, in addition to standard precautions, are used if a patient has a confirmed or suspected infection transmissible through respiratory droplets. PPE associated with droplet precautions are gloves, gown, and mask. The patient is also placed in a single-patient room. Influenza and respiratory syncytial virus (RSV) are indications for droplet precautions. **Airborne precautions** are taken when providing care to a patient with known or suspected infection transmissible via airborne route. The patient's respiratory particles are airborne for prolonged time periods and are carried by normal air currents. PPE for these patients an appropriate respirator with a level of N95 or higher. The most common airborne-transmissible infections are tuberculosis, measles, and varicella.

Security Measures

Within the healthcare facility, maintaining a strong **security system** is vital for patient and staff safety. The professional development nurse will likely be trained in and involved with the hospital's security team, playing an active role in promoting a safe environment.

There are many ways a hospital can be threatened. Examples include infant abductions, secure information breeches, violent person alerts, runaway patients, or bomb threats. For each type of threat, the facility will likely have a plan in place to act quickly and eliminate the potential for danger.

The professional development may be involved with a hospital security planning team, which meets to discuss potential threats and devise appropriate plans. This allows the nurse to voice their opinion and contribute helpful ideas for each potential situation. The security team can share key tips with the rest of the staff based on their training and experience, which is beneficial to the overall security of the facility. Planning, training, and drills all ensure that if a threat were to happen, the team is ready to respond.

Within the hospital, there are various methods of alerting the staff to a security breach. There may be alarm systems, announcements made over a PA system, or a text alert system on the staff's phones that notifies everyone of the situation. Many hospitals have **closed-circuit television security monitoring systems** that employ cameras and video screens to monitor high-risk areas, such as entrances and isolation rooms for violent patients. Certain security doors may be used to keep areas of the hospital off-limits to visitors or can close off areas of the hospital as needed.

Many hospitals use identification badges and bands to ensure only authorized persons and personnel are allowed in certain areas. For example, the parents of a newborn receive a special ID band identifying them as such, which ensures that no one else is permitted access to the baby and prevents abduction.

If the nurse receives a bomb threat over the phone, they should attempt to stay on the line with the person making the threat as long as possible. The nurse may alert other staff of the bomb threat to get the security team in action, while trying to collect as much data on the perpetrator as possible. This information can include sound of their voice, male or female gender, their location, the bomb location, and their motive. The nurse may even be able to deescalate the situation over the phone if they remain calm and collected, but the situation should be handed over to the experts on the security team as soon as possible.

Personal Boundaries

Boundaries in the workplace are an important part of maintaining professionalism. As a nurse, maintaining a professional attitude, demeanor, behavior, and appearance ensures a good working relationship with other colleagues. Healthy teamwork provides the best outcomes for patients. **Personal boundaries** are rules and limits that are set when forming relationships and interacting with others. Relationships at work should be kept professional. It is not uncommon for people to be unaware that personal boundaries are being crossed in the workplace, especially when there is an imbalance of power.

For example, a nurse is approached by a charge nurse assigning a new admission. The charge nurse touches the nurse's shoulder and states, "Hey, sweetie, I know you're busy, but I have to give you an admission." The charge nurse has crossed personal boundaries by touching the nurse and using endearments. It is often difficult to voice discomfort when another person crosses personal boundaries. Expressing discomfort should be done clearly, respectfully, and confidently. For example, the nurse might respond, "I will gladly take the admission. However, I am uncomfortable with you touching me or calling me sweetie. Please call me by my name." Setting these boundaries helps to prevent future occurrences. Should retaliation occur, the nurse should refer the concerns to a supervisor or manager.

Every workplace should establish a culture of safety. A culture of safety ensures that anyone can report misconduct, bullying, sexual harassment, or unwanted attention without experiencing retaliation. Sexual harassment in the workplace is defined as any unwelcome sexual behavior or remark by another colleague. Bullying in the workplace is characterized by a persistent pattern of mistreatment by other colleagues that can cause emotional, mental, or physical harm to an individual.

All facility employees should receive training on how to identify dangerous and unwanted behaviors, how to address them, and how to report them so they don't occur in the future. Safe reporting should be free of barriers. Employees should have a clear understanding of how and whom to report their concerns to. Employees should also feel safe and confident that their concerns will be investigated. Furthermore, they should be free of retaliation. Reporting unwanted behaviors can leave the employee feeling vulnerable and insecure. The main goal of reporting is to improve accountability and create positive change in work culture.

Sexual Harassment in the Workplace

There are two types of sexual harassment that occur in the workplace: quid pro quo and hostile work environment. The translation of quid pro quo is "this for that." **Quid pro quo sexual harassment** takes place when a superior conditions employment (e.g., promotional opportunity, raise, etc.) on sexual favors.

The type of sexual harassment known as **hostile work environment** takes place when sexual or discriminatory conduct creates a work environment that a "reasonable person" would find threatening or abusive (e.g., unwelcome advances, offensive gender-related language, and sexual innuendos). It is important to remember that male employees can also be victims of sexual harassment.

There are four well-known court cases that stemmed from sexual harassment in the workplace:

- *Meritor Savings Bank vs. Vinson*: The court held that sexual harassment violates Title VII. This case dealt with an employee who was plagued with unwanted sexual innuendos. The court said that the plaintiff did not need to prove concrete psychological harm, just an abusive or intimidating environment.
- *Harris vs. Forklift Systems, Inc.*: This case established the "reasonable person" standard for hostile environment sexual harassment.
- *Oncale vs. Sundowner Offshore Service, Inc.*: The court ruled that same-gender sexual harassment is actionable. This case dealt with all males working on an offshore oilrig, where a heterosexual male was threatened with rape.
- *Faragher vs. City of Boca Raton*: The court stated that employers can be held liable for supervisory harassment that results in an adverse employment action. This case dealt with female lifeguards who were sexually harassed. The city was held liable because the lifeguards' supervisors were not informed of the policy (it was not communicated effectively).

The following items are key elements to put in place in order to prevent sexual harassment from occurring in the workplace:

- Provide staff with a written, zero tolerance policy on sexual harassment that contains clear definitions and examples
- Provide a complaint procedure for staff to utilize
- Hold training sessions for employees and document attendees
- Investigate all sexual harassment complaints
- Follow through with corrective action (up through and including termination), if necessary
- Communicate the policy on sexual harassment to everyone in the company using multiple methods

Stress Management

Healthcare providers, like other service-oriented professions, are at a higher risk of experiencing burnout, compassion fatigue, post-traumatic stress disorder (PTSD), and other stress related health issues. The incident rate of stress-related disorders in healthcare professionals, especially nurses, increased significantly due to the COVID-19 pandemic. Burnout is a type of overwhelm and comprehensive exhaustion that occurs directly from work-related tasks. It is not considered a formal diagnosis like other mental health disorders. Symptoms include loss of interest in work, unhappiness at work, physical ailments, and symptoms that overlap with depression. Nurses may experience burnout from staff shortages, long work hours with no breaks, highly repetitive and taxing cases, administrative challenges, or limited professional and personal support.

Compassion fatigue, or secondary traumatic stress, occurs when people are constantly exposed to other people's traumas during the course of their workday. Symptoms are similar to that of burnout, depression, and anxiety, but they also include numbness and inability to empathize. Nurses experiencing compassion fatigue may find it difficult to sympathize with patients' suffering; they may outwardly show irritation and apathy, or they may blame the patient for their condition.

PTSD is a mental health disorder that occurs directly as a result of experiencing a highly stressful, scary, or otherwise traumatic event. Symptoms include recurrent, difficult thoughts, detachment, anger, and flashbacks of the traumatic event. Nurses may experience PTSD after difficult cases in which a patient does not survive or after interacting with violent and aggressive patients. These situations are highly taxing on their own, but chronic stress can lead to physical health problems such as hypertension, insomnia, and musculoskeletal pain.

Seeking professional counseling can be an important way to cope with stress, as counselors can tailor interventions to their clients' unique stressors. Caregiving professionals are accustomed to taking care of others during their workdays and may need to take care of their own families and dependents during their time away from work. Therefore, sustainable self-care is a crucial part of stress management for nurses. Nurses should seek out lifestyle behaviors that will nourish their well-being in the long run, such as getting adequate sleep, exercising, eating nutritious foods, drinking enough water, resting, participating in leisurely activities that are not related to work or caretaking, and spending time with supportive friends and family.

Self-Care

Self-care is a crucial part of maintaining a healthy personal and professional life as a nurse. Nursing is an emotionally taxing field, in addition to the physical and mental demands of the profession. Nurses are at significant risk for experiencing compassion fatigue and developing burnout. Research has shown that insufficient self-care practices contribute to both.

Caregivers can experience compassion fatigue in response to the distress of others, and as a result, they may feel overwhelmed and have difficulty coping. **Compassion fatigue** occurs because of a lack or deficit in the ability to separate oneself from the emotional experiences of others. It can manifest itself as emotional overwhelm, feelings of emotional detachment, or difficulty providing care for oneself and for others. **Burnout** is an adjacent state that is caused by chronic and total exhaustion (mental, physical, and emotional). Burnout symptoms can include fatigue, brain fog, depression, low frustration tolerance, and poor emotional control.

The key to addressing and preventing compassion fatigue and burnout is through self-care and building resilience. Self-care requires balancing personal needs with one's responsibilities to others. **Resiliency** is the ability to effectively respond, adapt, and grow in response to adversity. Ways to promote self-care and resilience include development of skills in the areas of emotional regulation, stress management, communication, and boundary setting. Additionally, it requires a holistic approach to preserving and maintaining personal wellness through mental, physical, emotional, and spiritual health activities.

Several evidence-based strategies have been shown to have a positive impact on self-care and resiliency. One way is by building compassion for oneself as well as gratitude. Strategies to achieve this include practicing positive self-talk, accepting that all humans (including oneself) make mistakes, treating oneself like a loved one or friend, writing or voicing things one is thankful for, and practicing mindfulness. **Mindfulness** refers to accepting reality in the moment without making judgements. Physical strategies for maintaining self-care include taking breaks, eating regularly, moving one's body, being outside, maintaining good sleep habits, maintaining social relationships and support systems, and journaling.

Self-care is unique to the individual. Perceptions have a tremendous impact on a person's reality; therefore, each nurse must develop a practice that feels fulfilling, healthy, and manageable for them. Development of personal self-care and resiliency strategies can be performed on one's own, but many hospital organizations are also developing programs to address the growing rates of compassion fatigue and burnout experienced by their staff. Nurses may participate in these programs, and they may also seek professional help through mental health and counseling services to support and facilitate self-care.

Nurse Resiliency and Well-Being

Nurse resiliency is a key characteristic in the prevention of burnout. The emotional toll and working conditions can become stressors for the nurse, especially in healthcare settings with high acuity patients or high turnover. Nurse resiliency is essentially the nurse's ability to overcome or adapt to adversities in the healthcare setting.

Nurse resiliency and well-being can be closely connected with the concept of emotional workplace safety. An important component of nurse resiliency is communication and positivity. If the workplace culture does not promote open communication, the nurse is less likely to report the feeling of pending burnout, resulting in worsening burnout and a likely decline in positivity.

How can the nurse promote their own resiliency and well-being? First, the nurse must recognize their own present or potential stressors. One nurse may feel overwhelmed with multiple patients but be flexible with their schedule, while another nurse may feel comfortable with multiple patients but be uncomfortable working back-to-back twelve-hour shifts. While these stressors may not always be resolvable, the nurse recognizing them is an important step in developing resiliency. Taking action to recognize and reduce stressors for physical, mental, emotional, spiritual, and social well-being is the most important form of nursing self-care. Common examples include regular exercise, getting adequate sleep, practicing relaxation techniques, and setting goals and boundaries.

Next, the nurse must feel comfortable utilizing any agency/facility resources present for combating burnout, promoting open communication, and furthering education. Nurse resiliency and well-being is a responsibility of both the individual nurse and the healthcare agency/facility.

Moral Distress and Moral Injury

Prominent causes of burnout in the nursing profession are moral distress and moral injury. The nurse feels moral distress when their moral code does not align with what is or is not happening. Moral injury occurs when the nurse can no longer cope with the moral distresses, leading to impaired psychological functioning.

For example, if the nurse is caring for a geriatric patient with a terminal illness, but the family is making the patient a full code, the nurse may have moral distress. Knowing the consequences of resuscitation on a patient, especially a geriatric patient that is actively dying, the nurse could feel morally torn between what is required and what they feel is ethical. The nurse may also feel distress when there is a staffing issue leading the nurse to not perform the level of care that they think is necessary.

Another example of an ethical dilemma is the practice of disaster triaging. With a mass casualty, patients are tagged based on their acuity level. While the nurse knows that it is necessary for the greater good by preserving time and resources, placing a black tag on a patient can be a devastating moral injury for the nurse. The best practice for the nurse experiencing moral distress is to first recognize it and then use available resources to work through the emotional turmoil.

Emotional Workplace Safety

A nurse is guaranteed to experience heightened emotions in one form or another throughout their professional career. Between the tasks, the patients, the environment, the administration, and so much more, the nurse will be subject to a wide range of emotional situations. Feeling overwhelmed from being new on the unit, frustrated by inadequate staffing, or sad because of a patient dying are all realistic feelings in the field of nursing. So how can the nurse manage these emotions effectively to actually improve patient care?

The key element in managing emotions for the betterment of patient care is the culture of the healthcare facility/agency. A culture with harsh reprimands and the silencing of issues can create an emotionally toxic workplace where staff members don't feel comfortable discussing issues, reporting errors, or even working as a team (out of fear and lack of trust). The nurse needs to ensure that the culture allows growth through asking questions, stating concerns, and promoting teamwork. Honesty, trust, and open communication are necessities in the workplace to ensure emotional workplace safety.

Personal Limitations and Seeking Assistance

Working in the hospital environment can be stressful, overwhelming, and physically demanding. The day-to-day activities involve more physical activity than in other care areas. Staff members are frequently on call and working overtime. The nurse is only able to provide the best patient care when they have also taken care of themselves. It is important to remain aware of physical, mental, and emotional health. The nurse should be aware of personal limitations, physically and mentally, and be cognizant of responsibilities that may put the nurse at risk. Whenever needed, the nurse should seek assistance.

Staff Empowerment

Recruitment and Retention

Recruitment refers to the act of bringing in and hiring new staff to a facility or unit. Retention refers to keeping staff long term. A balance between the two is necessary to maintain sufficient and safe staffing. There are several strategies nurse leaders can use to recruit and retain quality staff. Monetary incentives can be helpful for both recruitment and retainment. Sign-on and relocation bonuses may help recruit new staff from other locations. Offering quality benefits, retention bonuses, and retirement plans that increase over time can help with both recruiting and retention. Outreach programs through recruitment teams, job advertisements, and recruitment incentives for current staff can also help bring in new staff. However, the best way to bring in new staff and also retain staff is to promote a positive work environment with cohesive staff and supportive leadership. Nurses who enjoy their place of employment will stay and also encourage others to join them.

Employers can stay in touch with how their employees are feeling about the work environment by conducting what is known as **stay interviews**. During these interviews, topics including why employees came to work for the employer, why the employees have stayed at the employer, what would make the employees consider leaving, and what the employees would want to see changed are discussed. This allows management to make necessary improvements before they find themselves conducting exit interviews.

Finally, in a workplace that is serious about retention, open communication between management and employees about the company's mission and future goals is key. It is also important for management to show concern for employees' continued development and to promote from within when possible.

Exit Interviews

Individuals who are leaving a company are given an exit interview to uncover their reasons for parting ways with the organization. **Exit interviews** are typically conducted by a neutral party, such as an HR professional, rather than by the departing employee's direct supervisor. HR will typically summarize and analyze the data from exit interviews at regular intervals to share information with management regarding possible improvement opportunities.

Alumni Program

Employee engagement can continue even after employees have left the organization. One way is through an **alumni program** that allows HR to communicate with and keep up with former employees. There are several reasons to maintain an alumni program. First, former employees can be a valuable source of referrals and rehires because they are already familiar with the structure, culture, and skills involved with the company. Former employees may also later become clients, customers, or consultants for the company.

One way to ensure the effectiveness of such a program is to have a positive and professional process when employees leave the company. This ensures that former employees leave with a great impression of their former company, allowing them to act as ambassadors and relationship builders for the company even as they continue their careers elsewhere. Learning about an employee's future goals and securing their contact information before they leave sets the stage for future ongoing communication, which is also imperative. Personalized outreach messages—for example, information about entry-level positions for former interns versus consultancy opportunities for former specialists—ensure that communications are relevant and effective. Ways to evaluate the effectiveness of the company's alumni program include analyzing the number of rehires and how long they stay with the company upon rehire; analyzing the number and value of business connections made through former employees; and tracking the number of hiring referrals from former employees.

Professional Engagement

Professional engagement refers to having dedication to and feeling fulfillment within a job or career. It is one of the key factors in maintaining longevity of quality nurses. Professional engagement can be created internally within the highly motivated nurse but can also be encouraged through positive leadership and a positive work environment. Leadership can encourage professional engagement by promoting a culture of safety and by ensuring that staff are comfortable within their roles and are able to meet their own needs through appropriate pay and benefits. Leadership may also provide positive feedback which can further improve engagement. Professional engagement can also be encouraged by positive relationships between coworkers. Nurses are more likely to feel dedicated to their role when they feel safe, supported, and encouraged. Finally, and possibly most importantly, nurses are more likely to have increased professional engagement when they are able to engage positively with patients and see positive outcomes from their work.

Employee Engagement Data

Although HR can gain valuable insights into employee engagement by hearing from individual employees, conducting organization-wide studies allows HR to build a larger dataset. This provides an overall picture of how employees in the aggregate are engaging with the company, identify patterns, and highlight areas in need of improvement.

Generally, organizations collect data through **employee engagement surveys**. Some companies choose to work with third-party vendors that provide surveys and data analysis services. Some advantages of contracting out data analysis are the ease of implementation (no need for a company to design its own questions and response software) and the availability of benchmarking (third-party vendors work with many companies and have access to other datasets to provide comparisons of where other companies stand with engagement). Some companies choose to create surveys themselves, perhaps to save costs or have more control over the survey format.

Either way, even when working with a vendor that provides a survey template, management should review and select the types of questions. In fact, most surveys are structured as statements, and respondents are then asked to rank their level of agreement or disagreement (this discrete ranking response is called a **Likert scale**). Statements fall into common categories such as leadership (how leaders communicate with and motivate employees), alignment (how well employees' knowledge, skills, and abilities match their tasks), development (whether employees have opportunities for professional growth), facilitation (whether employees have access to the tools and resources they need to perform their jobs), and company culture (the personality of a company). The scores that employees assign to each statement can then be translated into quantitative data on engagement. Surveys also typically include a few open-ended response questions that allow employees to share comments or concerns that may not be covered by other parts of the survey.

After gathering data, the next step is for HR to analyze it. To make the data meaningful, there needs to be a point of comparison. For example, having similar or identical survey items every year allows HR to track if certain aspects of engagement are changing or remaining stable. However, HR also must judge whether any change is statistically meaningful. After pulling meaningful results from the data, the next step is to see what story they tell. This involves relating the survey results to other organizational metrics. For example, HR might notice that this year, there was a 10% increase in respondents who agreed with the statement, "I have many opportunities to challenge myself." HR finds that the highest positive responses came from the newest employees. Since HR implemented a new cross-training program for new hires last year, they might conclude that the program led to increased employee engagement in the realm of development.

In communicating the results of the survey, HR must look at the bigger picture of what the organization is trying to achieve and how employee engagement supports that goal. In the above example, HR might demonstrate how the cross-training program leads to more highly qualified employees who stay with the company longer, resulting in decreased hiring costs and increased customer retention. Employee engagement metrics should be considered in the context of overall business metrics.

Work-Life Balance

After taking the necessary time to recruit the right employees, it is important for companies to work to retain them. Employee turnover has high costs associated with it—lost time and lost productivity. There are many different ways that companies attempt to retain staff, and not one method works for all employees. For example, some employers feel that offering a competitive benefits package that includes health care, a retirement program, and life insurance is the best way to retain employees. However, sometimes low or no cost options that improve employees' work/life balance, such as flextime, telecommuting, and allowing employees to wear jeans to work every day (unless they are attending customer-facing meetings) are the best way to go. In addition, staff can be grateful for, and tend to stay longer at, workplaces that provide perks that are meaningful to them. Examples of these include on-site childcare, tuition reimbursement, dry cleaning pickup, and free doughnuts on Fridays.

Diversity, Equity, and Inclusion Advocacy

Response to Diversity

Characteristics of **diversity** include, but are not limited to, ethnicity, race, gender, religious preference, age, lifestyle, and values. According to the Synergy Model, patient needs and characteristics must be "linked" to nursing competencies to achieve maximum health. Nurses are aware that unmet cultural or diversity needs and preferences can adversely affect patient outcomes in much the same way that somatic illness affects outcomes; therefore, **cultural sensitivity** is an essential nurse competency. The development of cultural sensitivity and demonstrated appreciation of diversity by nurses is also viewed as a continuum in the Synergy Model. Novice nurses, who are learning to negotiate the institutional environment, may assess the patient's preferences but often continue to provide care that is consistent with their own belief system. As competent nurses gain life and clinical experience, they actively question patients to learn about and accommodate the traditions and customs of a diverse population, while helping the patient and family to understand the culture of the institution. Expert nurses are able to anticipate the needs of the patient and family by integrating cultural differences into the plan of care whenever possible. All of these nursing interventions work to alleviate the stress related to the acute care environment.

Research indicates that diversity in the workplace strengthens the workgroup by allowing consideration of multiple worldviews and a better understanding of the patient population served by the institution. Multiple viewpoints can also be an advantage in **conflict resolution**, especially when the conflict is related to diversity issues. The Synergy Model suggests that nurses become more sensitive to diversity issues with experience and that this sensitivity is applicable to the work environment as well as direct patient care. Attention to diversity issues also, however, requires institutional support for resource allocation and management. Depending on the specific needs of the patient population, services such as foreign language interpreters, appropriate food service, counseling services, and accommodation for religious observances must be considered. To optimize patient care, expert nurses assess the needs of the patient and family and provide access to the appropriate institutional resources.

The most significant threat to success in this process is **ethnocentrism**, which means that group members are unable to consider views that are contrary to their own beliefs. Alternative definitions in the literature view ethnocentrism as possessing false assumptions about another culture, which assumes that ethnocentric behavior is based on incorrect or incomplete information about other traditions and practices. Attention to diversity issues requires that providers proceed on the assumption that ethnocentrism is a universal human characteristic that must be addressed by the provision of appropriate information and instruction. In addition to understanding their own cultural views, nurses must be aware that many patients have preconceived views of "westerners" and their cultural norms, which may or may not be accurate, but can potentially affect the nurse-patient relationship. The resolution of ethnocentrism in a caring relationship requires acknowledgment of its existence and education as to the meaning of the traditions and practices.

Cultural Considerations

Patients will come from all backgrounds and cultures, and medical providers should be aware of the different cultural needs that may present themselves in a healthcare setting. **Culture** can encompass anything from a person's geographical location, race, ethnicity, age, socioeconomic status, and religious beliefs that influence the behaviors, traditions, and rituals that he or she chooses to engage in each day. It is important to note that cultural considerations will present themselves daily. Some patients may be unable to speak English and will need interpretive services. Some patients may request that only same-sex providers treat them. Some patients may need to keep culturally valuable adornments in place that could interfere with treatment (i.e., a metal symbol on a patient that needs magnetic resonance imaging, a procedure where metal poses an extreme danger). Respecting and attending to different cultural needs will provide the patient with a better healthcare experience, lead to increased patient satisfaction, and impact overall health outcomes (as patients will be more likely to seek out care if they feel comfortable doing so).

Medical providers can show that they consider cultural differences by kindly and compassionately asking patients to share cultural viewpoints, to share aspects of the medical system and services that make them comfortable or uncomfortable, and to continuously create rapport that allows the patient to feel comfortable in voicing their concerns. Medical providers should be mindful of any preconceived notions that they hold of certain cultures and, if possible, actively work to dispel these. Medical providers should also be mindful to not make presumptions, even if those presumptions come from an intention to be empathetic. For example, a patient who looks to be of Asian descent may have been born and raised in the United States and not identify well with any part of Asian culture. Finally, many healthcare organizations offer internal trainings that cover cultural considerations and cultural diversity. For staff that feel their knowledge and experience is limited in this aspect, these trainings can provide an avenue for personal and professional growth.

Having a diverse staff can be extremely beneficial when servicing a patient demographic that encompasses many cultures. Having a medical provider who is able to relate directly with a patient's culture can make the patient feel more comfortable and open. Additionally, a diverse staff can overcome common obstacles such as language barriers or lack of patient education. In this regard, healthcare organizations and nursing leadership should work to actively recruit a diverse workforce.

Gender Equity

Gender equity aims to provide all people with equal access to healthcare, regardless of gender or sexual orientation. Women report that they find health services less accessible, and studies indicate that women pay more for health services and health insurance premiums than men. However, men tend to have poorer health outcomes due to behaviors that may be influenced by social and cultural norms. For example, some studies indicate that men are more likely to feel stigmatized for seeking out mental health services and therefore have worse mental health outcomes than women. They also are less likely to practice hygienic behaviors that prevent disease transmission, such as handwashing.

People in the lesbian, gay, bisexual, trans, queer, intersex, asexual, and other sexual identities (LGBTQIA+) face significant health disparities that lead to poor health outcomes such as depression, suicidal ideation, and participation in risky behaviors. This appears to be due to a lack of education and understanding about these groups' health preferences and goals by healthcare providers. Additionally, many healthcare providers may harbor internal biases against these groups. People in the LGBTQIA+ community are also less likely to have access to health insurance through a spouse, as most employers do not recognize same-sex partnerships for insurance benefits. People who undergo gender transition undergo numerous health procedures in their lifetime that must be handled with sensitivity.

In order to achieve gender equity, healthcare providers must educate themselves on specific diseases faced by vulnerable populations, as well as specific health outcomes desired by these populations. For example, some healthcare providers may assume a young woman who does not want children may change her mind later in life and deny her a tubal litigation without acknowledging the patient's true health wants. Healthcare providers should consider any subconscious internal beliefs or stereotypes they may hold about patient populations, work to address them, and recognize culturally sensitive ways of delivering care.

Implicit Bias

Implicit biases are the stereotypes and unconscious assumptions that influence how an individual views other groups of people. These automatic judgments, which can be positive or negative in nature, form the lens through which people see and behave toward and interact with other people. Within the context of the healthcare setting, this can—and does—lead to inequity in patient-care practices.

The formation of unconscious bias occurs through a complex combination of factors. Individual experiences create memories and impressions, and the brain uses this data to identify patterns that become judgments and beliefs. Beliefs are also greatly influenced by input from family, friends, social groups, communities, and media. Then, our brains process that information and categorize it with the intent of helping us effectively manage our environment.

Unfortunately, this process is not perfect. As mentioned previously, bias is largely formed by personal and social experiences; therefore, social groups can perpetuate inaccurate or problematic biases (e.g., racism, sexism, classism, religious extremism, etc.). Additionally, our brains are biologically wired to identify problematic stimuli as a survival mechanism. In doing so, we tend to overmeasure negative stimuli and undermeasure positive stimuli in our daily lives. Moreover, our brains have an automatic tendency toward confirmation bias, which means that our brains tend to interpret new data in ways that confirm our previously held beliefs. Our brains minimize—and sometimes even forcefully reject—information that does not line up with what we believe. This can be seen in political discussions, with religious beliefs, or in conversations about human rights and equality. Yet another way our brains can come to incorrect conclusions is by making conclusions based on their current level of knowledge and awareness. Children interpret and understand the world in a vastly different way than adults. People from different social and cultural backgrounds will see and interpret experiences and other people in vastly different ways based on their experiences.

Impact on Patient Care

When viewed in the context of healthcare, implicit bias can have devastating consequences for patient-care and health outcomes. In the United States, data has consistently shown that certain populations (e.g., non-white, female, non-English speaking, disabled, obese, non-heterosexual, history of drug abuse) are at an increased risk for receiving suboptimal healthcare. This is an extremely complex and nuanced issue; however, healthcare provider bias is a major contributing factor to this inequity.

Provider bias can result in dismissal of patient concerns, which, in turn, can result in delayed or withheld treatment as well as worse health outcomes. One example of this would be delayed cancer diagnosis and treatment due to a female patient's reports of abdominal pain and changes in bleeding being dismissed by her male healthcare provider. Another example would be a nurse withholding ordering medications (without presence of contraindication) or not following up with the provider regarding inadequate pain management for a patient who has a history of drug use.

Minimizing the Adverse Impact of Implicit Bias

Consciousness accounts for just five percent of all of our total brain activity. This means that implicit bias is unavoidable. However, steps can be taken on an individual and organizational level to address and minimize its adverse impact on patient care.

On an organizational level, diversity in leadership and workforce is one strategy to manage implicit bias. This begins with hiring practices and promotion policies that value the input of individuals who represent different experiences, cultures, age groups, and interests. This helps to prevent biased decision-making or business practices.

On an individual level, caregivers must consciously begin to identify their own implicit biases by examining why they have these beliefs and critically examining their merit. This can allow individuals to recognize when subconscious thoughts are impacting their decisions and actions and can make them more accountable for their actions. Questioning our implicit biases and consciously focusing on the positive attributes of a situation or an individual can also begin to reprogram our subconscious belief systems, which can slowly impact those beliefs over time.

Federal Laws to Promote Outreach, Diversity, and Inclusion

Affirmative action aids employers in identifying imbalances in the workforce and assists them with placing a focus on hiring, training, and promoting groups of workers who are underrepresented. The following employers are required to have **affirmative action plans** (AAPs) in place (otherwise, having an AAP is voluntary):

- Employers with fifty or more employees and $50,000 in federal contracts
- Employers who are a member of the federal banking system
- Employers who issue, sell, or redeem U.S. Savings Bonds

The following sections contain detailed information about the major elements that make up an AAP.

Introductory Statement

An **introductory statement** is essentially a company overview that includes information concerning headcount, along with any significant employment changes that have taken place in the past calendar year. In addition, the company's policy on affirmative action and equal opportunity employment is also mentioned.

Organizational Profile

An **organizational profile** depicts the organization's staffing patterns, to determine if any barriers exist to equal opportunity employment. The organizational structure can be presented in a variety of formats (e.g., graphical chart, spreadsheet, etc.) to show the following information:

- Unit names
- Employees' job titles, gender, and minority status
- Total number of males and females
- Total number of males and females who are also minorities

Job Group Analysis

A **job group analysis** is a list of all titles that comprise each job group. Jobs are grouped according to those with similar content, responsibilities, salaries, and opportunities for advancement. This analysis represents jobs by functional alignment versus departmental alignment.

Job Group Analysis

Title	Salary	Total	Male Female	White	Black	Hispanic	Asian	Native Hawaiian	Indian	Two or More	Minority
Vice President Operations	28	1	1	1	0	0	0	0	0	0	0
			0	0	0	0	0	0	0	0	
Vice President Sales	28	1	1	0	0	1	0	0	0	0	1
			0	0	0	0	0	0	0	0	
Chief Financial Officer	29	1	0	0	0	0	0	0	0	0	1
			1	0	1	0	0	0	0	0	
Chief Operating Officer	30	1	1	1	0	0	0	0	0	0	0
			0	0	0	0	0	0	0	0	
Chairman	32	1	1	1	0	0	0	0	0	0	0
			0	0	0	0	0	0	0	0	
Summary of 1A – Executive		5	4	3	0	1	0	0	0	0	2
			1	0	1	0	0	0	0	0	

Availability Analysis

Organizations examine the internal (employees who are trainable, promotable, and transferable) and external (candidates in the reasonable geographical recruitment area) availability of women and minorities to determine their theoretical availability. External availability statistics can be obtained through state and local governments, which provide statistical data and may even publish it on their websites.

Utilization Analysis

The availability of women and minorities is compared with their current representation in each job group at the company. Companies typically define **underutilization** as the "80 percent rule." This rule is used to determine adverse impact in the employee selection process by comparing the rates at which different groups of people are hired for a job. Eighty percent was arbitrarily selected as an indication of underutilization. Then, for job groups where underutilization is found, reasonable placement goals are set (expressed as placement rates). It is also important to note that a company can have underutilization without experiencing adverse impact.

Other Required Elements

- Identify the individual who is ultimately accountable for the affirmative action plan
- List each identified problem area
- Detail the action-oriented affirmative action programs that will aid in reaching set goals
- Discuss how the affirmative action program will be monitored and reported to management
- Provide executive approval and signature on the affirmative action plan
- Create separate affirmative action plans for qualified, covered veterans and individuals with disabilities
- Ensure proper notices are posted on company bulletin boards about affirmative action and equal opportunity employment

Promote Outreach, Diversity, and Inclusion

A commitment to diversity and inclusion improves a company's relationship with its employees, customers and clients, and the community. Both a business case and a legal case can be made for engaging in diversity and inclusion initiatives. Additionally, the **Equal Employment Opportunity Commission** (**EEOC**) prohibits discriminatory hiring practices. Companies may also be subject to affirmative action laws in their states, and those that have contracts with the federal government must comply with several federal laws. Section 503 of the Rehabilitation Act of 1973, which applies to contractors with contracts over $10,000, requires those employers to take affirmative action for qualified individuals with disabilities. The Vietnam Era Veterans' Readjustment Assistance Act of 1974 (VEVRAA), later amended by the Jobs for Veterans Act, requires companies to have an affirmative action plan for veterans with service-connected disabilities and applies to contractors with 50 or more employees and contracts of $100,000 or over. Executive Order 11246 requires contractors with 50 or more employees and contracts of $10,000 or more to maintain an affirmative action program regarding women and minorities

One common way for companies to improve community outreach and develop a new generation of diverse employees is through an **internship program**. Having interns can be a win-win for the company and the community. People who are new to their field have a chance to develop their skills and learn more about the business. Meanwhile, the company can evaluate new talent and build a pool of prospective employees. Many companies hire full-time employees from previous interns, and these employees already have a great deal of loyalty to and knowledge about the organization. However, federal law should still be considered when designing an internship program. The FLSA establishes clear guidelines regarding wages and overtime pay for employees. Furthermore, for-profit companies planning unpaid internship programs must ensure that their interns are not in fact employees, utilizing a seven-point test created by the Department of Labor. Generally, the test evaluates whether unpaid interns are primarily gaining educational benefit, understand they will not be compensated, and are not displacing paid employees.

Organizations may also have **employee resource groups** (ERGs), which are formed by groups of employees who belong to similar demographic groups (e.g., an ERG for female employees or one for veterans). ERGs help employees to feel represented within the organization, build relationships, share experiences with others who understand their background, and give employers valuable insights into the unique needs and perspectives of a specific employee group.

Americans with Disabilities Act (ADA)

The Americans with Disabilities Act (ADA) was passed in 1990 to protect individuals with disabilities against discrimination in relation to aspects such as employment, pay, and benefits. The EEOC defines such disabled individuals as having a physical or mental impairment that limits one or more major life activities.

The ADA applies to companies and organizations with fifteen or more employees. The act dictates that unless a company or organization undergoes "undue hardship," they are required to make reasonable accommodations for any disabled employees. Examples of such modifications include improving existing facilities to make them more accessible or adjusting the circumstances under which a job is performed. It is important to know that disabled employees must still be able to perform the essential functions of their job positions, with or without accommodations, when hired.

Identifying reasonable accommodations is an interactive four-step process. First, barriers to the performance of the essential job functions must be identified for a disabled employee. Then, possible accommodations that may be helpful in overcoming the barriers are discussed. The feasibility of each of the accommodations is assessed, including if the accommodations are the employer's responsibility or will impose an undue hardship to the employer. Finally, the appropriate accommodations are chosen for the disabled employee. An employer is allowed to ask for proof of a disability if it is not obvious, along with information about the accommodation before deciding to make it. An employer cannot ask if an individual has a disability during a job interview. However, if a candidate comes to an interview in a wheelchair, the employer can ask the individual what type(s) of accommodations would be needed.

Examples of reasonable accommodations include the following:

- Modifying work sites
- Accessible facilities
- Flexi-time
- Flexi-place
- Providing readers and interpreters
- Modifying work schedules
- Assistive devices
- Reassignment (only available as a last resort)

Pregnancy Discrimination Act

The **Pregnancy Discrimination Act**, passed in 1978, was an amendment to Title VII of 1964. The act applies to all employers with fifteen or more employees and states that while pregnant women are working, they are to be treated in the same way as other employees who are performing their jobs. Therefore, pregnancy must be treated in the same manner as any other type of temporary disability.

Under this legislation, an employer:

- Cannot refuse to hire a pregnant woman
- Cannot force a woman to take leave or terminate her employment because she is pregnant
- Must give a woman a comparable position to the one that she held prior to her maternity leave (if the company already does so with employees taking short-term disability) upon her return to work
- Must provide a pregnant woman with reasonable accommodation(s) if she is unable to do her job and approaches her manager to that effect
- Cannot discriminate against a woman who has undergone an abortion

When a pregnant woman is interviewing for a job position, she is not required by law to disclose the fact that she is pregnant. If it is obvious that a female interview candidate is pregnant, a prospective employer can only state the job requirements for the position (ignoring the pregnancy) and ask the candidate when she is available to start work.

Uniform Guidelines on Employee Selection Procedures

The **Uniform Guidelines on Employee Selection Procedures**, passed in 1978, were designed to prohibit selection procedures that have an adverse impact on protected groups. Adverse impact occurs when the rate for a protected group is less than 80% of the rate for the group with the highest selection rate. This is also known as the 80 percent rule, or the four-fifths rule. Below are two examples:

Example 1:

Four hundred white candidates applied and two hundred were hired – 50%. One hundred Hispanic candidates applied and forty-five were hired – 45%. 80% of 50 is 40. There is no adverse impact here. If the number was lower than forty, there would be.

Example 2:

Sixty male candidates interviewed and thirty were hired – 50%. Forty female candidates applied and ten were hired – 25%. 80% of 50 is 40. Yes, there is adverse impact here, since there were only 25% females hired. Females must be hired at a selection rate of 40%.

Under these guidelines, procedures that have an adverse impact on women and minorities must be proven to be valid in predicting and/or measuring performance, so as not to be viewed as discriminatory. The "**bottom line" concept** was an outcome of these guidelines, meaning that an employer is not required to evaluate each component of the selection process individually if the end result is shown to be predictive of future job performance.

If adverse impact is found (which is not always intentional), the employer has alternatives:

- Abandon the procedure
- Modify the procedure to eliminate adverse impact
- Demonstrate job relatedness
- Conduct validation studies
- Keep detailed records
- Investigate alternatives with less adverse impact
- Show the business necessity associated with the need to keep the procedure (which is difficult to do)

Immigration Reform and Control Act (IRCA)

The **Immigration Reform and Control Act** (**IRCA**) was passed in 1986 and amended in 1990. This act was created to prevent discrimination against individuals based on national origin or citizenship on elements such as employment, pay, or benefits, so long as they are legally able to work in the United States. Employers are also required to verify new employees by having them complete an **employment eligibility verification form** (**I-9**) and receiving proof of lawful status within their first three working days. The back of the I-9 form lists each of the documents that can be used to show legality to work in the United States, verifying an individual's right to work and identity. Employers must retain I-9 forms for three years, or for one year after an employee's termination, whichever comes later. In addition, this act established civil and criminal penalties for hiring illegal immigrants.

Furthermore, the IRCA instituted categories for visas, such as immigrant visas or green cards. While permanent or indefinite visas are obtained through family relationships or employment, nonimmigrant visas are temporary. Another example is the H1-B visa, for which there is a yearly cap. This type of visa is set aside for certain kinds of working professionals who travel to the United States for a specified period of time.

Applying Communication, Collaboration, Negotiation, Consultation, and Conflict Resolution Methods

Communication Methods

There are five key principles for effective communication. The first is that telling is not the same as communicating. Communication involves the participation of both parties. Simply telling someone to do something is not effective communication. The other person must acknowledge the information and either ask questions, request clarification and further information, or communicate that they understand. This two-person exchange is communication.

The second key principle is that communication must be clear. It is not the responsibility of the secondary party to determine what the primary party meant by their communication. The primary party must make their communication clear without the need for interpretation.

The communicator should use simple, precise language. Care should be taken to avoid flowery, unusual, or ambiguous language when possible. The message cannot be adequately communicated if it is obscured by muddy language.

Communication requires the participation of both parties, which means that feedback is encouraged. If the receiving party did not fully understand the information, the primary communicator must be willing to hear and respond to queries, even when they are not positive.

The last principle is that direct communication is best. Communicate directly with the party who needs the information, whether that is in writing or via face-to-face conversation. Avoid having people pass verbal messages to others as those messages can get distorted or miscommunicated.

Even when these principles are followed, there can still be barriers to effective communication. The most obvious of these barriers are physical barriers. Distance, such as being on opposite sides of a room, and noise can make effective communication difficult. Similarly, trying to communicate in less-than-ideal surroundings, such as outside in bad weather, can cause misunderstandings.

There can also be psychological and social barriers, such as strained communication between employees who do not get along well or with employees who are intimidated by their managers. Fear, stress, distrust, and anger all inhibit communication. When tempers flare or when either party is feeling stressed, overwhelmed, or upset, it is best to wait to discuss the situation if at all possible. If communication must occur, both parties need to set their feelings aside in order to focus on the conversation and make the communication as effective as possible. In these situations, communicating in writing, such as via email, may be a better option than face-to-face.

Communication is also sometimes limited by semantics. What one party clearly interprets, another might find confusing. Using unfamiliar words or symbols, writing shorthand notes, or writing with poor penmanship can negatively affect communication. For example, if a manager writes notes for the next incoming nursing shift, but the manager's handwriting is illegible, the incoming staff may find it unreadable and incomprehensible. Thus, the communication was ineffective.

Communication Techniques

The nurse is responsible for being a patient advocate. The best way to truly advocate for a patient is not just to listen but to fully comprehend what the patient wants. To do this, the nurse must practice active listening. This form of listening requires the nurse to receive information by listening to the words, watching the body language, and gauging the feelings of the patient; process the information; and respond accordingly. Active listening not only improves the healthcare practice of patient-centered care but also helps to establish a trusting relationship.

Effective verbal communication is not just simply speaking out loud, but also speaking clearly in the language and form that the patient best understands. The nurse can speak clearly and concisely, but if the patient cannot understand the jargon the nurse used, the verbal communication is not effective.

Nonverbal communication encompasses body language, facial gestures, eye contact, and posture. The patient would not feel as comfortable sharing sensitive information with a nurse that is visibly disconnected with her arms crossed and poor eye contact. Nonverbal communication is the way that the nurse can physically show the patient that they are listening. Examples of nonverbal communication include the following:

- Posture: Slouching indicates disinterest, fatigue, and disengagement. The nurse should have erect posture, not only for the health benefit, but to show the patient they are engaged in their care.
- Position: The nurse should be facing the patient, both their face and body. Not facing the patient indicates the nurse does not care about sending a good message and that they do not care about their situation.

- Facial expression: It is not necessary for the nurse to have a big, bright smile on their face at all times, but a pleasant expression that is responsive to the patient's own facial expression gives off a positive energy that the patient may find encouraging.
- Territoriality/physical boundaries: Different cultures have different boundaries that are considered acceptable. The nurse should maintain a respectful distance from the patient, never too far away or too close for comfort. The patient's reaction is a good measure of whether the nurse is at an appropriate distance.
- Gestures: Most people use hand gestures to help communicate a message. The nurse may use hand gestures but must be aware of how much they are doing this. The nurse should avoid overgesturing, as this will take away from their overall message.
- Touch: Therapeutic touch is appropriate in certain instances with certain patients. This could involve touching their hand, putting one hand on their shoulder, or even a hug. Caution should be used when employing therapeutic touch, as some patients might find this uncomfortable. The nurse should use their best judgment on when this type of intervention is most appropriate and helpful.
- Mannerisms: Everyone has certain unique mannerisms, or a way they speak or gesture. The nurse should be aware of their own quirks and idiosyncrasies if possible and make certain they do not interfere with the patient's care or cause offense.
- Eye contact: Good eye contact is crucial to good patient care. Not enough eye contact shows lack of interest and boredom; too much eye contact can be construed as weird and scary. The nurse should be aware of their eye contact and use it as a listening tool to properly tune in to the patient's message they are trying to send.

Communication Types

There are multiple means that a company can use to communicate with its employees. Each method has its own potential advantages and drawbacks. Email makes it easy to get information to a lot of people very quickly. However, this communication method can result in employees suffering from "information overload" from too many emails, making it more likely that important information is overlooked. Also, there is a danger that confidential information may be accidentally communicated to the wrong people.

The **intranet** (internal website and computer network) has the benefit of eliminating risk of important information being accessed by someone outside the organization. Intranets can be very effective at communicating important ongoing information about the company, such as policies and procedures. In addition, companies often store necessary workplace documentation, such as HR-related forms, on an intranet. This allows employees to access that information when necessary. However, if outside parties need information on the intranet, they cannot access it. In addition, intranet communication is often "top-down" and does not allow for feedback from employees. It is also important to note that some intranet systems are not user-friendly, causing employees to be discouraged from using them.

Newsletters can provide a variety of information and have the potential to do so in an engaging, welcoming manner. However, newsletters can be labor-intensive. Since they are relatively infrequent (compared to the ease of sending an email), newsletters are not always useful for communicating urgent or immediate information. In addition, newsletters do not allow for formal two-way communication from employees (although this can be remedied by involving employees in the creation of the newsletter).

Finally, word-of-mouth communication can quickly spread information throughout a group of people. However, as in the children's game "Telephone," information can become muddled, misinterpreted, and downright unrecognizable as it is passed from person to person. A manager or supervisor has no control over misinterpretations and misunderstandings that can result from word-of-mouth communication.

Communication Strategies

There are numerous helpful communication strategies that companies can implement. For instance, a brown bag lunch program is an informal meeting including employees and management that is used to discuss company problems. The company-provided meal can help create a relaxed setting for exchanging ideas. Additionally, department meetings allow everyone involved to share solutions to company challenges.

Town hall meetings are formal gatherings for the entire company that are commonly referred to as "all-hands meetings." They tend to focus on sharing information "from the top down" concerning the overall organization. Thus, town hall meetings are not usually designed to allow feedback from employees about smaller detail issues. An open-door policy is used to establish a relationship where employees feel comfortable speaking directly with management about problems and suggestions. In essence, an open-door policy enables a supervisor to be a "human suggestion box." There are several potential roadblocks to a successful open-door policy. In certain situations, it can be difficult to create an environment where employees feel comfortable discussing problems in person. In addition, depending on the problem reported, it may not be possible to maintain confidentiality. However, in the right situation, an open-door policy can help companies identify problems quickly without having to wait for a formal meeting.

Management by Walking Around (MBWA), as the name suggests, involves having managers and supervisors physically get out of their offices and interact with employees in person. MBWA allows management to check on employee progress, inquire about potential issues, and gain other feedback without relying on employees to "make the first move" through an open-door policy or online suggestion form. This strategy prevents management from becoming isolated behind a desk and disinterested in employees' problems.

Communication Barriers

Prior to providing effective communication, the nurse will need to assess any communication barriers present. It is easy to just associate language with communication barriers, but the nurse will need to assess for more than that to ensure communication is both received and comprehended by the patient/family. Communication barriers can present in the form of a language barrier, cultural barrier, cognitive impairments or limitations, and physical impairments.

Language/Cultural Barriers

Language barriers can vary from completely different languages to mild accent differences. The nurse will need to become familiar with the facility/agency translation services. Each healthcare facility/agency will have an approved translation procedure to use. Using an approved interpreter can not only improve communication but can also provide cultural sensitivity/phrasing. Language barriers can also present with the use of slang or complex medical jargon.

Cultural barriers can present without a language gap. The nurse will need to be prepared to care for patients with varying cultural backgrounds without judgment. For example, some Asian cultures highly value stoicism when experiencing pain. If the patient states a verbal pain score of 10/10 and remains expressionless, the nurse will be responsible for communicating with the patient and treating the patient accordingly, as this is a cultural difference in reception and expression of pain.

Cognitive Impairments/Limitations

Cognitive impairments or limitations can occur due to neurological damage (e.g., CVA, TBI), a congenital disorder, or just the standard progression of childhood understanding. Cognitive impairments or limitations will require the nurse to establish the appropriate form and level of communication. For example, educating a five-year-old patient on an upcoming procedure will require the nurse to recognize the cognitive limitations present. The attention span, memory, and comprehension are not that of an adult, so the nurse will need to provide age-appropriate teachings.

Physical Impairments

Physical impairments include anything that would physically hinder the patient from speaking or hearing effectively. A common example is a hearing deficit that would require the nurse to speak clearly and slowly, without shouting at the patient.

Collaboration Methods

Collaboration occurs when interested parties work together to achieve a mutual goal. According to the Synergy Model, nurses collaborate with the patient, family, and other providers to satisfy the patient's healthcare needs. Several attributes of the process have been identified, including goal setting, problem-solving, communicating, and decision-making, which serve as an indication of the skills required of the individuals involved in the collaborative process. Some of the benefits of collaboration include improved patient outcomes, decreased healthcare costs, decreased length of stay, improved patient and nurse satisfaction, and improved teamwork. Collaboration related to patient care has been widely studied and is considered as both a process and an outcome, which occurs when no single individual is able to solve a stakeholder (patient) problem. Collaboration as a process is defined as a synthesis of diverse opinions and skills that is employed to solve complex problems. As an outcome, collaboration is defined as a complex solution to a problem that requires the expertise of more than one individual. This view of collaboration characterizes the process as a series of actions by more than one individual, which creates a solution to a complex problem.

Initially, all members of the collaborative team must identify their own biases and acknowledge the effect of these mental models on the decision-making process. In addition, members must also be aware that the complexity of the problem will be matched by the complexity of the mental models of the collaborative team members, which will influence the decision-making process. It is also essential for team members to recognize the elements of diversity in the group. For instance, while stereotyping is obviously to be avoided, there are gender differences that should be considered. Research indicates that men tend to be more task-oriented, and women tend to be more relationship-oriented in the problem-solving process; this means that consideration of both points of view is necessary for genuine collaboration.

Another requisite skill of the collaborative team is the development and usage of conflict resolution skills, which are required to counteract this common barrier to effective collaboration. Team members are required to separate the task from the emotions that are inherent in the discussion. Effective collaboration also requires that members of the team display a cooperative effort that works to create a win-win situation, while recognizing that collaboration is a series of activities that require time and patience for satisfactory completion.

Common barriers to effective collaboration include conflicting professional opinions, ineffective communication related to the conflict, and incomplete assessment of the required elements of the care plan. Research indicates that physicians tend to stress "cure" related activities while nurses tend to encourage "care" related activities, which means that some resolution of these differences is required for effective communication. Although the Synergy Model defines collaboration as a necessary part of the process that matches the patient's needs with the appropriate nursing competencies, it is also possible that the end product of the collaborative process may be the best possible solution for the patient and at the same time be totally unacceptable to the patient. Collaborative team members should also be aware that while successful collaboration improves patient outcomes, research indicates that genuine collaborative efforts are rarely noted in patient care, often because the group is unable to integrate the diverse mental models of the group members. This means the initial first steps of the process mentioned previously are essential to the success of the collaborative process.

Delegation of Tasks to Assistive Personnel

Nursing staff take on many responsibilities that can be delegated to other clinical and non-clinical colleagues. However, learning how to effectively and safely delegate tasks, while still making patients feel cared for, is a skill that can take time to develop. It requires knowing not only what the needs of the patient are, but also the strengths and weaknesses of assistive personnel and how to best communicate professional needs with them. It also requires personal development in becoming comfortable with outsourcing responsibilities, as the nurse who delegates still remains accountable for the patient.

Assistive personnel may be supervised by nurses, but clinical assistive staff can provide basic medical assistance such as monitoring patients' vital signs, assisting with caretaking duties, monitoring any abnormalities or changes in the patient, maintaining a sterile and safe environment, and any other request made directly by nursing staff. Non-clinical assistive personnel, such as front desk staff, can assist with patient communication (such as wait times), managing paperwork and ensuring it is complete, and performing any other administrative task that may support the nursing staff's cases.

When nursing staff choose to delegate tasks, they may feel worried about risking their own accountability or work ethic. However, relating with assistive personnel, understanding their strengths and weaknesses, understanding their interests, and remaining transparent about the needs that are present in the department can ensure that delegated tasks are a good fit for the person who is taking the responsibility. In this regard, nursing staff take on a leadership and managerial role that requires developing their problem-solving, time management, and interpersonal skills. Some effective tools for delegation can include standardized checklists that cover the procedure that is being delegated, formal and informal meetings about assistive personnel's comfort levels and interests in performing certain tasks, and matching professional needs with individual qualifications. When delegation is effective, it can help the entire department work in a more efficient manner. Additionally, both nursing staff and assistive personnel are more likely to feel like part of a cohesive team and less likely to feel overworked or undervalued.

Interprofessional Roles and Responsibilities

The difficult part of coordinating care and ensuring consistency is the number of interprofessional roles and responsibilities within the healthcare team. Each individual healthcare professional working toward the goals stated in the patient's care plan introduces the possibility of unintended overlap and miscommunication. The nurse's role in preventing these discrepancies is to understand who does what and why. That may sound generic, but understanding the dynamics of the healthcare team can help prevent lapses in patient care as well as provide the patient with a better healthcare experience:

Doctors

- Consists of medical doctors (MDs) and doctors of osteopathic medicine (DOs) Both MDs and DOs receive the same amount of training, but DOs specifically train with additional holistic models of care.
- Roles and responsibilities include diagnosing the patient, formulating treatment plans with additional diagnostics/therapies/medications, providing preventative healthcare, and providing information regarding healthcare decisions.

Advanced Practice Providers

- Consists of nurse practitioners (NPs) and physician assistants (PAs)
- Advanced practice providers can function with the same roles and responsibilities as the doctors, but may require oversight depending on the state's scope of practice.
- Advanced practice providers receive less schooling and clinical training than a doctor.

Nurses

- Consists of registered nurses (RNs) and licensed practical nurses (LPNs, also sometimes referred to as licensed vocational nurses [LVNs])
- Roles and responsibilities of the nurse include performing routine patient assessments, administering orders from doctors or advanced practice providers, being a patient advocate, providing patient education, and coordinating care.
- The difference between RNs and LPNs is the level of education and treatments provided. The RN is able to perform more complex medical therapies, while the LPN provides more direct patient care.

Nursing Assistants

- Roles and responsibilities include duties assigned by the doctor/advanced practice provider or nurse that are within the state's scope of practice (e.g., bathing, feeding, and toileting).

Medical Social Workers

- Roles and responsibilities include providing counseling, providing referrals for community resources, being a patient advocate, and using tools to assess the patient's well-being.

Additional Interdisciplinary Team Members

- Can consist of physical therapists, speech therapists, occupational therapists, respiratory therapists, dieticians, spiritual counselors/chaplains, healthcare specialists, or mental health counselors

Interdisciplinary Collaboration

Interdisciplinary rounding can provide an opportunity for team collaboration. Much like a clear hand-off process, interdisciplinary rounds reduce patient care errors, decrease mortality rates, and improve patient outcomes. Interdisciplinary rounds are an excellent place to discuss social service needs, nutritional care services, and transportation needs with all teams coordinating care for the patient in a single setting.

The patient's service needs may vary in depth for the inpatient stay and at the time of discharge; however, there should be an evaluation of these needs and a coordination of care for those services in which there is a need. Nurses document the action plan as it relates to services and requirements for the patient and collaborate with members of the interdisciplinary team to see that next steps are executed in a timely fashion. In many instances, rounding may not be possible due to the rapid pace and turnover of the medical environment, and thus, clear documentation will be needed to allow for synchronous care coordination.

Nurses, physicians, surgeons, nurse aids, physical and occupational therapists, mental health professionals, and medical assistants are just some of the members who may be collaborating on the care of one patient. Perception of power between these professionals can sometimes create a stressful environment that can also affect patient outcomes. Collaboration among team members is imperative so that patient safety does not become an issue. **Collaboration** involves joint decision-making activities between both disciplines, rather than nurses only following physician orders. Although each role may have a particular focus throughout the assessment and plan of care activities, they must jointly come together to formulate the best possible plan of care throughout the treatment period. Studies show that an attentive communication style between nurses and physicians has the most positive impact on patients.

Ongoing education of physicians and nurses may be a necessity to support a collaborative environment. In addition to continuing education and in-services, job shadowing can assist in promoting understanding and teamwork by exposing both the nurse and physician to one another's role.

Continuity of Care

If one imagines a patient's illness as a road, what would the ideal road look like? Smooth, no potholes, appropriate signage to guide and direct the patient from illness to wellness, right? In the real world of health care, the road the patient travels from illness to wellness often has bumps and miscommunications. Things do not go as planned, missteps are taken, and unexpected events or miscalculations unfortunately do occur.

All members of the healthcare team should be striving to provide patients with a high quality of care over time, or **continuity of care**. The patient begins their journey with an illness at a doctor's office, convenient care clinic, or an emergency room. From there, the road proceeds through various tests and procedures to diagnose and treat the illness. Management teams that include doctors and nurses provide input into this process and contribute resources. The patient is at the center of the continuity of care model. In continuity of care, the whole patient is treated, not just an organ or an illness. Ideally, the community surrounding the patient is also involved in promoting good health and high quality of life.

The roots of continuity of care lie in a meaningful, long-term relationship between the patient and the healthcare provider. This relationship ensures that the patient is known. Their needs are anticipated through regular check-ups and follow-ups after the illness has run its course. The idea is to form a firm bond of trust between the healthcare provider and the patient. This trusting relationship and deep knowledge of the case allow the provider to better advocate for the patient.

The physician or nurse practitioner coordinating care for the patient will look for ways to make the plan of care cost-effective for the patient. Tests and procedures are carefully weighed for their usefulness in the patient's case, looking for ways to eliminate wasteful healthcare spending.

The main idea behind continuity of care is to avoid what happens all too often in healthcare: **fragmentation of care**. The responsibility of the patient's case is often shifted from one entity to another over the course of an illness. Initially, the patient's case is handled in a primary care setting or perhaps an emergent care setting, depending on the illness. Then the patient may become hospitalized, at which point the hospitalist and various specialists step in and take over. At discharge, the patient's case is then handed over to their primary care physician and community centers. Due to this shifting of care, it becomes ambiguous as to who is overseeing the patient's care. The patient has a fragmented experience rather than a continuous one.

One issue faced by healthcare providers is not having the infrastructure to effectively coordinate patient care and avoid the problems associated with fragmented care. A case manager comes into play here because their role is perfect for coordinating the patients' care as they move through the system.

Primary care physicians face a hurdle when coordinating patient care because they have limited communication with the hospital team when their patient is admitted. Presently, there is often a team of healthcare providers called **hospitalists**, whose job it is to care for patients while they are in the hospital, but not pre- or post-admission. This is helpful because they know the ins and outs of the facility and have good communication with the hospital's specialists and surgeons. They can all work together to get the patient in and out of the hospital relatively quickly.

A **patient-centered medical home (PCMH)** comes into play pre-admission to prevent a costly hospital visit. The idea of a PCMH is to combat fragmentation of care and promote better continuity of care for the patient on their road to wellness. The PCMH is a model of care that is well-coordinated, proactive, and centered on the patient. In this model, a patient is paired with a personal physician to oversee their care. Their family and loved ones are recruited to assist in promoting a whole patient-focused wellness plan. The PCMH moves away from fee for service; instead, it focuses on fee for value, meaning the level of success in keeping the patient healthy determines how the healthcare team is reimbursed. The patient must regularly keep in touch with their primary care physician, a factor that has been associated with better patient outcomes.

Many communities are adopting the PCMH model of healthcare, attempting to promote a better continuity of care for patients on their road from illness to wellness.

Nurses are aware that the patient often requires continued reinforcement of the educational plan after discharge, which necessitates coordination with home care services. As facilitators of learning, nurses may be involved in a large-scale effort to educate all patients. The first step of any teaching-learning initiative is the assessment of the learning needs of the participants. Specific needs that influence the design and content of the educational offering include the language preference and reading level of the participants. Nurses must also consider the effect of certain characteristics, identified in the **Synergy Model**, on the patient's capacity to process information. Diminished resiliency or stability, as well as extreme complexity, are examples of characteristics that must be considered in the development of the educational plan. Nurses are also responsible for creating a bridge between teaching and learning in the acute care setting and the home environment. A detailed discharge plan, close coordination with outpatient providers, and follow-up phone calls to the patient may be used to reinforce the patient's knowledge of the plan of care.

Consultation Methods

Continuum of Care

Continuum of care refers to the healthcare team's ability to provide consistent services throughout the process of the patient's healthcare experiences. The healthcare team should be able to follow the patient throughout transfers of care and patient changes while providing the services needed over the patient's lifetime. There are multiple effective continuum-of-care models, but the main aspects include prevention, treatment, and maintenance.

Preventative healthcare can take the form of wellness checks, routine dental visits, and scheduled vaccinations, but the concept is evolving. It can mean education regarding heart health or weight management as well. Essentially, preventative healthcare is the attempt to prevent the need for further healthcare intervention.

This aspect of treatment is present in any healthcare environment, but it's most often found in EDs, urgent cares, specialty offices, and primary care provider offices. Treatment can take the form of medications, surgical interventions, therapies, or procedures.

The aspect of maintenance has the main goal of reducing the progression or symptoms of the disease process. Maintenance can include rehabilitation, therapies, medications, lifestyle changes, and education regarding compliance.

Referral Process

As patient advocates, nurses should be knowledgeable about referring clients when a need arises. The nurse is aware of many branches of the healthcare tree that are designed to assist with each patient's specific needs. A **referral** is a method by which the nurse contacts another member of the healthcare team to meet the patient's care needs in the most appropriate setting. This is part of care coordination and must happen throughout all stages of the client's continuum of care. Case managers play a key role in making appropriate referrals.

Referral occurs during the first stage of the nursing process: assessment. The nurse assesses the patient and identifies a need. For example, a school nurse may become aware of students who have learning or developmental disabilities. In these cases, the nurse may refer the child and their parents to a speech therapist, a language therapist, or a developmental therapist, depending on the case.

In the hospital environment, the nurse may recognize the need for an auxiliary team and refer the client to them. Such **auxiliary teams** include the palliative care and hospice team, respiratory therapy, physical and occupational therapy, and speech/language therapy. **Community resources** should be used when appropriate, such as extended-care therapy, social service support, and shelters for the homeless and disadvantaged. Patients may also need spiritual care, in which case clergy can be requested to make a bedside visit.

With any referral, the nurse must follow the appropriate protocols and remain within their scope of practice. Other members of the health care team, such as physicians and nursing management, should be consulted. Doctor's orders must be obtained where necessary.

After the referral has been made, it is vital that the nurse or case manager evaluates the patient for their response to care. Evaluation is a key component of the nursing process. Without evaluating for effectiveness, the process is incomplete. Only after evaluation has shown effectiveness and the patient is on their way to recovery can the plan of care be deemed successful.

Conflict Resolution Methods

Conflict with Patients or Family Members

Nurses sometimes must contend with aggressive and violent behavior from patients or their family members who may be distressed. An aggressive or violent patient can be characterized by the exhibition of any nonverbal behaviors or verbal communication that intend to cause conflict, harm, pain, or injury. An aggressive or violent patient may invade personal space, make verbal threats or obscene gestures, mimic or follow through with physical threats, speak unnecessarily loudly or in a hostile manner, or be generally abusive in some other verbal or physical way. The causes motivating these behaviors are variable. Patients may show aggressive or violent behavior due to a psychiatric or physiological issue, such as drug abuse, delusions, head injuries, and infections of the brain. However, aggressive or violent behavior can also be a result of the patient's personal background and history, such as family upbringing, socioeconomic status, and current personal stressors.

While mediators are available for complex situations, the nurse will need to be prepared to practice basic mediation techniques. It is important for the nurse to remain consistent, not allowing varying emotions to dictate the care they provide. Effective mediation practices include the following:

- Discussing conflicts in detail to verify understanding
- Identifying root issues
- Establishing goals for conflict resolution
- Context reframing

Nurses should assess each patient for potential aggressive or violent behavior. This can include looking for known risk factors on intake forms (e.g., medical and psychological history, documented history of violence or substance use, history of detention or imprisonment, or personal stressors such as unemployment). This can also include assessing the patient directly and taking note of appearance, mental and physical state, pupil size, level of perspiration, mood, tone of speaking, and any comments made by the patient that could indicate current feelings of hostility or anger.

Nurses should be knowledgeable of their healthcare setting's policies and local laws as they relate to managing or sedating aggressive or violent patients. To protect the safety of medical personnel, the patient, and other patients in the vicinity, if a patient becomes visibly aggressive or violent, physical restraint may need to be provided by a dynamic team from the facility. In some cases, it may be necessary to administer antipsychotic medication or sedation.

Nurses should keep the following principles in mind when handling conflict or communicating with family members:

- Recognize that the family is the constant in the patient's life while the service systems and personnel within those systems fluctuate.
- Be aware of family strengths and individuality and having respect for different methods of coping.
- Encourage and facilitate family-to-family support and networking.
- Share complete and unbiased information about the patient's care with family members on a continuing basis in a supportive manner.
- Design accessible healthcare delivery systems that are flexible, culturally competent, and responsive to family needs.

Conflict with Staff Members

Staff conflict occurs when team members have different views or thoughts on an issue. Conflict on the job can be disturbing and anxiety-provoking. However, it is an inevitable part of working as a team.

Recognizing and reporting conflict involves the following steps:

- *Defining the conflict*: Conflicts occur when two or more people have differing attitudes or viewpoints. Conflict can be helpful when it is resolved in a healthy manner, equally fulfilling to both parties, and results in closure.
- *Evaluating the various factors that can provoke conflict*: Arguments, a lack of trust, workflow disruptions, impaired interpersonal relationships, criticism of others, and frustration are examples of issues that can incite conflict.
- *Recognizing the variations of personality types*: It is imperative to embrace the various ways team members think and feel and how these diverse factors will affect the outcome of the conflict.
- *Distinguishing types of communication*: Team members can display a wide range of communicative techniques during any type of interaction. However, conflict can cause people to behave in varying ways, such as becoming guarded or aggressive. It is important for team members to be aware of this possibility.

Here are a few ways to resolve team conflict:

- *Collaboration and Open Communication*: Working together and maintaining an open exchange between team members helps to cultivate relationships among group members. By encouraging the conflicting parties to actively participate in the resolution, a more in-depth understanding of the dispute can be achieved.
- *Compromise and Negotiation*: Maintaining a level playing field encourages both parties to remain confident but not belligerent, promoting equality between team members. Discussing the issue rationally allows team members to focus on common goals and interests, rather than individual parties and their diverse opinions. As a result, the conflicting parties can separate themselves from the conflict and issue at hand.
- *Mediation*: Sometimes one-on-one communication with each team member is required in order to discern each person's concerns, beliefs, and opinions. Once this occurs, the team can investigate resolving the conflict via methods that are satisfactory to all involved.

There are six stages of team conflict resolution:

1. Clarifying the disagreement and making sure both sides agree on the topic of the issue.
2. Establishing a common goal agreed upon by those involved in the conflict.

3. Discussing the various techniques the team can use to gain a common understanding.
4. Defining the issues that are in the way of reaching the common goal.
5. Coming to an agreement regarding the best way(s) to resolve the conflict.
6. Agreeing upon a solution and deciding the responsibilities of each member.

Furthermore, it is important to remember that every conflict and team dispute is unique. Keep the following in mind when deciding how to approach a situation:

- *Acknowledge personal reactions of team members*: Every team member may have a totally different response to conflict and how it is being handled by the team. These include being evasive, dominating, accommodating, collaborative, or cooperative.
- *Choose useful conflict resolution techniques*: When a conflict arises, it is important to be aware of the fact that team members will have varying principles and priorities on how to settle it. Therefore, selecting the best technique for resolving conflict will depend on each situation and those involved.
- *Recognize the benefits and drawbacks of team conflict-resolution strategies*: These include dealing with the issue, thinking it through, discussing it in person, using a mediator, apologizing when needed, and communicating clearly and effectively.
- *Be aware of situations that typically require employee disciplinary action*: Since conflict can disrupt the workflow of the whole team and covers a wide range of behaviors, sometimes disciplinary action is required.

De-escalation Techniques

De-escalation in healthcare can be a complicated balancing act between empathizing with the individual and establishing boundaries of mutual respect. There are a few techniques that the nurse should feel comfortable practicing in the event that a patient, family member, or even coworker needs to be de-escalated.

First, the situation should be taken to a private area with a safe exit for the nurse at all times. Not only can the stimuli from a public environment worsen agitation, but it can also create a situation in which an altercation is more likely to occur.

Next, the nurse needs to focus on maintaining a calm demeanor. Regardless of the individual's level of anger, the nurse should always maintain a non-threatening posture and calm voice. Using active listening and empathy, the nurse can attempt to de-escalate the individual.

Lastly, the nurse needs to ensure that firm boundaries are in place. The concept of respect will need to go both ways, and it is appropriate for the nurse to calmly reiterate the consequences to certain actions.

Group Facilitation

Interprofessional/Interdisciplinary Teams

No employee works alone. The unit or department is staffed by a team, and everyone, from the nurse executive and managers to the nurses and the staff, is part of that team. Managing a team means understanding the **team dynamics**—everyone's work styles, values, and goals—and how everyone works together to care for the patients.

It is important to understand that a group is not a team. A group of people can work in the same place, but they are not a team unless they can work together toward a common goal. Members of a team are engaged with one another and actively collaborate together to solve problems. They show respect for one another and keep the goal—providing the best care for the patients—always at the forefront.

It is the responsibility of the managers to create a cohesive team and cultivate a successful team dynamic within the unit or department. The first aspect of this is creating a common goal and developing a plan for reaching and maintaining that goal. Goals can be set for daily tasks or longer-term projects within the unit, department, or organization. Regardless of their scope, goals should be established using the **SMART** acronym: Specific, Measurable, Achievable, Relevant, and Time-Bound.

SMART Goals

A specific goal includes detailed information about who is expected to do each task or who will be impacted by each task. The goal should be precise, clear, and free of jargon, confusing, or ambiguous language. A basic, specific goal might be that nurses should visit all of their patients on the unit within the first hour of their shift.

The team's goal should also be measurable, meaning that it can easily be determined whether or to what extent the goal was reached. If a nurse has ten patients and visits only eight of them during the first hour of their shift, the nurse has reached 80% of the goal.

Goals should also be attainable. Setting goals that a team is wholly unable to achieve creates tension, anxiety, and feelings of hopelessness and inadequacy not only within the team but also for each individual member of the team. Unattainable goals can eventually lead to job dissatisfaction and result in losing employees. Instead, set goals that the team can achieve, even if they must put in more work or effort to get there. It would not be reasonable to ask a nurse with ten high-needs patients to complete visits to all of them within too short a time frame. The nurse will just become anxious and frustrated, and patient care could suffer.

Goals for the team should be relevant. Goals should make sense to the team, encourage better patient care, and allow the department to run more smoothly and efficiently.

The last aspect of SMART is that goals should be time-bound. There should be an end date by which the goal should be met. The team should have time to work toward achieving the goal, with enough urgency to make them strive to improve but not so urgent as to create stress and anxiety.

Roles and Responsibilities

For any team to be successful in a task, it is important that they have clear roles and responsibilities. Each role may have specific responsibilities attached to it. These roles may be important in the day-to-day management of the unit so that delegation and task management can be streamlined. However, establishing set roles and responsibilities is especially important when a high-stress emergency situation may occur. For example, if a patient is having a life-threatening emergency, it is important to know which nurse will be documenting interventions, which nurse will be assisting with interventions (such as CPR, medication administration, etc.), which nurse will provide communication with additional resources (e.g., doctors, house supervisors, etc.), and who may take on a leadership role directing the emergency situation. Establishing these roles before an emergency happens can reduce anxiety during the emergency and improve chances of success in overcoming the situation as a team.

While each team member on a unit may have individual roles and responsibilities, the roles and responsibilities of the individual nurse may change over time. As nurses gain more experience and knowledge, they may take on new responsibilities and leadership roles. For example, a nurse may gain a new skill and become a resource to the unit in being the expert on performing said skill. More knowledgeable and experienced nurses may become preceptors, mentors, or educators. Nurses may also choose to step into new roles. For instance, nurses may establish a practice council focused on making quality improvements to unit patient care practices.

Team Dynamics

Once the team is established and working toward a common goal, the managers need to carefully assess the team dynamics, or how the members of the team interact with one another and collaborate together to achieve their common goal. It takes time and care to build a team that works together, communicates well, and collaborates effectively to provide superior healthcare to its patients. Common pitfalls must be avoided. One such pitfall is the "us" versus "them" mentality that can develop when things don't go as planned. For example, if a nurse neglects to complete a task that then falls on the next shift to finish, it can create negative feelings. It is important that everyone understands their role and is accountable for their responsibilities.

Managers can help alleviate these feelings by encouraging clear communication. Scheduling shifts that overlap slightly allows for staff on differing shifts to communicate with one another. A short meeting where the outgoing team can brief the incoming team on previous events and current patient status updates creates a sense of unity and collaboration between the different shifts. Furthermore, it reminds everyone that they are on the same team and working together to provide the best care for their patients.

Team Conflict Resolution

Despite everyone's best efforts, there will inevitably be conflicts that must be resolved. Ideally, team members will be able to communicate with one another and resolve minor issues between themselves, but that is not always the case. Nurse executives and managers must be prepared to assist in finding a mutually agreeable solution to conflicts.

The first step to **conflict resolution** is fully understanding the situation. Managers must be willing to listen to their employees. They must take the time to meet with the employee one-on-one, without other distractions, and actively listen to the employee's concerns. The manager should refrain from any judgment and instead seek to fully understand the situation, employee's feelings, and position within the conflict. Once the manager has heard from the initial party, the same time and consideration should be given to the other person, to hear their side of the situation.

Once the manager fully understands the conflict, they can determine the best path forward. Ideally, both parties should be involved in reaching resolution, with equal and due respect given to everyone. Sometimes the manager needs to act as a mediator, allowing the two parties to talk to one another, understand each other, and resolve their differences. Other times, the manager may need to resolve a dispute by deciding on which particular action to take. In all cases, though, the employees need to feel heard, understood, and valued throughout the resolution. They need to know that the resolution is in the best interest of the team and the patients.

Leveraging Diversity

Humankind is a unique mix of demographic differences in ethnicity, race, socioeconomic situation, gender, sexual orientation, and religion. **Diversity** can also come in the form of attitudes, ideas, beliefs, and experiences. In other words, people come from many different walks of life, and the healthcare team must be ready to manage patients from every background and situation. To this end, a diversified team can better relate to its patients, and patients feel more comfortable when they feel as though their team understands them and can relate to them. In addition to patient comfort and satisfaction, a diverse team leads to more innovative thinking and unique ideas for problem-solving. Generating creative and exciting ways to solve problems and meet team goals can invigorate the whole team, building on their sense of unity, respect, and appreciation for one another.

There are specific elements that managers can implement to foster a diverse work team and inclusive environment. First, management must create a safe space where everyone is valued, questions are welcomed, and the whole team is committed to understanding one another. In addition, managers should be aware of their own implicit biases and work to overcome those. The workplace policies and procedures should be reviewed to ensure that they are not adversely affecting any particular demographic, and employees should feel free and comfortable to bring any concerns to their managers.

Managers should also require a diverse pool of recruits when looking for new hires. Human resource departments and employee search firms should understand the needs and requirements of the team, both from a skilled professional standpoint as well as from a diversity and inclusion perspective. Managers should also ensure that everyone has equal access to professional development opportunities, while utilizing the unique knowledge, skills, and ideas of each team member to strengthen the team as a whole.

Focus Groups/Meetings

Staff Advocacy

Professionally, nurses advocate for policies that support and promote the practice of all nurses regarding access to education, role identity, workplace conditions, and compensation. The responsibility for professional advocacy requires nurses to provide leadership in the development of the professional nursing role in all practice settings that may include acute care facilities, colleges and universities, or community agencies. Leadership roles in acute care settings involve participation in professional practice and shared governance committees, providing support for basic nursing education by facilitating clinical and preceptorship experiences, and mentoring novice graduate nurses to the professional nursing role. In the academic setting, nurses work to ensure the diversity of the student population by participating in the governance structure of the institution, conducting and publishing research that supports the positive impact of professional nursing care on patient outcomes, and serving as an advocate to individual nursing students to promote their academic success. In the community, nurses may collaborate with government officials to meet the needs that are specific to that location.

Professional Networking

Professional behaviors in nursing are meant to advance both the profession of the individual and also create better opportunities within nursing as a whole. Networking and participation in professional organizations are necessary to create connections between nurses and to provide professional opportunities that would not be possible without working together.

Networking refers to the act of forming relationships and contacts that could potentially provide one with future opportunities. This can be done on the unit between fellow nurses, by maintaining a positive relationship with leadership, and also by seeking outside relationships through professional organizations and community events. Networking requires forming a bond, but also expressing one's personal goals so that others within the relationship know how to help if an opportunity arises. Networking might help a nurse move up into a leadership position or find another job within their profession if change is needed. Working together in this way can help improve career satisfaction and stability within the nursing profession.

Similar to networking, participation in professional organizations allows nurses to work together to form a community and make improvements within the profession. One example that is common in some states and healthcare facilities is participation in nursing unions. When working in unions successfully, nurses can advocate for improved staffing standards, higher pay, and better work environments. This can improve career satisfaction, nursing job retention, and the level of care available to patients. Nurses can also get involved in practice counsels meant to improve quality of care on their unit and in their hospital. For example, a wound-care practice counsel could work together to track how certain interventions are affecting outcomes of patients with pressure sores and advocate for improvements to practice where needed. Finally, nurses can also participate in outside organizations, such as specialty organizations, to obtain continuing education, improve their personal practice, form bonds with others in the specialty, and even advocate for improved practice in the specialty as a whole.

Professional Development

Professional Standards, Certification, and Credentialing

Each healthcare facility/agency will be responsible for following the regulations set forth by local, state, and federal laws and guidelines. The healthcare facility will follow these laws through the implementation of policies and procedures. For any nursing skill or practice, each healthcare facility will have a specific policy/procedure to follow, of which the nurse will likely be assessed for understanding and competency. Policies and procedures are created, reviewed, and revised by the healthcare facility's quality assurance/improvement team. Below are the common healthcare regulatory and accreditation agencies:

Healthcare Facility/Agencies

- Quality Assurance Team: Includes compliance specialists, administrators, and QA healthcare personnel

Local Agencies

- Varying local agencies responsible for public health measures and emergency response planning

State Agencies

- State Board of Nursing **(BON)**

Federal Agencies

- Occupational Safety and Health Administration **(OSHA)**
- National Institute for Occupational Safety and Health **(NIOSH)**
- Environmental Protection Agency **(EPA)**
- Department of Health and Human Services **(HHS):**
    - Centers for Medicare and Medicaid Services **(CMS)**
    - Center for Disease Control and Prevention **(CDC)**
    - Food and Drug Administration **(FDA)**
    - National Institutes of Health **(NIH)**

Accreditation Agencies

- Assurance (NCQA)
- Commission on Accreditation of Rehabilitation Facilities (CARF)
- Council on Accreditation (COA)

Nursing Professional Practice Model

The nursing professional practice model is a cultural framework for nursing care defined by most healthcare facilities/agencies. The model is put in place within the specific facility/agency to give the nursing staff professional guidelines for communication, care, and collaboration with the facility/agency's values in the forefront. While each healthcare facility/agency will have a different set of values, the general framework for a successful nursing professional practice model is typically the same. The five general subtopics of a nursing professional practice model include the following:

- Core professional values
- Professional relationships
- Professional recognition and compensation

- Care delivery system
- Management/administration

The keys for a successful professional practice model require the following:

- Nursing involvement in the creation, review, and revision process
- Evidence-based research and literature
- A graphic or visual to depict the model
- Routine evaluation to evolve with the changes within the organization and general healthcare environment

A nursing professional practice model not only provides the nursing staff with a framework of good nursing practice, but also an opportunity to buy in to the culture. In a large healthcare facility, cultural practices have to be routinely assessed and reinforced.

For example, the administration within a hospice inpatient facility highly values the nurse frequently spending time with the patient (e.g., giving emotional support, conversing with the patient and family). This facility also has a nurse-to-patient ratio of 1:5 with controlled substances being administered frequently. In this situation, there may be a gap in the priority values and the reality in the clinical setting. The administration may value quality time, but the clinical staff may be unable to provide that level of care with the current workload. In this situation, the nurses may state that the nurse-to-patient ratio will need to change to allow more quality of time with each patient.

Professional Practice Standards

Maintaining professional practice standards is another important role of the professional development nurse. They must follow standards that have been set forth by professional nursing bodies, such as the ANA. One way that professional development nurses can achieve this goal is through participating in **professional development** opportunities alongside their staff. They can also maintain professional practice standards by providing skill competency sessions and continuing education opportunities. Each of these components promote and facilitate quality nursing care delivery.

Professional Practice Evaluation

Personal and collective growth in the field of nursing requires ongoing evaluation of professional practice. This occurs on individual, group, organizational, and global levels throughout the field of nursing. Performing this necessary critique identifies strengths and weaknesses and allows for ongoing advancement of the profession.

General areas of evaluation can focus on many performance aspects. Aspects of **professionalism** (e.g., appearance, behavior, communication, and leadership style) can be addressed as well as the level of adherence to applicable standards or policies. Another performance category could be related to growth and development, including completed continuing education or advanced certification (e.g., becoming an Oncology Certified Nurse). Other areas of evaluation include engagement with professional organizations, committees, quality improvement projects, or community involvement. Additionally, contributions to the field of nursing or healthcare (e.g., professional writing or political involvement) can be considered.

On a personal level, nurses perform self-reflection and planning to determine how they feel about their performance and potential areas for improvement. They can formulate professional goals and plan the development necessary to achieve those goals. At a team or organizational level, nurses also receive feedback from peers and leadership. **Peer feedback** identifies how colleagues perceive the performance of their coworkers. **Leadership feedback** often provides a more global view of performance through comparison of personal performance to averages of larger groups (e.g., the unit, hospital, or region). Organizations also receive feedback in the form of surveys from employees as well as the organization's customers. Each level of evaluation provides opportunities to examine growth pathways and formulate development plans.

Upon identifying an opportunity for improvement, it is critical to follow up with a plan for development. Goals should be specific, time-bound, and identify resources necessary to achieve the goal. On an organizational level, this can include referencing education materials, enrolling in professional or organizational groups or counsels, or breaking goals down into smaller steps. Lastly, re-evaluation must occur at regular intervals to follow up on previous goals. This provides external accountability for completing the steps and achieving the stated goals.

Certification and Credentialing

Each state and territory in the United States has a Nurse Practice Act, under which a **board of nursing** must be established. This board regulates nursing standards, credentials, education requirements, best practices, and licensure within the state or territory. Each area's board of nursing ensures that once standards for licensure are met, they are meticulously maintained throughout one's nursing career in order to uphold high safety and quality standards. If a nurse fails to maintain standards established by their area's board of nursing, they may lose licensure or undergo other disciplinary and corrective actions. If nurses choose to move jurisdictions, they may need to pass requirements for the new jurisdiction. Nurse practice acts and boards of nursing are in place in order to ensure that all forms of nursing, which can take place in a range of settings and with a wide demographic of patients, exhibit competence, skill, quality, and care in all contexts.

Mentoring Processes

Mentoring and coaching refers to the act of providing guidance and support to another. This can be done through the teaching and encouraging of new staff and nurses by more experienced staff and nurses. These resources are vital to integrating the newer generations of nurses into the nursing profession and can promote further benefits such as a more positive work environment, improved care practices, and even career advancement. Nurses can be mentors and coaches at any stage of their professional career and can also have or need mentors and coaches at any stage. These mentor/mentee relationships can establish organically as one nurse guides and encourages another naturally as they work together and form a positive working relationship. Nurse leaders can also encourage mentorship through establishing mentoring programs by recruiting nurses and helping to match them with nurses who may need more support in their role.

Reflective Practice

Reflective practice refers to the act of looking back upon one's practice or work to understand a particular situation better and then using this reflection to improve their practice. Reflection can be more appropriate in certain situations, and understanding when and how to reflect is necessary for this practice to be successful. Reflective practice may also involve making changes to one's practice and then further assessing how those changes worked. In addition, reflective practice can be promoted by positive nurse leaders and mentors. Reflective practice can create better outcomes for patients when integrated into nursing practice.

There are many situations when the nurse may find that reflection is helpful and even necessary. Most commonly, reflective practice may be implemented following negative situations. If there are mistakes made during a procedure, complications following a procedure, or a patient expresses unhappiness with the care they have received, it can be beneficial to look back on what may have gone wrong. Identifying where a fallout may have happened and then considering how it could be avoided in similar situations in the future is a necessary form of practice improvement and education for the nurse. This can also be done in positive situations. When the nurse reflects on how actions taken in a situation were successful, those actions can then be further applied to promote more positive outcomes.

Once the nurse has reflected upon how a particular situation proceeded, the nurse can then take action to potentially implement changes for future situations. After these changes are implemented, reflective practice is further used to determine the successes and/or failings of said changes. The nurse may reflect on whether the changes made a difference in outcomes, and if these outcomes were better or worse than before the change was implemented. Here's an example of this: when a nurse reconstitutes a medication, he notices that the pressure in the bottle causes some of the medication to spray out when drawn up, leading to waste and the patient not receiving all of the medication. The nurse might try a new method of mixing and drawing up the medication, such as first drawing air out of the bottle to reduce the pressure. The nurse should then reflect on whether or not his new technique prevented medication waste. The nurse may even employ the knowledge and experience of those in leadership or mentor roles to help solve this problem. When nurse leaders and mentors promote a nonjudgmental environment that allows for constructive feedback and quality improvement, they can play a vital role in promoting reflective practice in the nursing profession.

Reflective practice is not always purely an individual action; it can involve the entire healthcare team. Often after a particularly difficult situation with unclear outcomes, the team may come together to debrief on what went well, what could have improved, and what to do moving forward. These can be especially common following situations involving close teamwork and high levels of stress, such as codes or procedures with unexpected complications. However, reflective practice can also be applied to day-to-day activities and changes. Reflective practice can be an important part of quality improvement measures within a unit.

Professional Empowerment

Professional empowerment refers to a professional's internal motivation to strive for excellence within their role. Within the nursing profession, this idea of excellence may mean becoming an expert in certain skills, advancing one's education or career station, or providing the best possible patient care experience to all who enter the hospital. Excellence may look different for each nurse. Some will find great motivation, for example, in staying within their current role and becoming competent mentors to their peers. Others may see excellence as advancing their education to management or advanced practice levels. All are valid and necessary for success within the nursing profession. While professional empowerment may look slightly different for each individual nurse, nurses can improve their own empowerment by setting professional goals and finding satisfaction in achieving their desired outcomes. Nurse leaders also promote professional empowerment by encouraging autonomy within roles and encouraging a positive environment dedicated to improvement and excellence.

Practice Quiz

1. Two of Olivia's staff are having a dispute about which responsibilities are whose. What can she do to resolve the situation?
   a. Request that HR revise and clarify the job descriptions
   b. Establish a protocol within the department for handling job disputes
   c. Schedule a meeting with herself and the two employees to clarify the responsibilities of each person
   d. Tell the two employees to sit down and resolve the issue themselves

2. Which of the following are some of the differences that create diversity within the workplace?
   a. Gender
   b. Ethnicity
   c. Religion
   d. All of the above

3. How can a diverse nursing team better care for patients?
   a. Patients feel more comfortable when they feel as though their nurses can relate to them.
   b. A diverse team creates less potential for conflict.
   c. Different people have different styles of bedside manner.
   d. Patients like people with different personalities

4. What is one thing that managers and professional development nurses can do to foster a more diverse workplace?
   a. Increase professional development opportunities and requirements.
   b. Create a safe space where everyone is committed to inclusiveness and understanding one another.
   c. Set a schedule to change up team groupings every week.
   d. Strictly adhere to department policies and procedures.

5. What is the first stage in effective resolution of staff conflict?
   a. Agreeing on a solution that will prevent the conflict from reoccurring
   b. Clarifying the topic of disagreement with the affected parties
   c. Determining who started the conflict
   d. Defining barriers to reaching a common goal of resolution

See answers on the next page.

Answer Explanations

1. C: The most immediate and effective solution is to schedule a meeting with all three parties to resolve the confusion. Once that is done, then a request can be put in to HR or upper management for a revision to the job descriptions, Choice *A*, if necessary. Choice *B* can be helpful in the long term, but it would not immediately fix the current problem. Telling two people who are already at odds that they have to fix the problem themselves, Choice *D*, often just creates more conflict and can lead to resentment.

2. D: There are many different factors that can create diversity within a team. Gender, ethnicity, and religion are all examples of diversity that can exist amongst team members.

3. A: Patients feel more comfortable when they feel as though their nurses understand them and can relate to them, which leads to better care and a better experience for the patient. While all teams have the potential to experience conflict, Choice *B*, diversity does not necessarily make this more or less likely. It is also true that different personalities will care for patients differently, Choices *C* and *D*; however, that is not a characteristic of diversity.

4. B: Creating a safe work environment where everyone is committed to understanding one another helps to foster a diverse team and an inclusive environment. While continuing education, Choice *A*, is important, it is not usually a factor in creating diversity. Changing up team groupings, Choice *C*, can actually create a more divisive environment. Adhering to the department's policies and procedures, Choice *D*, is generally a good practice, unless it goes against diversity and inclusion efforts. Instead, existing policies and procedures should be reviewed to ensure that they are not adversely affecting any particular demographic.

5: B. The first stage in staff conflict resolution is to clarify the disagreement or conflict and make sure the involved parties agree on what the problem is before moving forward. Choice *A*, agreeing on a solution, is the last stage of conflict resolution. Choice C, determining who started the conflict, is blame-based and not part of effective conflict resolution. Choice *D*, determining barriers to resolution, is a stage of conflict resolution, but is not the first stage**.**

Ethical, Legal, and Regulatory Standards

Professional Standards and Ethics

ANA Nursing Scope and Standards of Practice

The Nursing Scope and Standards of Practice publication by the American Nurses Association outlines the ethics, skills, and competencies to be followed by professional nurses at any stage of their vocation. The document establishes the foundation for the obligations, duties, promises, and ideals expected of the nursing profession from their peers and the public.

There are ten provisions that comprise the Code of Ethics, with the most recent added in 2025. The first three provisions focus on the nurse's relationship with and duty to respect the patient, their families, and advocates for the patient's preferences and wishes. The nurse's influence may range from a single individual to the community to global encompassment.

Provision four relates to a nurse's own practice, with accountability and responsibility in the promises made by healthcare professionals. These include promoting health, engaging in evidence-based practice aimed at improving health outcomes, and reducing the risks that can lead to illness.

Provisions five and six provide direction on self-guidance and care through respect of one's own work and professional fortitude. These tenets encourage autonomy over the nurse's professionalism, focus on the ethical environment within the nurse's locus of control, and support the health of the nurse and the nursing collective.

The final three provisions promote advancement of the nursing profession through development of standards, knowledge base, and policy while also collaborating and building strong relationships with other disciplines. These provisions recognize that nursing cannot function independently. Nurses must integrate within the multidisciplinary team to advocate for patients, reduce inequalities, and create conditions that promote the well-being of humans and the environment.

Ethical Decision-Making Model

The ethical decision-making model for nursing is a step-by-step process for approaching situations where there is concern that the decisions being made are not in the best interest of or alignment with patient preferences. According to the 1991 Patient Self-Determination Act, patients have the right of self-determination, or the right to make their own decisions about the types of healthcare they will or will not accept. This applies when a patient becomes incapable of making their own decisions and has an established durable power of attorney for healthcare to make the choices that align with the patient's pre-determined wishes. When these difficult situations arise, the following framework can provide guidance. The ethical decision-making model is composed of seven steps:

1. Define the problem
2. Understand the issue within the Code of Ethics
3. Analyze and prioritize the facts
4. Create possible interventions
5. Evaluate effects of each intervention
6. Determine and implement the chosen intervention

This road map can assist with determining the best course of action when there are concerns that the patient's ethical principles are compromised. Ethical issues can be a great source of stress to the patient, caregivers, and clinical staff. It is important to be prepared to take action when the patient's autonomy, beneficence, fidelity, or justice is at risk. The solution can involve review by the facility's ethics committee, legal counsel, or appointment of a court-appointed guardian depending upon the severity of the ethical issue.

Code of Ethics

Advocacy

The American Nurses Association (ANA) provides this definition of nursing practice:

> "The protection, promotion, and optimization of health and abilities; prevention of illness and injury; facilitation of healing; alleviation of suffering through the diagnosis and treatment of human response; and advocacy in the care of individuals, families, communities, and populations."

The ANA also addresses the importance of advocacy in its Code of Ethics, specifically in Provision 3:

> "The nurse promotes, advocates for, and protects the rights, health, and safety of the patient."

The ANA Code of Ethics further states that nurses must advocate

> "with compassion and respect for the inherent dignity, worth, and uniqueness of every individual, unrestricted by considerations of social or economic status, personal attributes, or the nature of health problems. "

Advocacy is a key component of nursing practice. An **advocate** is one who pleads the cause of another; a nurse is an advocate for patient rights. Preserving human dignity, patient equality, and freedom from suffering are the basis of nursing advocacy. Nurses hold a significant role that gives them the opportunity to care for patients in every way: meeting their needs, addressing concerns, and working to achieve positive outcomes. Additionally, they aid in communicating with physicians and serve as a guide through the complexities of the medical system. Nurses educate the patient about tests and procedures, while maintaining awareness of how culture and ethnicity affect the patient's experience. Throughout the process, nurses strictly adhere to all privacy laws.

Advocacy is the promotion of the common good, especially as it applies to at-risk populations. It involves speaking out in support of policies and decisions that affect the lives of individuals who do not otherwise have a voice. Nurses meet this standard of practice by actively participating in the politics of healthcare accessibility and delivery. They are educationally and professionally prepared to evaluate and comment on the needs of patients at the local, state, and national level. This participation requires an understanding of the legislative process, the ability to negotiate with public officials, and a willingness to provide expert testimony in support of policy decisions. The advocacy role of nurses has the potential to address the needs of the individual patient, society, and members of the nursing profession.

In clinical practice, nurses represent the patient's interests through active participation in the development of the plan of care and subsequent care decisions. Advocacy, in this sense, is related to patient autonomy and the patient's right to informed consent and self-determination. Nurses provide the appropriate information, assess the patient's comprehension of the implications of the care decisions, and act as patient advocates by supporting the patient's decisions. In the critical care environment, patient advocacy requires the nurse to represent the patient's decisions even though those decisions may be opposed to those of the healthcare providers and family members.

Professionally, nurses advocate for policies that support and promote the practice of all nurses regarding access to education, role identity, workplace conditions, and compensation. The responsibility for **professional advocacy** requires nurses to provide leadership in the development of the professional nursing role in all practice settings that may include acute care facilities, colleges and universities, or community agencies. Leadership roles in acute care settings involve participation in professional practice and shared governance committees, providing support for basic nursing education by facilitating clinical and preceptorship experiences, and mentoring novice graduate nurses to the professional nursing role. In the academic setting, nurses work to ensure the diversity of the student population by participating in the governance structure of the institution, conducting and publishing research that supports the positive impact of professional nursing care on patient outcomes, and serving as an advocate to individual nursing students to promote their academic success. In the community, nurses may collaborate with government officials to meet the needs that are specific to that location.

The nurse must function as a moral agent. This means that the nurse must be morally accountable and responsible for personal judgment and actions. Nurses who practice with moral integrity possess a strong sense of themselves and act in ways consistent with what they understand is the right thing to do. **Moral agency** is defined as the ability to identify right and wrong actions based on widely accepted moral criteria. The performance of nurses as moral agents is dependent on life experiences, advanced education, and clinical experience in healthcare agencies. Moral agency can often be difficult to decipher when managing complex patient situations. When ethical dilemmas arise, such as handling end-of-life and refusal of treatment cases, the care team must work together to make the best care decisions possible with the patient in mind.

The role of moral agent requires nurses to have a strong sense of self and a clear understanding of the definition of right and wrong; however, nurses must also be aware that these perceptions of right and wrong will be challenged every day. The nurse can expect to encounter difficult situations where the moral action related to the patient's right to self-determination is opposed to the moral action with respect to competent patient care.

Ethical Considerations

Healthcare providers routinely face situations with patients where they must analyze various moral and ethical considerations. In the emergency department for example, **ethical dilemmas** can arise without much time to process resolutions. Quick judgment and action are often necessary to care for patients who may not be fully sound in body or mind.

Nurses are held to the American Nurses Association's **Code of Ethics**, which outlines moral and ethical guidelines for nursing practice. Above all else, nurses have the responsibility to do no harm while serving as advocates, minimizing injury, and protecting the overall health and functioning of their patients. It is important to consider the patient holistically when applying these values. Holistic considerations may include how the patient views quality of life, their family values, affected family members, legal considerations, and logistical considerations, such availability of time and medical resources. When patients are unable to make decisions autonomously or provide consent to treatment, nurses should act from these responsibilities to make wise and compassionate decisions on the patients' behalf.

Dilemmas that can arise for nursing staff include situations where the patient may have cultural or personal beliefs that prevent lifesaving treatment. For example, a female emergency patient may not want to be treated by any male staff, or a patient that needs a blood transfusion may not accept this procedure due to religious beliefs. In cases where the patient is able to directly communicate their wishes, the nurse may need to defer to the patient's wishes in order to preserve the patient's autonomy.

Alternative means of care, such as finding available female medical providers to assist with the female patient who does not want to be treated by male staff, may be required in these scenarios. It may mean withholding treatment that the patient refuses. If the patient's life is in question and rapid medical action is necessary, nursing staff must consider the patient's wishes in the plan of care. Ethical considerations like these will vary by case and patient, and will depend on the severity of the case, the medical and personal history of the patient, and the judgment of the nurse in question. In all cases, it is ideal if the nurse and patient can communicate openly about the potential options to determine the best course of action.

Code of Ethics

Similar to the scope of practice, the nursing code of ethics can slightly vary between healthcare agencies. With that being said, there are certain ethical practices that are consistent for all practicing nurses. The Code of Ethics for Nurses with Interpretive Statements gives the nurse a list of ethical practices to utilize for all patient care. The Code, created by the American Nurses Association (ANA), includes the following practices:

- Practicing with compassion and respect
- Providing care with the patient being the primary responsibility
- Providing care being a patient advocate
- Keeping up to date with nursing scope of practice to provide safe patient care
- Ensuring self-care to prevent burnout and provide safe, efficient patient care
- Working towards any advancements or improvements in safe patient care
- Working towards furthering education
- Ensuring effective interdisciplinary collaboration for improvement of patient care
- Promoting social justice and nursing integrity/values

Organizational Recognition

The Joint Commission

The Joint Commission is a nonprofit accrediting organization that certifies healthcare organizations and programs in the United States. Its primary goal is to improve the quality, safety, and efficacy of patient care. The Joint Commission sets industry standards that healthcare facilities must meet to receive accreditation, which ensures quality of care and compliance with safety regulations and establishes emergency preparedness protocols. The organization evaluates hospitals, clinics, nursing homes, ambulatory care centers, and other healthcare providers through in-depth on-site inspections and ongoing monitoring. The Joint Commission emphasizes patient safety, infection control, role competency, and effective communication. Accreditation by the Joint Commission is often a requirement for facility funding and insurance reimbursement. Through promoting continuous improvement and accountability, the organization strives to enhance healthcare delivery and clinical excellence across the United States with standardized, safe, and quality care.

Magnet Designation

Nursing Magnet Designation is a superlative recognition awarded by the American Nurses Credentialing Center (ANCC) to healthcare organizations that meet and exceed benchmarks for excellence in nursing practices and patient care. Achieving Magnet status signifies a commitment to high-quality care that is evidence-based and peer-reviewed. ANCC advocates for striving to create a supportive and innovative work environment for engaged nurses. Hospitals with Magnet designation score higher for improved patient outcomes and nurse satisfaction and have a lower attrition rate. The designation process involves a rigorous evaluation of factors such as nursing leadership, professional development, collaboration, and organizational innovation. Magnet hospitals emphasize empowering nurses, promoting research, and maintaining a culture of continuous improvement. This recognition not only enhances a hospital's reputation but also attracts top nursing talent, ultimately benefiting patient care. Overall,

Magnet designation serves as a hallmark for nursing excellence, encouraging healthcare organizations to prioritize nursing standards, work-life balance, and optimal patient outcomes.

Risk Management

In a healthcare facility, human lives are the focus of services provided and risks are inherently present in the work. These risks include lawsuits, malpractice claims, financial loss, and harm (whether intentional or unintentional) to the patients. Effectively managing risk in order to reduce the probability of a negative outcome encompasses a number of theoretical and analytical steps.

Identifying potential causes of risk can come both from theoretical brainstorming, as well as reviewing concrete evidence. Key stakeholders can examine existing processes and hypothesize how they may present risk. Additionally, reviewing documented instances where risks came to fruition can bring attention to what the healthcare facility and providers should avoid. Documented instances can be those that occurred at another facility, which can serve as a learning lesson for the industry, or they can be instances that occurred internally, such as a filed patient lawsuit or complaint. Regular risk assessments, similar in nature to an audit, can pinpoint areas of risk. These should be system-wide and conducted at regular intervals, with extra assessments conducted any time a new system is implemented or a new healthcare regulation comes into effect.

Once potential causes of risk have been identified, stakeholders should objectively identify which have the possibility to cause the most overall harm, whether it is to the organization, to medical staff, or to patients. These should then be listed in order of urgency, and individual solutions should be discussed. The PDCA cycle of process and quality improvement can be a useful tool when determining an effective yet streamlined solution, as it encompasses many of the qualities that a risk-mitigating solution will need.

Finally, a system should be in place that allows all medical staff to voice areas of risk that they see on the job. As the front line in many of the processes that take place in a healthcare facility, medical staff are able to provide valuable insight regarding risk. Medical staff should feel comfortable reporting causes of risk in the workplace, and a standardized procedure for reporting risks should be in place. In the event that a negative outcome due to preventable or unavoidable risk does occur, it is important that all staff members know how to best respond to the event in order to mitigate its effects on the organization's reputation, business operations, staff members, and patients.

Risk-Management Concepts

Failure Mode Effect Analysis

Failure mode and effects analysis (FMEA) is a systematic method to discover all the ways something can go wrong in a process and then address each of those possibilities. The failure mode is the way something might fail. The effects analysis concerns the consequences of the failure. The overall goal of this system is to identify potential failures and prevent them from happening. FMEA is a team-based tool that includes the following:

- Identifying the steps in the process
- Failure modes (What could go wrong at each step?)
- Failure causes (How could the failures happen?)
- Failure effects (What would the consequences of each failure be?)

Once these have been identified, the next steps are to determine the likelihood of the failure occurring, the likelihood of catching the failure, and the severity of consequences if the failure occurred. Then the potential failures are ranked by risk level so the team knows which to address first.

The FMEA tool can be used at several different junctures, but is best used before a new process is launched to predict potential failure. It can also be used when an existing process needs improvement, when existing processes are being used in a new manner, or when an existing process is being modified.

Let's walk through an example. Say a provider initiates a new drug therapy for a patient. The steps in the process are identified. First, the provider initiates therapy; second, the administration of medication begins; third, the provider monitors the patient's initial response to the new medication; etc. Then potential failures for each step would be identified. So, for the first step (provider initiates therapy), possible failures could include that the order wasn't entered into the electronic health record (EHR) or that the provider did not check the five rights of medication administration. These possible errors would be identified for each step mentioned earlier. Then the team would identify how these mistakes could occur. Maybe the provider got called away to an emergency and could not enter the order, maybe the wrong patient was pulled up on the EHR and the order was entered under the wrong patient's record, or maybe the wrong medication was entered for the correct patient. Next the team would determine the consequences of each failure and rank them in order of severity. If the medication was not ordered, there would be a delay in care. If the medication was urgent, not administering it could have serious consequences. The same applies if the wrong medication or patient was chosen. Along with the severity ranking, the team would evaluate the likelihood of catching these errors before they happen. Lastly, strategies would be developed to prevent these errors from happening. Most EHRs have safety checks built in when prescribing medications. Nurses must scan the patient and the medication before administering. The five rights of medication administration are frequently reviewed on the unit. By breaking up a process into steps and then identifying and preventing potential pitfalls, the workplace and the patients become much safer.

Root Cause Analysis

A **root cause analysis** is a powerful tool to address individual incidents of system failure in a way that creates broad and lasting change. Root cause analysis assesses all factors that contribute to the system failure and attempts to identify the fundamental cause or causes of the failure. This singles out the most effective target for change to prevent future failure.

Root cause analyses are non-punitive. They address the *why* and *how* of a problem, approaching the problem within its system rather than as the failure of an individual. A non-punitive leadership response to errors is vital in healthcare because it fosters transparency and reporting of errors and near-misses. If a staff member is afraid of punishment or retribution, they will have a greater incentive to remain quiet or even cover up errors, which is a serious threat to patient safety.

Root cause analysis involves individuals at all levels and in all systems at the point of failure. The participation of the individual or individuals most closely involved with the actual system failure is crucial, as they will often have the clearest view of the causes that need examination.

Root cause analysis may, and often does, identify more than one root cause. The goal of the process is to identify a clear cause-and-effect chain between the root cause and the failure. This information can be presented as insight to help leaders and staff take action to prevent similar system failures in the future.

In a root cause analysis, healthcare leaders must use flexible and holistic thinking to go beyond what may seem obvious. They must resist the inclination to assign blame and consider the implications of all contributing factors, including those that are outside their scope of expertise or practice.

Healthcare is a highly complex enterprise. Potential for error is ever-present, and healthcare leaders cannot rely solely on the vigilance of individual staff members to prevent errors.

Just Culture

Just culture is a philosophy that encourages transparency and accountability across many levels of an organizational system. Individuals have responsibility for outcomes in the organization, as do established policies and procedures that guide decision-making and behaviors across the organization. Just culture aims to drive ethical decision-making while acknowledging that a myriad of variables can contribute to poor outcomes. Patient outcomes are affected by the nurse's direct patient care; however, they are also influenced by leadership decisions, hospital-wide policies, federal regulations, and other factors outside of the nurse's control. Instead of blaming people for workplace situations that go wrong, just cultures aim to improve problematic processes.

Just cultures acknowledge that human error is possible with even the best standardized operating procedures in place. When a patient experiences poor outcomes, the situation is sometimes attributed to a mistake made by the nurse. The nurse may be terminated from their role or punished in another way. However, continuously replacing nurses rather than addressing the root cause of errors is a costly and inefficient resolution. Just cultures can be cultivated by establishing the expectation that all individuals within an organization have shared accountability for ensuring patient outcomes and by encouraging open communication from staff members across the organizational hierarchy. For example, entry-level staff members should feel comfortable expressing to senior leadership how system flaws may be contributing to poor patient outcomes.

Frontline workers should feel comfortable reporting when they believe they have made an error on the job, rather than delaying resolution out of fear for their job security or punitive responses. Comparatively, senior leadership should understand frontline roles so that they can best identify gaps and make prompt process changes. Organizations should regularly review standard operating procedures with input from all staff members to identify gaps and opportunities for process improvement that could lead to better patient outcomes.

Finally, although just culture focuses heavily on improving whole systems rather than solely blaming individuals for healthcare errors, the philosophy encourages personal responsibility where possible. Individual employees should not intentionally work carelessly or with disregard for patient outcomes. Federal regulators now look for just culture practices within hospital safety standards, typically through indicators such as employee reporting standards, risk assessment frameworks, communication standards between healthcare providers and patients, and corrective action and prevention plans that focus on process improvement.

Incident Reporting and Escalation

Adverse event reporting can be commonly associated with legal formalities and repercussions, but it serves as a prominent resource for quality improvement measures when used correctly.

First, the nurse must understand what defines an adverse event. An adverse event is a situation where an undesirable clinical outcome occurs related to the care provided, while not being related to the underlying disease process or condition. Types of adverse events in healthcare include medication errors, falls, equipment errors, and nosocomial infections.

Next, the event must be properly reported, not only for the benefit of the patient affected by the adverse event, but also for future patient safety measures. For example, if a fall occurs related to an equipment error, reporting this adverse event can result in quality improvement measures such as in-services on equipment usage and fall prevention.

Patient Safety Culture

A patient safety culture is an environment in which nurses can admit to mistakes without being punished. The goal is to allow nurses to report to strategize prevention measures and teach other nurses ways to avoid the same mistake. Patient safety culture is one of actability, accountability, and learning.

Speak Up

Speak Up is The Joint Commission's patient safety program, which encourages patients and family members to participate in their healthcare. Speak Up is a mnemonic that stands for Speak up, Pay attention, Educate yourself, Advocates can help, Know about your medicine, Use a quality healthcare organization, and Participate in all decisions about your care. Information is available via posters and videos on topics such as vaccinations, new parents, and surgery. The program's goal is to empower patients to become autonomous in their healthcare decision making.

High Accountable Organizations

High Accountable Organizations, also known as Accountable Care Organizations, are groups of providers or hospitals that work together to ensure the best patient care. This includes providing high-quality care, reducing medical costs, and improving health outcomes. These programs originated from the Center for Medicare and Medicaid Services. High Accountable Organizations may focus on a specific geographical location or special population, like people with diabetes. This model allows providers to holistically look at a patient's health history and services that have been provided at other facilities. For the patient, this means less repeat testing and services.

Near-Miss Reporting

Near misses are events during which a medical mistake was almost made but was corrected before any harm was done to the patient. An example would be a nurse almost administering the wrong medication but realizing the error before it was given to the patient. Reporting allows institutions to identify weaknesses and correct them to prevent the near miss from happening again. It is important to learn from near misses to prevent errors that result in harm to patients which are called **adverse events**. The object of reporting is not to be punitive but to improve processes for better patient care.

Adverse Event Reporting

If there is an unanticipated or **adverse event**, the nurse should follow the facility's policies and procedures for reporting and documentation. One of the first activities after the patient is stable should be to inform the respective manager or charge nurse of the event. The facility may also have internal processes to follow that serve to mitigate any potential legal consequences.

For example, one of the more common reportable events that a surgical nurse will be involved in is an **incorrect count**. In the event of an incorrect count, the circulator should make attempts to recover the missing item. The circulator should also follow the facility's policies and procedures; at some facilities, X-ray may not be required for needles smaller than a certain size because they are typically not visible on the X-ray. If an intraoperative X-ray is required for a potentially retained object, the team should ensure that the integrity of the sterile field is maintained because the X-ray may be performed prior to full closure of the incision.

Following reasonable attempts to recover the potentially retained object, the circulator should complete the necessary documentation in the patient's chart, such as which count is incorrect, what actions were taken to recover the object, and who was notified. In addition to the documentation in the patient record, the facility's policies may require reporting of the incident in an internal system. This allows the facility to gather additional data that may not be appropriate for the patient record. In the event of a retained foreign object, the facility can use this information to determine if all appropriate actions were taken.

Peer Accountability

As a nurse, it can become difficult to balance the day-to-day responsibilities like nursing procedures, documentation, interdisciplinary communication, and providing education. While these short-term responsibilities are of vital importance, the nurse must not forget the importance of their own ethical responsibilities.

Peer accountability is one of those ethical nursing responsibilities, as the main goal is providing safe and effective patient care. Peer accountability often gets misconstrued as tattling or whistleblowing, when in reality it is simply a chance for continuing education and improved patient safety. The goal is not to get someone in trouble but to fix the issue at hand. For example, if a nurse witnessed another nurse not using proper aseptic technique when inserting an indwelling urinary catheter, further education would need to be provided for the nurse to provide safe catheter care.

Incident Command Structures

Chain of Command

In any workplace environment, an established chain of command is vital to streamlining communication and improving efficiency. In healthcare, the chain of command can get confusing with so many disciplines and titles and with the frequency of changes. Each individual nurse will need to become familiar with their specific employer's nursing chain of command, but there are general guidelines that the nurse in any clinical setting should recognize:

Chief Nursing Officer (CNO)

- Top tier of nursing leadership, working aside the CEO of the healthcare facility/agency
- Oversees all aspects of nursing care within the healthcare facility/agency

Director of Nursing (DON)

- Administrative nursing with a more hands-on leadership role
- Reports directly to CNO

Advanced Practice Registered Nurse (APRN)

- Includes nurse practitioners (CRNPs), nurse specialists (CNSes), nurse anesthetists (CRNAs), and nurse midwives (CNMs)
- Provides direct patient care in coordination with MDs and/or DOs

Nurse Manager/Unit Manager

- Manages the nursing staff within an entire unit/department (e.g., nursing manager for all nursing shifts within the Medical ICU)

Charge Nurse

- Manages the nursing staff within a nursing shift (e.g., charge nurse for the day shift at the Medical ICU)
- Provides direct patient care with assigned patients

Registered Nurse (RN)

- Associate's or Bachelor's degree in nursing
- Provides direct patient care with varying complexities

Licensed Practical Nurse (LPN)

- Diploma/certificate in practical nursing
- Provides basic nursing care in communication with the RN

Nursing Assistant

- Provides assistance with appropriate ADLs
- Obtains vital signs within scope of practice

Hospital Incident Command Structure

Hospital incident command structure refers to the structure of command in place to coordinate the handling of an emergency situation. This can be a collaboration between many departments, both within an individual hospital and when working with outside organizations, such as emergency services and government. Depending on the severity of the emergency incident, this command structure may even go all the way up to the federal level. These emergencies can be natural disasters, such as storms or earthquakes, or caused by humans, such as terrorist attacks or mass shootings. Whatever the cause may be, it is important for the hospital to have an incident command structure and for staff to understand what to do in these scenarios.

Generally speaking, the incident command structure comprises the head command, who is then in charge of leading those responsible for things like logistics, operations, finances, and communication. The goal is to be able to bring in any available resources to react to emergency events. The person in command is also responsible for planning ahead so that the hospital and any involved community organizations are prepared, possibly even preventing potential emergencies from happening. After the response to the emergency, the command will then work on hospital and community recovery, working to rebuild to the normal state of affairs that was present prior to the event.

During an emergency event, it is expected that the roles of individuals involved may change depending on the needs of the incident command. Nurses who normally work at the bedside may be responsible for tasks such as decontamination of HAZMAT patients, triaging mass casualties, or even assisting with the flow of patients or visitors. Nurses must also be prepared to potentially take on more roles than usual due to limited resources to meet a greater need.

In order to prepare for emergency events, it is the nurses' responsibility to understand the hospital incident command structure and know generally what is expected of them in these situations. Nurses should know how they will be contacted or how emergency information will be relayed to them. They should also know what roles they may have to perform and should expect to be flexible depending on needs. Finally, the best way to be prepared is to participate in available practice drills and be a part of the incident command planning process.

Emergency Response Plans

In the case of an emergency, a nurse must be prepared to recommend certain clients for an immediate discharge, activate the **emergency response plan**, and participate in disaster drills. Each facility must have plans for emergency situations, and the nurse may be part of such planning.

Disasters can be internal or external. Examples of **internal disasters** include fires; violence in the workplace; failure of utilities, such as water or electricity; and electrical outage or flooding caused by weather disasters such as tornadoes, hurricanes, or earthquakes. An **external disaster** can include a serious community event in which a population sustains many injuries. Such events can include mass shootings, train wrecks, and airplane crashes. Acts of terrorism or bioterrorism can affect a facility both internally and externally. Likewise, weather events can affect a healthcare facility both internally and externally, depending on the extent of damage that occurs.

An example of an act of terrorism that caused a massive influx of patients to local hospitals was the Route 91 shooting in Las Vegas. This was an external event that caused the activation of certain emergency response plans to deal with the influx of incoming patients. Such events must be discussed as a potential occurrence in each facility. Healthcare facilities must put plans in place to deal with such catastrophes in a smooth, coordinated manner to effectively care for the maximum number of patients.

The hurricanes Irma and Harvey that struck the Gulf states in 2017 are an example of an external weather situation that directly affected those communities with electrical power losses, flooding, destruction of property, and injuries and illness related to the flooding and high winds. The healthcare system must be ready for these situations with an effective emergency response plan.

One of the first steps when activating an emergency response plan is to discharge patients who are medically stable enough to clear beds for incoming patients. Facilities only have a set number of beds available for patients. When the influx of patients is greater than the number of beds available, a crisis arises. When a **catastrophic event** occurs, nurses are part of a triaging process that determines whether certain patients can be relocated to open beds for incoming patients. Unstable clients will stay put; they are at the top of the rung of patients to stay. Stable patients may be discharged only if it is likely they will remain stable without ongoing nursing and medical care. On the bottom rung, below unstable and stable clients, are ambulatory and self-care clients. These are patients who are walking around and able to independently care for themselves outside of a hospital facility. Ambulatory and self-care patients will be discharged to clear beds for incoming disaster patients.

Mass Casualty

Healthcare systems must develop procedures for mass casualty events that cause surges in patient admittance. Mass casualty events can quickly result in understaffing and other resource depletion. Examples include natural disasters, pandemics, acts of terrorism, and situations of extreme violence. A disaster management plan that integrates all available healthcare resources in a region (such as large hospitals, small medical offices, and volunteer healthcare personnel) can support a coordinated and comprehensive response. Communities should proactively ensure that such a plan exists and can be logistically deployed well before a mass casualty event occurs.

Several best practice frameworks, including the National Response Framework and the National Incident Management System, can be adapted locally to promote coordinated responses in the case of patient surges. The CDC has developed a resource calculator for various mass casualty events that helps a hospital system predict how many patients will be seen in the first hour after a specific type of event and the rate at which patients may arrive thereafter. This modeling tool can also help healthcare systems predict what resources may be needed after specific events and prepare a localized plan accordingly. Factors to consider may include from where to call additional personnel, the amount of personal protective equipment to have on hand, plans for triaging patients, methods for establishing makeshift healthcare centers, and addressing community recovery after the mass casualty event.

Mass casualty events not only affect the physical health and well-being of a community; they also take a psychological toll on community members and first responders. Community recovery may include mental health services for first responders, financial aid from the state or federal government, and long-term health supports for community members directly involved in the event. Healthcare systems can prepare for mass casualty events by regularly drilling their proposed plan and using these sessions to identify gaps that may be present during a real event. Gaps that present themselves in real situations include disproportionate admittance to a single hospital (e.g., the one closest to the scene of the event), language barriers, back-up staff that are unable to serve, widespread contamination, miscommunication, or harm caused to healthcare facilities themselves. For example, in many natural disasters, healthcare facilities may lose power or become inaccessible.

Natural Disasters

Natural disasters refer to destructive events resulting in property and infrastructure damage; injuries to people, animals, and livestock; and ecological devastation. Natural disasters are often mass casualty incidents. They include events such as hurricanes, floods, earthquakes, avalanches, blizzards, landslides, volcanic activity, tornados, heat waves, wildfires, and windstorms. Medical facilities normally have protocols in place to address potential natural disasters that could occur in the surrounding geographic area. These protocols address not only organizational procedures to follow in the event of a natural disaster, but also how to house and/or evacuate victims of specific types of natural disasters. For example, a coastal hospital will likely have procedures in place for hurricanes and flooding, while a hospital near a fault line will likely have procedures in place for an earthquake.

Consider the importance of the nurse's adaptability to crises with reference to assisting patients and families impacted by natural disasters. Upon deployment to an area destroyed by torrential rains and subsequent flooding, a nurse could encounter families in need of not only immediate medical care, but ongoing crisis intervention. In conditions such as these, patients are often overwhelmed by their physical pain as well as concerns for how to meet their basic needs for food, shelter, and clean water. Disaster relief relies on medical triage to determine the appropriate level of care needed by patients and is typically assessed based on a four-tier model:

- Black/blue is reserved for the deceased.
- Red is reserved for immediate care such as chest wounds or gunshots.
- Yellow is reserved for those with stable wounds or head injuries.
- Green is reserved for minor injuries such as fractures or burns.

In this situation, the nurse must be prepared to rapidly assess the patient's level of injury and the most expedient treatment needed for stabilization and move on to the next case within minutes. Does the patient or anyone in the family maintain a specific medication regimen to manage chronic illnesses? Have any doses of required medications been missed? Are any assistive devices such as hearing aids or canes needed? It is important to note that the nurse will need to focus on the medical stabilization of patients in this stage rather than delving into psychosocial and emotional trauma.

During disaster-relief efforts, nurses are normally dispatched to both acute care and follow-up care zones. Once immediate medical needs are addressed, patients are transferred to a safe holding area. This space is set aside for psychosocial triage, where patients' basic emotional and physical needs are met. Social workers and chaplains are readily available to debrief survivors. Consider the example of a nurse working with a family impacted by the previous illustration. Having lost their home and belongings and facing recovery from minor injuries, they have been transferred to the holding area for processing.

The nurse in this example would receive a brief synopsis from triage, but only regarding injuries and treatment. In this stage, the nurse would obtain a brief social history, information on chronic disease, and feasible relocation options. Then, the nurse will need to begin guiding the patients through processing the emotional trauma of the incident. Are all family members accounted for? Does anyone in the family unit manage any mental health conditions that have been triggered? What, if any, legal or illegal substances are used or abused by anyone in the family unit? These questions are to help determine if the survivors' emotional responses are directly related to the recent trauma.

Responses to acute traumatic events often mirror the typical response of those who have experienced chronic trauma. The nurse must also assess patients for underlying mental health conditions that may have been exacerbated. In this instance, the most appropriate nursing diagnosis would include ineffective coping. Typical nursing interventions would require the nurse to work with the patient to access previously successful ways of navigating traumatic events, presenting viable options for the next steps, and allowing the patient the time to process the best response to the traumatic event.

Disaster Preparedness

The nurse plays a key role in disaster preparedness and designation of roles to team members, which is necessary for successful execution of each emergency response plan. During a fire, for example, the nurse must competently implement all four elements of the **RACE** acronym, as follows:

- **R**: Rescue all those in danger, including patients, visitors, and staff.
- **A**: Activate the alarm after those in danger have been cleared.
- **C**: Contain the fire in the smallest possible area. This is accomplished by closing all windows and doors, preventing the fire from spreading.
- **E**: Extinguish the fire if it is small enough and the nurse can do so safely.

Concurrent with knowledge of the RACE acronym during a fire is knowledge of how to use a **fire extinguisher**. There are five main types of fire extinguishers: Type A, Type B, Type C, Type AB, and Type ABC. Type A extinguishers are used for common solids, such as paper, mattresses, and clothing. Type B extinguishers target oil, gasoline, and grease fires, common in kitchens. Type C extinguishers fight electrical fires. Type AB extinguishers combines the roles of Type A and Type B, while Type ABC extinguishers combines all three. Type ABC is most common due to its ability to extinguish all types of fire sources. This is likely the type of extinguisher located within a hospital facility for that reason.

When attempting to use a fire extinguisher, the nurse must remember the acronym **PASS**, which describes the following steps for effective use:

- **P**: Pull the pin to begin using the fire extinguisher.
- **A**: Aim directly at the bottom of the fire.
- **S**: Squeeze the trigger to release the spray.
- **S**: Sweep, moving from side to side across the base of the fire. This will effectively extinguish the fire.

Along with knowing their role when fire threatens the safety of patients, the nurse must also know what to do when the hospital's utilities fail. Electricity powers many life support machines for patients, such as oxygen delivery systems and mechanical ventilation machines. Most hospitals have back-up **generators** to keep these machines going when the power goes down. The nurse must alert maintenance and management immediately if the power goes off. Many hospitals have special red outlets into which important patient machinery should be plugged for just that reason.

There are times in the workplace when the nurse may encounter violence, harassment, or aggression. The source of these behavioral conflicts may be a visitor, fellow staff member, or patient. Causes of **workplace violence** may include delirium and disorientation, especially in hospitalized patients with illness and medication side effects in play. Visitors and family members may become disruptive for any number of reasons, including misunderstandings about care during high-stress and emotionally charged healthcare situations involving a loved one. Whatever the cause, the nurse must work to deescalate the situation verbally, enlisting help from team members and hospital security staff when needed.

Each healthcare facility will have explicit guidelines that must be followed in the case of a **weather emergency**, such as a hurricane, tornado, or earthquake. Closing windows, doors, and curtains, as well as moving patients to the appropriate predetermined safe place, are all part of the nurse's role during these situations.

For each of these emergencies, a chain of command needs to be established long before a catastrophic event occurs. A **chain of command** clearly defines who is in charge during the disaster, how information will be communicated, and the roles of each team member. **Emergency drills** are an excellent chance to rehearse each role and ensure that things run smoothly and efficiently in the event of a disaster.

Analysis of Gaps in Practice that Indicate Potential Risk Management Issues

Risk Factors

Nurses must acknowledge patient safety risk factors and ensure processes to prevent them. Common types of risk factors that can lead to patient harm include pharmacological (ensuring the five rights of medication administration), environmental (reducing fall and infection rates), equipment (verifying equipment is working properly), and demographic (verifying patient by name and date of birth).

Environmental Risk Factors

Environmental risk factors include anything in the patient's surroundings that can cause harm. This includes the patient's room, infection control, fire safety, and more. Several factors go into ensuring a patient's room is safe and best equipped to prevent falls. One is rooming patients that are more likely to fall, those who are noncompliant, and those with psychiatric conditions or dementia closest to the nurse's station. This allows the nurses to monitor these patients more closely. Another is moving any tripping hazards in the room, including phone chargers and items or spills on the floor. Nurses should also follow policy for setting bed alarms and having patients wear nonslip socks and fall risk bracelets. For infection control, nurses should follow standard precautions including wearing appropriate PPE. No matter the risk to the patient—whether from fall, fire, or infection—the nurse should prevent the risk from occurring, assess the surroundings, then either remove the danger or remove the patient from danger.

Equipment Risk Factors

Common patient safety risk factors that concern equipment include improper decontamination of equipment and equipment that is not labeled properly. Pathogens are present on equipment that is used on multiple patients, such as portable X-ray machines, ultrasound devices, and even stethoscopes. Hospital-acquired infections are harmful to patients and costly to facilities. Nurses should ensure that equipment has been properly sanitized before each use. Another area of concern is untagged equipment, such as IV bags and lines, fire extinguishers, and damaged equipment. When a patient has several IV lines, they should all be properly labeled and include the date the tubing needs to be changed. In an emergency, knowing which line goes to which bag is vital. Damaged equipment should have a label indicating it is damaged and should not be used on patients. This equipment should be stored in a separate location from the functioning equipment.

Pharmacological Risk Factors

Pharmacotherapeutic intervention selection is a form of clinical judgment that is based on the findings of the nurse's comprehensive assessment. The selection of pharmacotherapeutic interventions is based on: indications for the therapy; contraindications; cost and compliance; efficacy; adverse effects; dose; duration; and patient directions. The patient's pharmacokinetic response to any drug is related to the patient's inherited metabolic pathways, comorbidities, and the drug characteristics for all prescribed and over the counter (OTC) drugs. The potential for altered drug metabolism can also be the result of the binding of one or more prescribed drugs to liver enzymes, which can decrease (inhibition) or increase (induction) excretion of the drugs through that same enzyme pathway. Inhibition is more common than induction, which potentially results in an adverse drug reaction (ADR) due to increases in the plasma concentration of the drugs. The risk for ADRs also exists when two drugs compete for the same enzyme pathway. These potential sources for ADRs are not always predictable. This means that the nurse will be aware of common ADRs while maintaining close monitoring for patient-specific reactions.

The risk of ADRs resulting from pharmacotherapeutic interventions is greatest for elderly patients. More than 50 percent of patients receiving Medicare take five or more prescribed drugs every day. However, the majority of younger adults report at least occasional use of OTC medications that contain aspirin, acetaminophen, ibuprofen, or naproxen. Many patients underestimate the importance of reporting this use to their care provider, which increases the risk of interactions with prescribed medications. In addition, physician groups have recently requested decreases in the amount of acetaminophen that is contained in OTC combination drugs such as cold and headache preparations. The current levels can potentially result in liver failure even when the patient complies with the recommended dosage schedule. This risk exists for the elderly, patients who consume alcohol, and those patients with undiagnosed susceptibility for this adverse reaction.

The World Health Organization (WHO) and the FDA maintain information related to all reports of drug interaction. The FDA Adverse Events Reporting System (FAERS) also publishes revisions to the black box warnings on all drugs administered in the United States. Identified drug interactions are classified as major, moderate, or minor, according to the documented adverse effects of the interaction. In general, major interactions mean that the combination of drugs should not be used, while the drugs that result in moderate reactions should be used with appropriate caution. Drug interactions are also classified as **pharmacokinetic reactions** (PK reactions) or **pharmacodynamic reactions** (PD reactions). PK reactions refer to drug interactions that occur in one of the four kinetic phases. PD reactions refer to drug interactions that alter the body's response to the drugs.

There are two kinds of contraindication for a pharmacotherapeutic intervention: absolute and relative. An **absolute contraindication** means that the administration of the drug or combination of drugs can result in life-threatening adverse effects that must be avoided. A **relative contraindication** means that the potential for adverse effects should be weighed against the expected therapeutic effect. An absolute contraindication can be related to the reaction of one or more drugs with another drug or with certain patient populations, such as pregnant women, patients with renal failure, and people with other drug allergies. An example of an absolute drug-to-drug contraindication is that warfarin cannot be given with aspirin; one drug potentiates the effect of the other, resulting in an increased risk for bleeding.

Absolute contraindication for pharmacotherapeutic interventions in pregnant women is associated with **teratogenicity**, which is the risk for birth defects due to maternal exposure to the drugs. Patients with renal disease are at risk from the drug interactions because most drugs are excreted by the kidneys, and when there is any degree of altered renal function, the plasma concentration of the drugs, and therefore the risk of adverse effects, will be increased. Patients with identified allergies are at greater risk for hypersensitivity reactions to other drug therapies. Many of the recommended contraindications are contained in condition-specific protocols such as oral contraceptive use, smoking cessation, and obesity therapy. For example, absolute contraindications to oral contraceptive therapy include a known or suspected pregnancy or a history of thrombotic disease. Relative contraindications include the presence of hypertension and current smoking history. In children, there is an absolute contraindication for the use of aspirin in patients recovering from a viral infection due to the risk of Reye's syndrome, which is rare but often fatal.

Another issue that is associated with the selection of pharmacotherapeutic agents is the use of off-label use of drugs, which means that the drug is being used for a treatment that has not been approved by the FDA. This practice is common in the treatment of cancer when a drug that has been evaluated for the treatment of one form of cancer is used to treat a different form of cancer without being evaluated by the FDA for that specific use. These new therapies can be related to adverse reactions that may be unpredictable. This practice is common in pediatric populations, especially in children with rare diseases because there is insufficient research data to support the providers' clinical decisions.

The **selectivity** of a drug may also be defined as the propensity of a given drug to affect the desired receptor population over others in the body; thus, a highly selective drug reduces the likelihood of possible side effects. **Potency** is a measure of the dosage necessary to produce a standard effect; a more potent drug can be administered in smaller doses than a less potent one. One safety measure of a drug is the **therapeutic index**, which compares the lethal dose of the drug to the therapeutic dose of the drug. Drugs with higher therapeutic indexes are thought to be safer to administer than those with low therapeutic indexes.

This measure is criticized for the use of death as the definition of undesirable adverse effects, and a portion of the supporting data is derived from animal, not human studies. However, it does provide a means of comparing the acceptability of two drugs. The efficacy of a drug is also affected by the **placebo effect**, which is the patient's positive or negative perception of the results of the drug that are not related to the therapeutic outcomes associated with the drug. The availability of generic drugs can also influence the drug selection. Although the inactive ingredients may vary, name brand and generic drugs must contain the active ingredients in the same dosage, potency, and route of administration. The formulation of injectable generic drugs is most often exactly the same as that of the name brand drug.

Genetic Risk Factors

A **genetic risk assessment** estimates an individual's risk for the development of chronic and rare diseases that are genetically linked. This assessment only identifies a statistical probability, not cause and effect, because diseases that result from variants in multiple genes as opposed to a single gene increase the complexity of estimating the risk. There is a wide variation in the degree to which the genetically-linked diseases contribute to the possibility of expression of the disease in the offspring. For instance, the genetic risk associated with the development of melanoma is 21 percent whereas the risk associated with type 1 diabetes is 88 percent. There are two categories of risk: absolute risk and relative risk. **Absolute risk** means that if the patient has a one in ten chance of developing a disease in their lifetime, that person has a 10 percent risk for that disease. **Relative risk** compares the risk for two groups for the same disease. For instance, the risk of breast cancer is higher for descendants of Ashkenazi Jews who emigrated from Eastern Europe than for the average female population in the United States.

There are family patterns that increase the risk for the development of diseases including having multiple first-degree relatives with the same condition, having a relative diagnosed with the condition before the age of 55, having a relative with a disease that is more common in the opposite gender, and having more than one genetically linked disease in the family. The genetic pedigree, which is a visual representation of the patient's family tree, may be used to assess the patient's genetic risk factors. Providers must also support patients and families as they decide whether or not to access formal genetic testing. The Genetic Information Nondiscrimination Act (GINA) and the Health Insurance Portability and Accountability Act (HIPAA) of 1996 provide some protection against discrimination due to the findings of the testing. There also can be ethical questions related to reproductive planning and family dynamics. The patient should be encouraged to seek professional counseling when considering genetic testing. The patient should also understand that direct-to-consumer genetic tests may or may not provide reliable information for the patient's unique circumstances and that none of the commercial products provides counseling.

Behavior and Lifestyle Risk Factors

The Centers for Disease Control (CDC) identifies and tracks four lifestyle risk factors: poor exercise habits, inadequate nutrition, smoking, and excessive alcohol intake. Each of these lifestyle behaviors increases the risk of chronic diseases such as HTN, stroke, and respiratory disease. The research clearly implicates smoking as a factor in the development of all of these conditions; yet, adults and young people continue to smoke. The government has enacted age restrictions on the sale of tobacco in addition to imposing a significant tariff that is included in the price of cigarettes, and commercial companies market a wide array of prescription and nonprescription smoking cessation products. There are commercial and medical weight loss programs that provide one-on-one and peer support and twelve-step programs for all forms of addiction. The nurse is responsible for supporting patients' plans to change by providing the necessary information prior to the change in behavior and then supporting patients as they initiate and maintain the changed behavior.

The patient should understand that persistent change requires effort continued over time and that even modest reductions in lifestyle risks will have some effect on the progression of chronic diseases. In other words, the patient does not have to run a marathon to gain some benefit from regular, light exercise. Modest dietary improvement and increased activity can lower blood pressure and lipids; however, smoking cessation requires total abstinence to be effective in reducing the development or progression of chronic illness. The nurse will monitor the patient's medication needs as these risk factors are addressed to be sure that medication doses are reduced as necessary. It is not uncommon for patients who eliminate smoking, increase exercise, and improve their nutritional status to be able to discontinue or limit their use of antihypertensive drugs, oral hypoglycemic drugs, or antilipidemic drugs. A patient who has accurate health-promoting information, contacts for needed community resources, and the support of the provider will have the greatest chance for successful change.

Host Risk Factors

Host risk factors, or **host factors**, are terms that refer to a patient's susceptibility to certain diseases. Several factors can affect the probability that someone will develop an acute or chronic illness. Assessing these factors via a health history interview followed by a physical assessment can direct the advanced practice nurse to develop a treatment plan that will prevent possible complications. Microorganisms thrive when they invade the body and overpower the immune response. The first line of defense in the body is the skin. When the skin is broken, it opens up a pathway for microorganisms to enter the body and cause illness. Assessing the patient's skin integrity is an important component of a physical assessment. Patients who have skin integrity issues are more at risk of developing infections. To survive, the body must maintain an acid-base balance. The pH levels vary throughout the body. The stomach is highly acidic, whereas the large intestine is more basic. In females, vaginal pH is moderately acidic. When pH levels in these areas change, microorganisms can grow.

For example, when the vaginal pH turns alkaline, there is an increased risk of developing bacterial vaginosis (BV), which can cause itchiness, discharge, and discomfort. The immune response is activated when a microorganism enters the body. Cell mediators alert the body that there is a potentially harmful organism present. White blood cells (WBCs) help fight off infection in the body. When patients have decreased levels of WBCs, they are more susceptible to infection due to a delayed or weakened immune response. Medications can alter a patient's immune response. Corticosteroids, a class of anti-inflammatory drugs, suppress the immune system. They are helpful in autoimmune illnesses in which the body attacks its own immune system. However, a practitioner should always balance the risks and benefits of suppressing immunity. Age is an important host factor for susceptibility. Older adults go through age-related changes, such as loss of skin elasticity, a decrease in sphincter control of the bladder, and a decreased cough reflex. These changes can increase the risk of skin, urinary tract, and pulmonary infections.

Demographic Risk Factors

It is important for the nurse to know which diseases or conditions ethnic and racial groups are prone to. The white population is more prone to atrial fibrillation than people of other races. The Hispanic population has high rates of obesity and diabetes; in individuals from Puerto Rico, there is an increased incidence of HIV infection and AIDS.

Obesity and type 2 diabetes are common in African Americans, and the death rate from HTN, stroke, HIV infection, and AIDS is higher than the rate in the non-Hispanic white population. Asian Americans have an increased incidence of tuberculosis, and hepatitis B infection occurs more commonly in recent immigrants to the United States. Asian Americans also have an increased rate of chronic obstructive pulmonary disease (COPD), in spite of the fact that smoking rates among Chinese and Japanese Americans are lower than average. Native Americans have a high incidence of alcoholism; recent pharmacologic research indicates that altered metabolic pathways may contribute to this finding. As with the Asian American population, the nurse will be aware of the frequent use of herbal preparations in the Native American population as well.

Patients at Risk for Readmissions

One of the healthcare team's primary goals is to prevent the need for patient readmission and to recognize those patients that are at a higher risk of readmission. Readmission is defined as the readmission of a patient to an acute care facility with the same chief complaint within thirty days of discharge. While not all readmissions can be avoided, there are some steps the healthcare team can take to recognize risk factors and provide the necessary resources.

Certain Disease Processes

Disease processes with complexities (especially progressive diseases) increase the need for readmissions, even with adequate treatment and education. These disease processes can include CKD, heart failure, COPD, sepsis, CVA, and MI.

Patient Demographics

Patient demographics that increase the likelihood of a readmission include advanced age, male gender, and lower-income individuals. The patient's education level can also be an issue regarding comprehension of medical treatment.

Inadequate Healthcare

Inadequate healthcare refers to gaps in interdisciplinary communication and poor discharge instructions. If the patient is discharged without proper follow-up, extensive discharge information, and a clear understanding of the path forward, the likelihood of readmission is high.

Social Determinants

Social determinants of health (SDOH) are nonmedical factors that affect a patient's health and well-being. These factors include socioeconomic status, transportation, political climate, and racism, among others. For example, if a patient does not have running water, how can they perform hand hygiene before a dressing change? Screening for these factors helps ensure patient safety and well-being. When screening patients for SDOH, ensure that resources are in place to give to patients or refer them to. For example, if a patient is facing food insecurity, the nurse should have resources for food banks and food assistance programs ready.

Noncompliance

Lastly, patient noncompliance with the medical treatment plan increases the likelihood of readmission. The nurse can assist in the prevention of noncompliance by thoroughly reviewing the importance of each aspect of the treatment plan (e.g., taking furosemide as ordered to prevent another heart failure exacerbation).

Care Bundles

A **care bundle**, developed by the Institute for Healthcare Improvement, is a succinct set of evidence-based practices to improve patient care for common treatments that pose risks. One example is a central line bundle that has five steps to prevent catheter-related bloodstream infections. Bundles are helpful because they pull together multiple ways of performing a task into one evidence-based process to promote uniformity. The goal of the bundle is to provide the highest possible patient care and outcome.

Bundles have specific formats that are slightly different from checklists and algorithms. Bundles have a stepwise approach in which each step must be completed before moving to the next to achieve the optimum outcome. They are based on Level 1 evidence-based practices, which compare randomized controlled trials to ensure the nurse is using the best data to perform the procedure. Additionally, bundles provide black-and-white, yes-or-no distinctions that leave no gray area up for interpretation. Lastly the bundle must be completed by one healthcare team in one setting. Care bundles are to be repeated as needed until the service is no longer required.

Another example of a bundle is the ventilator bundle, which was created to prevent ventilator-associated pneumonia, a common hospital-acquired infection. Through research, it was found that doing the following four interventions may prevent or delay the onset of this type of pneumonia:

- Administering deep vein thrombosis prophylaxis
- Administering gastric ulceration preventative medications
- Elevating the head or bed to between 30 and 45 degrees
- Assessing whether the patient can breathe on their own daily

Sentinel and Reportable Events

A discussion in ethical nursing must also include the practice of professional reporting and appropriate resources. Medication errors, procedural errors, abuse, unsafe conditions, and medication diversion are just a few of the reportable incidents the nurse may face in practice.

Reporting will differ in each situation based on the type of incident and the facility/agency guidelines (in compliance with state/federal regulatory bodies). The following points review the typical response to a reportable incident and the subsequent resources to utilize:

Medication administration errors and procedural errors

- Each facility/agency will have an incident reporting system
- Sentinel events are mandatory to report in certain states

Abuse

- Nurses are mandatory reporters of any form of patient abuse
- State and facility/agency guidelines will be specific to the patient population (e.g., the elderly, children, etc.) and the reporting agency

Unsafe conditions

- Unsafe staffing and work conditions are to be reported to the specific state board of nursing

Medication diversion

- Reporting diversion of controlled substances will vary based on where or by whom the diversion occurs (e.g., coworker, patient's family member/friend)
- Reporting to facility/agency reporting system in both circumstances with potential for involvement with DEA, state board of nursing, state pharmacy board, and potentially law enforcement

Nurses are mandated to report certain findings or suspicions, such as child abuse, elder abuse, and human trafficking. Regardless of whether the nurse thinks the patient's claims are true or if there is any proof, they must report. Sometimes patients will divulge this information on their own, but often the nurse must assess for these risks and for social determinants of health.

Abuse and Neglect

Patients can arrive at a clinic or hospital as a result of experiencing abuse or neglect. They may also arrive for some other reason but show signs of having been abused or neglected. Nurses must be able to identify when patients have been experiencing abuse and neglect and know how to provide care while ensuring that the situation is escalated to the necessary authorities. Abuse and neglect most commonly result from domestic violence between partners, violence against children by their parents or caregivers, or against elders by caretakers. Abuse may be physical, emotional, financial, or sexual.

While abuse refers to intentional assaults, neglect refers to inadequate caretaking that endangers someone. This may include not feeding, bathing, or otherwise assisting a person who is unable to take care of themselves. Signs of neglect include poor hygiene, malnourishment, and the presence of bedsores. Neglect may take the form of withholding necessary medications or mobility supports (e.g., a walker) or exposing the person to unsafe situations.

Identifying potential abuse and neglect should be a component of the intake process. Nurses should note any visible signs and ask the patient questions about their care. Nurses should be aware of visible signs of abuse, including bruises, burns, injured limbs, trauma near the patient's private areas, disrespectful treatment by caretakers, and fearfulness shown by the patient near certain visitors. Nurses may consider directly asking the patient about specific instances of abuse. Patients may not feel comfortable answering these questions, and nurses should allow them time and privacy away from their caregivers to complete intake. After intake, a physical examination can also provide clues about patient abuse and neglect.

Physical abuse involves injuries to the body from force, such as punching or kicking. If the nurse notes various bruises or cuts in various stages of healing without explanation, it may be a sign of physical abuse. *Sexual abuse* is when sexual contact is made without the consent of one party, including rape, coercion into doing sexual acts, and fondling of genitalia. The nurse should look for unexplained bruises or bleeding around the perineal area, new difficulty sitting or walking, or increased agitation as potential signs of sexual abuse. *Emotional* or *mental abuses* are not quite as obvious as physical abuse as the damage inflicted is internal or hidden. Emotional and mental abuse is usually caused by verbal assault. The abuser may belittle and criticize the victim to the point that the victim feels worthless, insecure, and afraid. If the nurse senses an uncomfortable relationship between an informal caregiver or family member and the patient, this should be monitored, investigated, and reported if abuse is suspected. Financial abuse most commonly affects elders who may have decreased cognitive or physical functioning. In financial abuse situations, relatives, friends, or other caretakers may steal money from the patient, forge the patient's signatures on financial documents, or otherwise give themselves legal authority with unjust cause (e.g., claiming that a patient is not healthy enough to make personal decisions and needs a power of attorney). If the nurse suspects that checks and other financial means meant for the patient are being rerouted and misused by a caregiver, this abuse should be reported right away.

If either abuse or neglect is suspected, evidence should be documented in the patient's medical chart in case an investigation occurs. If the nurse suspects abuse or neglect, they are mandated to report it to the appropriate entity. The charge nurse and/or nurse manager should be notified, so the appropriate action can be taken to right the situation. There are also hotlines that can be called, such as the National Center on Elder Abuse (1-800-677-1116).

Human Trafficking

Most trafficking victims are women or young men. Many victims are accompanied by their trafficker, which can complicate the processes of identifying and helping them. They generally show signs of physical and mental abuse. A red flag that warrants further attention is when a patient is accompanied by someone who appears overly involved in the case but does not seem to be genuinely concerned about the patient; this is often the trafficker. Their identification may indicate no relation to the patient, but they will insist that they are a friend or romantic partner. They may control all of the patient's personal identification and insist on paying in cash. The trafficker may be highly resistant to letting the patient go anywhere alone with the healthcare provider, yet this is the best way to identify whether someone is a trafficking victim and help them out of the situation. Many victims are seen for medical issues that do not result from trafficking activities but from delays in receiving routine care. For example, a woman who is being trafficked may become pregnant and not receive prenatal care until she is in an emergency situation.

Most healthcare facilities have specific policies and procedures in place to identify and screen trafficking victims. Screening processes should be age appropriate and sensitive in order to help the victim in the most dignified and compassionate manner possible. In most states, adult victims must choose whether they want an intervention. However, all healthcare providers can anonymously and safely report any suspicions of possibly trafficked individuals to the necessary authorities. Intervention can be a traumatic event for the patient and must be handled cautiously, while also ensuring that it is performed quickly and that the trafficker is restrained. Social services, legal services, and law enforcement are often a part of any intervention, making it a highly complex and collaborative initiative.

Reportable Diseases

The provider, hospital, or laboratory are required to submit state-identified reportable disease information with personal identifiers to the local authorities to facilitate disease control. Reportable diseases are selected by surveillance case definitions that provide state and local public health officials with precise criteria to be used for these decisions. The local health authorities can voluntarily submit notifiable disease information without personal identifiers to the Centers for Disease Control (CDC). The formal report to CDC is submitted through the CDC's National Notifiable Diseases Surveillance System (NNDSS). The CDC also reminds providers that the reporting mechanism is not to be used in the diagnosis or the treatment of an infectious disease. The CDC aggregates national data related to the incidence of any one of approximately 120 notifiable diseases that are categorized as infectious, noninfectious, or as representing an outbreak due to a food source. These diseases are reported to protect the health of individuals and to defend against threats to public health.

Workplace Violence Events

Workplace violence in nursing refers to threats or actual incidents of violence, aggression, intimidation, harassment, or force. Workplace violence can occur by former or current colleagues, by someone from the nurse's personal life, or by individuals who have no relationship to the nurse or workplace. Statistically, nurses experience a higher rate of workplace violence, most often from patients they are treating or from someone affiliated with the patient. Nurses are most likely to report experiencing physical assault (e.g., kicking, hitting, pushing, hair-pulling), being screamed at, being spit on, and needing to restrain patients. This is perhaps due to the fact that they are regularly dealing with mentally unwell populations or patients that are heavily medicated from procedures; in fact, psychiatric nurses experience the most incidents of workplace violence among all nursing specialties. Additionally, healthcare settings may cause extreme feelings of stress and fear in patients, their friends, and family, especially if they are worried about the patient's prognosis or financial issues. They may be unable to healthily express or cope with such extreme feelings; therefore, they become hostile.

Workplace violence in specific healthcare settings has been associated with high turnover and staff shortages. Additionally, nurses who experience workplace violence often have to take one or more days off from work to recuperate. Not only are these experiences taxing and scarring for affected healthcare professionals, but they are also extremely costly for the healthcare facility. Hiring, training, firing, providing severance, and other human resources tasks are expensive for the organization.

Nurses may also feel uncomfortable about reporting incidents, as they may believe that doing so goes against their nursing oath to protect the patient or fear that it could jeopardize their job security. Such situations can have long-lasting negative health effects on nurses; they may fear going to work or experience stress disorders after a violent situation occurs. Healthcare workers who experience workplace stress are more likely to experience job-related fatigue, burnout, medical errors, and poor patient outcomes. Some healthcare systems have begun to make administrative changes to address workplace violence, including the presence of metal detectors, security escorts, alarm systems that nurses can activate when needed, and system-wide surveillance and monitoring of patients. Additionally, more hospital staff members are receiving training on de-escalation techniques.

Regulatory Requirements for Reporting Death

When a patient dies in certain unusual or sudden circumstances, the hospital is legally required to notify and cooperate with the local coroner's office, who will examine and investigate the deceased patient. These **coroner's cases** are required to be reported in cases when an individual dies suddenly or because of an accident, suicide, homicide, or occupation-related circumstance. Additionally, suspicious deaths or deaths associated with medical treatment and care are legally required to be reported.

After calling to report the death, the hospital must comply with all requests for information made by the coroner's office. HIPAA privacy laws require that hospitals may disclose private health information to coroners and funeral directors without the necessity of consent from family or the patient. Healthcare providers are also required to leave any attached medical devices in place (e.g., IV catheters, endotracheal tubes, etc.) and any medications that were administered around or at the time of death. The coroner's office coordinates collection and transportation of the deceased patient, and an autopsy is performed. The death certificate is required to be signed within 48 hours and is completed by the physician caring for patient at the time of death, the coroner, or the medical examiner, depending on the circumstances of the death.

Audits

An **audit** is an inspection of a specific aspect of an organization. Audits can be conducted on procedures, finances, incentives, product counts, or any other area of the business that can be monitored. Audits may be conducted internally or by an external, independent body; most effective organizations perform both types regularly. Audit activities may include checklists of certain processes that must be in place, benchmark score comparisons, and evaluation practices. Internal audits allow organizations to be prepared for external audits. Non-compliance of standards found by an external auditing body, especially if it is a regulatory agency, may result in fines, disciplinary action, intensive monitoring, or a shutdown of the organization.

Safety Rounds

In addition to daily rounds from the provider, nursing **safety rounds** are another opportunity to address patient safety. Safety rounds can be performed by the bedside nurse or by a patient safety team. Their frequency depends on the facility. This approach partners the family members with nurses to watch out for patient safety. Since family members are often with the patient for extended periods of time, they are in a great position to notice subtle changes in the patient's disposition that could impact the patient's safety.

Safety Huddles

A **safety huddle** is a short (ten- to fifteen-minute), interdisciplinary debrief of patient safety concerns that were faced yesterday and anticipated ones that may be expected on the current day. This is a way to improve communication between team members and raise awareness around areas of patient concern. It is not a forum to solve safety issues—that responsibility goes to managers or safety committees—but rather to make sure the healthcare team is on the same page regarding patients' safety. This opportunity for communication lessens the chances of near misses and patient harm. Huddles foster problem identification and team collaboration, thereby increasing patient safety.

Controlled Substance Audits

Drug diversion is an issue in any setting where controlled substances are available and can be stolen for personal use. Addiction is the most common reason for drug diversion in healthcare settings. Unfortunately, nurses can be vulnerable to drug addiction, which can become worse due to their unique ease of access in the workplace. Some studies indicate that approximately 10% of nurses abuse drugs, and they are more likely to abuse prescription drugs (such as methamphetamines, opioids, and sedatives) than the general population. Nurses are mostly likely to divert drugs by not giving them to the patient for whom the medications were intended, replacing desired prescriptions with alternate medications, taking leftover medications for personal use, or dispensing more than what is needed for a patient and keeping the extra for personal use. Signs that a nurse may be impaired due to substance abuse include erratic behavior, dilated pupils, and noticeable shifts in working ability (e.g., working significantly more shifts or missing work).

Drug diversion is harmful for the nurse, and it seriously jeopardizes the quality of care received by patients. Additionally, drug diversion situations leave a healthcare facility vulnerable to lengthy and resource-intensive legal battles with patients and their families. Therefore, regular administrative processes and quality systems must be in place that can promptly detect drug diversion. From a human resources and administrative perspective, these may include procedures such as background checks for drug-related offenses, pre-employment and random drug testing, and intensive individual rehabilitation processes when drug diversion is detected. From a quality systems perspective, drug management may include highly secured drug storage, video monitoring systems, and sophisticated data collection software that align drug disposal from legitimate prescriptions with expected remaining totals.

Regularly auditing the supply of controlled substances in a facility should be a critical part of any healthcare organization's quality management system. Several quality and public health agencies, including the CDC, recommend prompt reporting drug diversion to licensing bodies rather than allowing for any internal leeway or rehabilitation time. Licensing bodies typically conduct a hearing of the case and may require their own rehabilitation processes, an extended period of time where the nurse is not allowed to work, or a permanent loss of licensure. The relapse rate for nurses who are found guilty of diverting drugs, even when required to complete professional counseling and rehabilitation, is relatively high.

Narcotic Medication Management

Narcotic medication management has its own set of guidelines, including distribution and documentation of narcotic usage. The potential for narcotic abuse guides strict documentation of narcotic chain of custody. Most institutions use a central form of medication dispensing, such as a Pyxis system. Pyxis is managed by the institutional pharmacy and is stocked by pharmacists and pharmacy technicians. Access to Pyxis is granted to those approved to remove and use the medications; generally, nurses and anesthesiologists.

When a narcotic is removed from this system, the narcotic count is verified by the person removing the narcotic, and the narcotic is then removed and administered to the patient. If the person initiating narcotic removal discovers an incorrect narcotic count, the Pyxis system shows the last transaction involving the medication, including the name of the person who removed it and the prior narcotic count. The discrepancy must be resolved at that point, or the issue is turned over to pharmacy and/or hospital security. If a narcotic is removed from the system and the full dose is not administered to the patient, the narcotic must be wasted with another licensed person (such as nurse or anesthesiologist) witnessing the waste. This is documented either on paper or in the Pyxis system.

Reporting Medication Errors

Medication errors can cause significant patient harm if not addressed promptly. Nurses have the responsibility to report medication errors, should they occur. Every healthcare facility should have a protocol for reporting medication errors. Errors can be reported internally within the facility or to a couple of organizations, including the Institute of Safe Medication Practices and the US Food and Drug Administration (FDA) via their MedWatch reporting system. An incident report is used to gather information related to the event, not as a means to discipline an employee. For quality improvement purposes, the information is then used to analyze factors that led to the error.

Medication errors can occur during any stage of administering treatment. Medications administered to the wrong patient occur as a result of failure to verify a patient's identity by using their full name, date of birth, or other specific identifiers. Administering the wrong medication to a patient should also be reported. Three medication checks must occur to ensure the correct medication is administered. These checks occur during preparation, dispensing, and returning of the medication. Other medication errors include administering the drug via the incorrect route, administering the incorrect dose, and administering the medication at the wrong time based on the provider's prescription.

Reporting

Reporting critical patient information in a timely manner and using the correct order in the chain of command are legal obligations of nurses. Failing to report important information could result in serious ramifications and punitive action for the nurse, such as loss of employment and licensure. Furthermore, it can result in patient harm or unresolved conflicts that escalate into larger issues. Preventing patient harm and potential conflicts both start with accurate and timely reporting.

A basic definition of a **report** is the relaying of information that one has observed or heard. When this report is given to an authority figure who can intervene, it should contain the patient name, situation, time of event, and circumstances surrounding the event.

Handoff Reporting

As one shift ends and another begins, there is a **handoff report** that is given from the outgoing team to the oncoming team. The nurse who has completed the shift will tell the nurse beginning the next shift all pertinent information related to each individual patient. Throughout the shift, the exchange of smaller pieces of information continues to take place to keep all members of the healthcare team equally informed.

In the handoff report, the nurse should strategically relay information in a simple, concise manner that is easily understood by the oncoming nurse. It can be easy to get carried away with reporting and include every little detail of the day, opinions about patients or other coworkers, and stories of particular conversations or interactions that occurred during the shift. These superfluous details should be limited, and the report should be kept to the essential items only.

The communication experience during the hand-off process should be a work of art that demonstrates all of the characteristics of a clean exchange of information among professionals. **Hand-offs** not only allow for the dissemination of information from one profession to another but serve as an opportunity for the receiving professional to ask questions and identify concerns. They act as a means to protect the patient from harm and enable professionals to provide a high level of continuity of care.

Patients are most susceptible to an adverse event during the hand-off time frame, as with most transitions in care. The reasons for the enhanced risk are closely related to organizational behavior and patterns during the process that may influence the hand-off process. For example, common distractions that arise in a perioperative environment include patient volume in the receiving unit, the need to maintain a rapid and "efficient" pace during the turnover phase, and reduction of abrasion with surgeons.

The hectic pace of the healthcare environment increases the risk for mistakes and inexplicable communication errors. According to one study, sentinel events occur as a result of poor communication practices that take place during the hand-off process. Nurses can become complacent in this exercise because it is very much part of their routine activities. Organizations must follow a standardized method for hand-off communications to reduce the danger of any impact to patient safety. This standardized approach is a requirement of The Joint Commission.

The requirement dictates that professionals must allow adequate time to exchange information and ask questions and to allow for responses. The benefit of following a standard practice helps to reduce errors and potentially avoid exclusion of pertinent data. Nurses can follow a consistent method for the following:

- Documentation practices
- Review and discussion of critical information
- Adequate preparation and delivery of patient care

A standardized shift handoff procedure can provide a seamless transition between two different medical staff members who may be providing care for the same patient. It can provide detailed and crucial information about the patient and the case; equally important, it can serve as a tool that indicates that official responsibility has moved from one provider to another. This provides a clear mechanism for providing accountability for the individual who is overseeing specific tasks between staff members.

Internal handoffs occur within the same healthcare facility, including, but not limited to, shift handoffs and inter-department handoffs (e.g., a physical therapist is working with a patient in the orthopedic surgery ward). All established healthcare facilities will have their own internal handoff protocols. This can include procedures such as formal handoff training for new staff, continuing training for established staff, verbal handoff protocols, written handoff forms, and stringent repercussions for staff members who fail to meet handoff standards.

External handoffs occur between two separate healthcare entities or during a transition of care. Unless the two systems involved have similar procedures, external handoffs can be compromising situations for the patients and prone to errors.

Errors in handoffs can occur when procedures are not standardized—that is, they do not occur in the exact same manner and convey the exact same information each time a handoff occurs. Developing formal, written standard operating procedures can eliminate the occurrence of various human errors. Standardizing a process may include (but is not limited to) a written checklist, a process flowchart, a meaningful acronym, or an audit tool for staff members to follow. Additionally, errors in handoffs can occur when established standard operating procedures are ignored, written poorly, or are too broad for the scope of the procedure. Errors in handoffs can also occur if medical staff are rushed, are unsure of the team members they are working with, or receive incorrect information anywhere along the duration of a patient's stay.

Bedside Report

Giving the change-of-shift report at the bedside is a practice that every nurse should adopt for the improvement of patient-centered care. Not only can this form of report save time by including the patient/family in all handoff information, but it also reduces the risk for medical errors. Performing a bedside report can also allow both nurses to be hands-on with relaying assessment information.

Interdisciplinary Team/Group (IDT/IDG)

Interdisciplinary communication ensures patient safety. Although documentation in the EMR provides quick access to the patient's clinical history, any immediate concerns should be verbally communicated to the appropriate provider. The interdisciplinary team is composed of professionals within various disciplines and specialties. The nurse must be knowledgeable of the roles and responsibilities of each health care team member to ensure purposeful communication.

Interdisciplinary meetings can be formal or informal but will require structure to be effective. Some healthcare facilities like to do bedside IDT meetings, while others prefer a more formal structure such as using a meeting room. The importance of this type of information sharing cannot be overstated. Every aspect of the patient's care—physical, emotional, spiritual, financial, mental, and social—will be discussed in this setting of information sharing. Changes in the patient's level of care, medications, and therapies will be discussed, along with pertinent discharge planning, social/community resources, and any spiritual or cultural concerns/needs.

Transfer of Care

When possible, a face-to-face discussion will take place between the team transferring the patient and the staff receiving the patient. A patient qualifies for transfer to a different unit once their health status stabilizes and transfer of care does not create a safety risk. Nurses must document all transfers of care within the patient's medical record.

Here is an example of an SBAR intraoperative hand-off to the PACU:

Components of an Intraoperative SBAR Hand-Off to PACU	
Situation	• Patient name • Surgical Procedure (including site) • Anesthetist provider name • Surgeon name
Background	• Anesthesia administration • Medications and dosage (including antibiotics) • IV fluids/sites • Blood type/products • Specimens (type, location, quantity, tests requested) • Estimated blood loss • Urine output • Surgical sites • Dressings, tubes, drainage (including location) • Unexpected or adverse events in the OR
Assessment	• Hemodynamic stability • Respiratory/airway/oxygenation status

Components of an Intraoperative SBAR Hand-Off to PACU	
	• Pain status and pain management • Body temperature (i.e., hyperthermia or hypothermia) • Neuro status • Monitoring (e.g., equipment, lines) • Special needs (e.g., autism, disabilities) • Safety risks
Recommendations	• Implement postoperative orders • Allow for time to answer questions of PACU staff before, during, and after transfer of patient • Actively support patient transfer activities (including lines, equipment, and patient) • Address any known family concerns • Discharge from the PACU once stable

SBAR Method

Some organizations employ the **SBAR method** to help guide communication. SBAR is an acronym for situation, background, assessment, and recommendation. An SBAR report starts with the situation: why is this communication necessary? The background is a brief explanation of the circumstances leading up to the situation. The assessment details the present issue at hand, while the recommendation provides guidance on the best course of action.

The advantages of using SBAR include the following:

- Enhancement of situational awareness
- Promotion and utilization of critical-thinking skills
- Predictable and reliable communication
- Provision of a framework that reduces bias commonly seen with organizational hierarchy and experience
- Expansion of collaborative interactions between nurses and physicians
- Advancement of collaborative discussions in nurse-to-nurse exchanges

Situation

For the situation, the nurse identifies what is happening with the patient. The overview should be concise. It is a succinct statement of the problem. Examples of situation details include the following:

- Demographics (patient and surgeon names, other physicians, age, admission date, surgery date)
- Problem
- Patient stability

Background

In reviewing the background, the nurse provides information about the patient's clinical background that is applicable and relevant to the patient's current situation. He or she is answering the question, "What got us to this point?" Examples of background information details include the presentation history.

Assessment

For the assessment component, nurses should describe findings and provide an analysis of possible options and considerations. Examples of assessment details include the following:

- Procedure-specific assessment
- Vital signs
- Temperature (route of temperature)
- Blood pressure (e.g., cuff or arterial line)
- Monitoring
- Hemodynamic pressure
- Pulse (e.g., apical or peripheral)
- Respiratory status
- Breath sounds
- Oxygen saturation
- Mechanical ventilator settings
- End-tidal carbon dioxide
- Monitoring
- Lab results
- Neurological function (e.g., level of consciousness)
- Intake and output (e.g., intravenous [IV] fluids)
- Location(s) of IV access
- Pain
- Pain rating
- Sedation level
- Dressings and drains
- Condition of the skin
- Drainage (type, color, amount)
- Scores
- Scores associated with the procedure itself
- Monitors and readings (including cardiac monitor)

Recommendation

Finally, the recommendation aspect of the hand-off report should serve as a discussion among professionals about what should happen next. This discussion focuses on next steps and concerns. It is an excellent opportunity to identify if there is a need to update the plan of care or notify the surgeon or physician of any findings, medication adjustments, and pending laboratory data.

Read-Back/Repeat

Some organizations incorporate an additional R, which is known as the read-back or repeat. This extra step is where staff can read back orders to ensure that there is a mutual understanding of the need.

It is a sequential process that challenges individuals only to include pertinent and relevant data. The recipient of the information validates their understanding of the information. This clarification period gives the communicator an opportunity to clarify details if necessary or to take any essential action.

The SBAR method allows nurses to spend less time writing. This effect, in turn, increases the amount of time they can focus on patient care. Studies demonstrate that use of the SBAR technique reduces the risk of adverse events, including death, and increases communication among nursing staff. It has become an industry best practice according to The Joint Commission, and as a result, organizations use electronic tools that reflect the SBAR framework to comply with The Joint Commission on Accreditation of Healthcare Organizations' National Patient Safety Goals.

S

Situation

I am calling about ....

The patient's Code status is ....

The problem I am calling about is ....

e.g. I am concerned the patient is going to arrest

I have just assessed the patient personally:

Vital signs are: Blood Pressure .... / .... Pulse ....

Respiration .... Temperature ....

I am concerned about the:

Blood pressure because it is	**over 200** or	**less than 100** or	**30 mmHg below usual**
Pulse because it is	**over 130** or	**less than 40 and symptomatic**	
Respiration because it is	**less than 8** or	**over 30**	
Temperature because it is	**less than 96** or	**over 104**	
Urine output because it is	**less than 25 ml/hr** or	**200 ml/8hrs**	
O_2 because it is	**less than 88% on 6/liters**	**nasal cannula**	

Other ....

B

Background

The patient's mental status is:

Alert and oriented to person, place, and time		
Confused and	cooperative or	non-cooperative
Agitated or	combative	
Lethargic but conversant and able to swallow		
Stuporous and not talking clearly and possibly not able to swallow		
Comatose	Eyes closed	Not responding to stimulation

The skin is:

Warm and dry	Pale	Mottled
Diaphoretic	Extremities are cold	Extremities are warm

The patient **is not or** **is on oxygen**

The patient has been on .... (l/min) or (5) oxygen for .... minutes (hours)

The oximeter is reading .... %

The oximeter does not detect a good pulse and is giving erratic readings.

A

Assessment

This is what I think the problem is ....

"Say what you think the problem is"

The problem seems to be cardiac infection neurologic respiratory

I am not sure what the problem is but the patient is deteriorating

The patient seems to be unstable and may get worse, we need to do something

R

Recommendation

From Physician ....

Transfer the patient to Critical Care	Come to see the patient at this time
Talk to the patient or family about Code status	Ask a consultant to see patient now

Are any tests needed:

Do you need any test like CXR ABG EKG CBC BMP

Others ....

If a change in treatment is ordered then ask:

How often do you want vital signs?

How long do you expect this problem will last?

If the patient does not get better when would you want us to call again?

Information Sharing

Information sharing can be overwhelming for even the most experienced healthcare workers. With a high caseload of patients, varying acuity levels, and only so much time in the day, gaps in communication can easily occur. This is why using communication tactics for sharing pertinent information is so important. The nurse should be prepared to practice both informal and formal types of information sharing.

Standardized Communication Tool

A standardized communication tool sets the same parameters for requested information each time an instance of communication occurs. By asking for specific answers to the same set of questions, regardless of who is sending information and who is receiving it, standardized communication tools aim to reduce variability in communication, incomplete or partial communication, and irrelevant communication. In the medical setting, standardized communication tools are associated with improved quality of care, improved patient outcomes, and improved patient satisfaction. Electronic medical records, the SBAR hand-off technique, and safety checklists are examples of standardized communication tools.

Standardized Communication Plan

Standardized communication plans are a component of National Patient Safety Goals. Clear verbal, non-verbal, and written communication between healthcare providers is essential for patients to receive high quality care. Communication is especially crucial during patient transitions, such as nursing shift changes, as these periods are when patients are most likely to experience adverse outcomes. The Joint Commission recommends the SBAR communication technique when one healthcare provider is sharing information about the patient to any other provider. SBAR stands for Situation (why the communication is taking place), Background (the status and medical history of the patient), Assessment (the speaker's perspective of the problem), and Recommendation (what action the speaker believes would be most beneficial to the patient).

Closed-Loop Communication

Closed-loop communication is commonly seen in the surgical setting, where the surgical team will frequently reiterate instructions given and ensure follow-up to prevent surgical errors, retention of surgical instruments, and postoperative infections. While this is a vital practice in the surgical setting, the healthcare team should also utilize this type of information sharing in routine practice. See the figure below for a visual of how this cyclical communication tool works in practice. It is important for the nurse to practice the check-back communication to "close the loop" and verify that the information obtained is consistent with both parties.

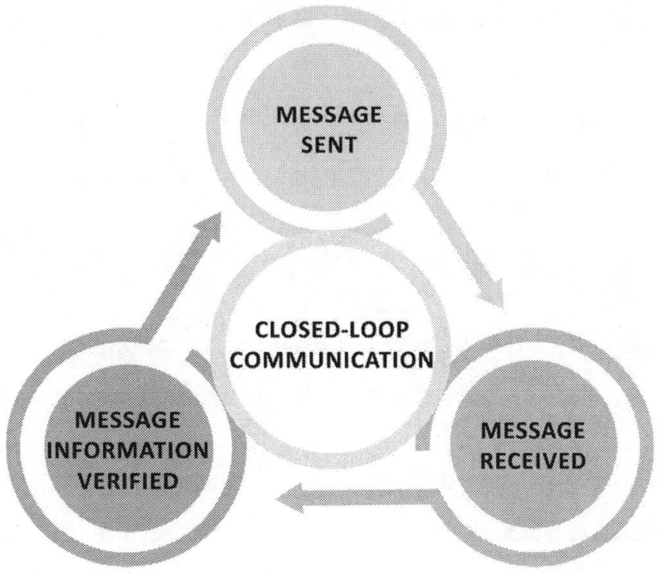

Read-Back for Verbal Orders

Read-back occurs when staff reads back orders to ensure that there is a mutual understanding of the need. It is a sequential process that challenges individuals to include only pertinent and relevant data. The recipient of the information validates their understanding of the information. This clarification period gives the communicator an opportunity to clarify details if necessary or to take any essential action.

Ideally, verbal orders should only occur when the provider is physically unable to write out the orders due to an emergency or other extenuating circumstances. Verbal orders must be carefully read back to the provider to ensure accuracy. The verbal order process includes receiving, reading back, documenting, and executing the order. During the read-back, the nurse must repeat the order that was given as it is interpreted. The provider must then confirm the read-back with the nurse.

After the verbal order has been given, the nurse must document the date and time of the order as well as the provider's name. After the emergency situation has passed, the provider must review the verbal order for accuracy and sign the order, including the date and time. Verbal orders must be physically signed by the provider within 24 hours of being given to the nurse.

Legal and Compliance

Legal Implications

Nurses must uphold and answer to certain legal rights and responsibilities within their profession. From simple tasks like managing a patient's property, to more complicated issues such as reporting abuse and neglect, the nurse has a legal responsibility to act.

Nurses need a knowledge of the common legal terminology in their practice. The following is a list of terms the nurse should know:

- **Common law**: Based on legal precedents or previously decided cases in courts of law
- **Statutory law**: Based on a state's legislative actions or any other legislative body's actions
- **Constitutional law**: Based on the content of the Constitution of the United States of America
- **Administrative law**: Passed down from a ruling body, such as continuing education requirements mandated by each state's nursing association
- **Criminal law**: Involves the arrest, prosecution, and incarceration of those who have broken the law, including misdemeanors and felonies
- **Liability**: Involves accountability for one's actions from a legal standpoint
- **Tort**: Refers to nursing practice violations, such as malpractice, negligence, and patient confidentiality violations
- **Unintentional tort**: Examples can include negligence and malpractice in certain situations
- **Intentional tort**: Examples can include false imprisonment, privacy breaches, slander, libel, battery, and assault

Sensitive Information Protection

Patient privacy and **confidentiality** are constant concerns for all healthcare providers. Given the sensitivity of medical procedures, the healthcare team must maintain strict patient confidentiality. Under the Health Insurance Portability and Accountability Act (HIPAA), a patient's information is required to be protected and kept confidential regardless of the form, including electronic, written, and spoken communication. **Protected health information** (**PHI**) should be shared only on an as-needed and minimum necessary basis. When discussing patients or cases in settings where other personnel may overhear the conversation, the medical team should be careful not to include any PHI that may violate the patient's confidentiality. Additionally, when information is displayed electronically to families and visitors in waiting rooms, patient names should be avoided. HIPAA violations can have negative consequences for the providers and/or the facility.

The nurse plays an important role in keeping a patient's health information private. Sharing personal details—such as a patient's name, condition, and medical history—in an inappropriate way violates the person's right to privacy. For example, a nurse telling a friend who does not work in the facility that the nurse took care of the friend's aunt, without the aunt's consent or knowledge, is considered a violation of privacy. Another way a nurse could violate privacy is to access a patient's medical record when they are not actually caring for them. For example, if a celebrity has been admitted to a different unit, and the nursing assistant accesses the celebrity's electronic health record, then they are in violation of HIPAA. Those who are caught violating HIPAA could lose their jobs and face other punitive actions. Nurses should also ensure that other staff members, as well as patients, understand the confidentiality requirements of the facility, state, and country.

Electronic Access Audit/Activity Log

Most of the patient's health information will be logged in an electronic health record (HER). Anyone who accesses this information will be tracked and monitored. Most institutions will conduct routine audits to see who has been accessing which records and if they were authorized to do so.

Use and Disclosure of Personal/Protected Health Information (PHI)

- Consent/Authorization to Release: A patient is usually asked to sign a consent to release PHI before receiving treatment. This allows the healthcare provider to release their information for treatment, payment, and healthcare operations, abbreviated to TPO. **Treatment** is all care given to the patient by the healthcare provider; **payment** involves claims, billing, and collection by insurance companies; and **healthcare operations** involves educational purposes such as training new CMAs. Healthcare operations does not include using patient information for research; a different consent must be signed for that purpose.
- Drug and Alcohol Treatment Records: Certain patient health records regarding the treatment of drug and alcohol addictions are specifically protected by federal regulations. Violation of the confidentiality of these records could result in a criminal penalty to the offender. There are certain emergency situations in which this information may be shared as well as research purposes in which release of information is allowed.
- HIV-Related Information: HIV-related information is protected by law. Reports on diagnoses and treatments are to be kept private and confidential by healthcare providers. The reason this information is kept confidential is that persons with an HIV-AIDS diagnosis may face discrimination because of some people's unfair prejudices.
- Mental Health Records: Part of HIPAA provides special protection to mental health records. For example, though mental health information is largely grouped together with general health information about a patient, psychotherapy notes have special safeguards that keep them confidential. In the case of minors with mental health issues, there are specific guidelines that dictate who can be talked to about which issues, such as discussing a teen's medication regimen for mental illness with a legal guardian or parent.

Copyright Law

Copyright law affects nurses, especially in academia and research roles, as it protects their creative works (e.g., educational materials, documentation, and findings). In professional roles, nurses are often responsible for providing input and developing policies, manuals, or instructional content within their roles as organizational staff, which is a form of intellectual property (IP). There must be an awareness of who owns the right to the product. Copyright ensures that the original work is not copied or used without permission, safeguarding their professional contributions. Additionally, copyright laws must be followed when using materials created by others (e.g., articles, images, or videos) through proper citations, recognition, and licensing compliance. Understanding copyright law prevents legal issues and promotes ethical use of resources in patient care and education. Awareness of copyright law empowers nurses to protect their work and utilize resources responsibly, maintaining professionalism and legal compliance in healthcare settings.

Plagiarism

Plagiarism, as in all professions including healthcare roles, involves presenting someone else's work, ideas, or research as one's own without proper acknowledgment. It undermines professional integrity, compromises patient trust, and can lead to severe academic and legal consequences. In nursing roles at any level, maintaining honesty is crucial, as it directly impacts patient safety and the quality of care. Common forms of plagiarism include copying text, failing to cite sources, and paraphrasing without attribution. To prevent plagiarism, nursing students and professional nurses can practice superlative research and writing habits by properly citing sources, utilizing paraphrasing while giving credit, and understanding ethical guidelines related to use of others' literary works. Educational institutions and healthcare organizations emphasize the importance of originality and integrity to uphold professional standards. Recognizing the significance of academic honesty in nursing promotes a culture of trust, accountability, and ethical practice, ultimately enhancing patient outcomes and the credibility of the nursing profession.

Intellectual Property

Having awareness of intellectual property (IP) considerations protects a nurse's own work and contributions to science and the field of nursing. This includes understanding of rights related to original education materials, research, and clinical innovations developed through their work. Proper attribution and securing rights prevents unauthorized use or plagiarism. Nurses involved in research or creating content must also adhere to confidentiality agreements and privacy laws like HIPAA to avoid infringing on patient or institutional IP. Collaborations with healthcare organizations may involve licensing or transfer of rights; therefore, understanding of contractual obligations is vital. Protecting IP fosters innovation, ensures professional recognition, and supports ethical practice. Conversely, nurses must respect others' IP rights, avoiding infringement through plagiarism or unauthorized use. Overall, awareness of IP considerations enables nurses to ethically manage their intellectual contributions, promote healthcare advancements, and comply with legal and organizational policies.

Integration of Legal and Regulatory Requirements

Regulatory and compliance standards mainly refer to the laws and policies that are in place to ensure safe and quality care within a healthcare facility. Specific requirements may vary from state to state. For example, some states require certain nurse-to-patient ratios, while others do not have any legal staffing requirements. There are also federal regulations, such as requirements for doctors and nurses to meet licensing standards and policies that protect patients, such as HIPAA (Health Insurance Portability and Accountability Act) and EMTALA (Emergency Medical Treatment and Labor Act). Hospitals may be monitored for compliance by government officials and by independent accrediting bodies depending on availability and resources of the hospital. It is important for nurses to understand these regulatory and compliance standards to maintain their licensure, avoid potential legal action, and maintain the health and safety of their patients.

Nursing Scope of Practice

Another responsibility of the nurse is to work within their own scope of practice. So the main questions become: what is the nursing scope of practice, and how does the nurse stay up to date on changes?

Nursing scope of practice simply means what the nurse can legally and ethically practice based on competency through active licensure and any testing required. Federal regulations are geared towards the general practice of safe patient care and advancements in practice, while each state will have a specific set of laws that will be defined in the Nursing Practice Act (NPA). Standards of nursing practice will be thoroughly defined in this document to give the nurse in each state a specific scope of practice. Each facility will also have a set of regulations that the nurse should know.

For example, federal regulations and certain state laws approve of an LPN initiating a peripheral IV as long as competency tasks have been completed. With that being said, if the specific agency does not approve of LPNs initiating a peripheral IV, the scope of practice of the LPN within that agency will be to not initiate peripheral IVs. For this reason, the nurse will need to ensure the use of federal, state, and agency resources to ensure appropriate and ethical nursing practice. Following nursing regulatory bodies (NRBs), the state board of nursing (BON), and agency policies and procedures can help the nurse know, and practice within, the approved scope.

Evaluating the Appropriateness of Healthcare Provider's Orders for a Patient

Nurses are responsible for executing two types of tasks: independent and dependent. Those considered independent are patient duties that do not require a doctor's order and can be performed within a nurse's scope of practice; those that are dependent are patient duties that can only be administered as per instruction from a doctor or other independent licensed practitioner.

When receiving an order, the nurse is required to make sure it is thorough, appropriate, and executed quickly. Nurses should never act on any orders from a healthcare provider that are unclear or inappropriate. Instead, the nurse should follow up on any order that seems uncertain by contacting the provider right away for an explanation.

For an order of restraints to be considered complete, it must at least include why the order is needed, the kind of restraint required, the length of time it should be used, patient actions that necessitate its usage, and the signature of the person who ordered it. Medication orders must designate the name of the patient along with the drug name, dosage, administration instructions, frequency, indication, and a signed confirmation of the person who ordered it. Any part of this process that deviates from these requirements or seems incorrect requires intervention from the nurse.

Federal Employment Laws

Family Medical Leave Act (FMLA)

The Family Medical Leave Act (FMLA) was passed to allow eligible employees to take up to twelve weeks of job-protected, unpaid leave during a twelve-month period for specific family and medical reasons. Employees are covered under this act if their employer has at least fifty employees—full- or part-time—working within seventy-five miles of a given workplace. Additionally, the employee must have worked for their employer for at least twelve months and for a total of 1,250 hours over the past year.

FMLA covers leave for the following reasons:

- The birth of a child, adoption, or foster-care placement
- The serious health condition of a spouse, child, or parent
- The serious health condition of the employee, one requiring inpatient care or continuing treatment by a healthcare provider
- Qualifying exigency leave, or leave to address the most common issues that arise when an employee's spouse, child, or parent is on active duty or call to active-duty status—e.g., making financial and legal arrangements or arranging for alternative childcare
- Military caregiver leave or leave to care for a covered service member, such as the employee's spouse, child, parent, or their next of kin, with a serious injury or illness. Employees are to be granted up to twenty-six weeks of job-protected, unpaid leave during a twelve-month period to care for a covered service member.

Instead of taking all of their leave at once, employees can choose to take FMLA leave intermittently or in blocks of time for specific, qualifying reasons as approved by their employer. One reason for doing so would be for an employee to attend medical appointments for their ongoing treatment and testing for a serious health condition.

Spouses who work for the same employer must share the amount of FMLA time they take for the birth of a child, adoption, or foster care placement or for the serious health condition of a child or parent. The total amount of leave taken by both spouses must add up to twelve weeks for the reasons stated above or twenty-six weeks for the care of a covered service member.

Employers also have the right to require employees to take unpaid FMLA leave concurrent with any relevant paid leave, such as sick time or vacation time, to which the employees are entitled under their current policies. In addition, a week containing a holiday still counts as a full week of FMLA, whether or not the holiday is considered to be paid time.

Employers are required to maintain an employee's group health care coverage while they are out on FMLA leave when the employee was covered under such a plan prior to leave. Once an employee's FMLA leave has ended, they are to be reinstated to their original job or to an equivalent job with equivalent conditions of employment, pay, and benefits.

Employers who fail to comply with the FMLA act may face both civil and criminal penalties. Also, if the Department of Labor finds that an employer did not post FMLA rights and responsibilities notices in the workplace, then a penalty of $211 can be assessed for willful failure to post.

Americans with Disabilities Act (ADA)

The Americans with Disabilities Act (ADA) is a federal law that prevents discrimination based on disability. This law requires employers to provide reasonable accommodations to employees with a disability. For example, an employer may accommodate a disabled employee by building a wheelchair accessible ramp to enter and exit the building. Additionally, the ADA stipulates that public entities be accessible for disabled persons. The ADA does include both mental and physical medical conditions, and temporary conditions may qualify as a disability. ADA protections apply to every aspect of job application procedures, employment, and promotions.

National Labor Relations Act

Employees may choose to be represented by a labor union. However, there are other forms of employee representation as well. The National Labor Relations Act of 1935 (NLRA; also known as the Wagner Act) is administered by the National Labor Relations Board (NLRB) and protects the rights of private sector workers to join labor unions. Additionally, it constrains employee representation in nonunionized companies. Nevertheless, nonunion employee representation plans can be found in many organizations where employees want a voice in the workplace. Like unions, these groups allow employees to advocate for fair treatment and improved employment conditions while also creating a channel for communication where employees can give input into the decision-making process.

However, the decisions ultimately rest with management. Unlike unions, nonunion employee representation plans keep all decisions and bargaining within the organization. One example of this type of body is a works council, which generally represents employees on a more local level than a trade union. A works council operates within an organization to improve communication between employers and employees and to increase employees' bargaining power. In the United States., a works council must be elected by employees without interference by the employer in order to be recognized as lawful. In other cases, employees may also choose to be represented by legal counsel or a governmental body to assist in negotiations or resolving disputes.

Additional Regulations

Other important regulations include the Fair Labor Standard Act (FLSA) which establishes rules such as minimum wage and overtime pay, standards for child labor, and definitions for exempt and non-exempt employees. The Occupational Safety and Health Act of 1970 created the Occupational Safety and Health Administration (OSHA), which ensures that employers provide a safe and healthy workplace. Examples of OSHA regulations include eliminating or reducing hazards when possible, providing free safety equipment, informing employees about chemical hazards, providing comprehensive and comprehensible safety training, keeping records of work-related injuries and illnesses, and displaying the official OSHA poster describing employees' rights and employers' responsibilities.

Nursing Licensure

An important part of professional nursing practice is understanding and operating within applicable laws and regulations. Nursing professionals are held to very high standards due to the delicate nature of the work they perform. Additionally, healthcare providers are subject to legal ramifications within their practice and must be aware of how to protect themselves from potential liability.

A foundation of nursing practice is to obtain and maintain nursing licensure as well as to follow the practice standards outlined by one's State Board of Nursing. The **State Board of Nursing** provides guidance for nursing education programs, state testing, provision of appropriate nursing care, and management of misconduct by licensed nurses. These provisions are outlined in the state's **Nurse Practice Act**, which outlines statutory laws governing legal nursing responsibilities.

There are many other legal materials that impact nursing practice as well. For example, common laws are previous legal decisions that set precedents for future proceedings. **Common law** can have significant influence on malpractice decisions and lawsuits involving patient rights. Additionally, the **Health Insurance Portability and Accountability Act** (**HIPAA**) legally governs the safe use of protected patient information. The **Patient Bill of Rights** is yet another binding document that outlines various protected rights for patients, including informed consent and the right to refuse. In non-hospital settings, nurses are protected by **Good Samaritan laws** to reduce legal liability for acts performed during emergencies. Also, nurses are governed by The Centers of Disease Control and Prevention (CDC) health codes to protect and maintain public safety. These codes outline standards of mandatory reporting (e.g., cases of abuse and communicable disease) and standards of ensuring public safety (e.g., safety education and immunization).

In personal practice, nurses must consider how to protect themselves if they are required to defend themselves within the legal system. Patients and caregivers could potentially file lawsuits if they feel standards of care or patient rights were not upheld. Some of the more common issues brought against nurses can include any of the following: forced physical touch (assault), not performing standards of care (breach of duty), unlawful use of restraints (false imprisonment), privacy breach (HIPAA violation), not performing the typical standard of care action that would be reasonably expected (negligence), or being the direct cause of harm (proximate cause).

Nurses can legally protect themselves in many ways. Proactive steps include maintaining all required licensure and training associated with state laws. Additionally, nurses can purchase malpractice insurance to financially protect themselves if they are involved with a legal case. Nurses have a duty to understand and follow all laws pertaining to nursing practice in their state, and they also have a duty to uphold standards of care and patient rights as outlined by their organization. Accurate, concise, objective, and timely documentation practices also help to provide evidence of appropriate nursing care. Lastly, developing and maintaining trusting relationships with patients and caregivers can help to lessen legal risks.

Regulatory and Compliance Standards

Nurse leaders have an important role when it comes to the implementation and delivery of safe, high-quality care and maintaining **regulatory compliance** within their organizations. In order to achieve these responsibilities, professional development nurses must have a thorough understanding of the regulatory and compliance standards that govern healthcare practices. These standards are in place to protect patients and staff as well as maintain the integrity of an organization. Professional development nurses must abide by these standards as they navigate the complex landscape of healthcare. Examples of regulatory and compliance standards include licensing and accreditation, quality and patient safety standards, infection control, and medication safety and management.

Organization Licensing and Accreditation

One crucial area that nurse leaders must focus on is **licensing** and **accreditation**. Healthcare organizations are required to obtain and maintain appropriate licenses and accreditations to function. It is the responsibility of nurse leaders to ensure that their facilities are meeting the requirements set forth by regulatory bodies, including state health departments. Some of these requirements include adherence to professional practice guidelines, staffing ratios, and safety standards within the facility. Since requirements are ever-changing, nurse leaders must stay up-to-date on such requirements to maintain organizational and corporate compliance.

Quality and Patient Safety Standards

Nursing professionals must maintain the highest quality standards for patient safety within their healthcare organization, including implementation of **quality improvement** practices. They should also follow quality standards that are set forth by organizations, such as the **National Committee for Quality Assurance** (**NCQA**). Standards outlined by this organization include patient-centered care, evidence-based practice, and patient safety. When nurse administrators have robust quality improvement programs in place, data can be analyzed to identify areas of improvement or concern. Overall, these actions help meet quality and safety goals or standards.

Infection Control

Infection control is arguably one of the most important concepts in healthcare. Nursing professionals are obligated to ensure compliance with infection control standards within their organizations. They can do so by staying up-to-date with guidelines and procedures set forth by health organizations, such as the **Centers for Disease Control** (**CDC**) and World Health Organization (WHO). They must also enforce guidelines and procedures outlined by these organizations in their facilities. Another responsibility of the nurse administrator includes infection prevention, which can be accomplished through staff education via online modules or professional development days. The nurse administrator can also utilize surveillance methods to monitor healthcare-associated infections within the organization. Additionally, nurse managers may utilize random monitoring of staff infection control methods, such as hand hygiene practices.

Medication Safety and Management

Patient well-being is closely aligned with safe medication practices. Nursing professionals are responsible for facilitating **medication safety** within their respective healthcare organizations. To do so, they must abide by medication management standards. Examples of such standards include proper medication storage and handling, appropriate reconciliation processes, education on safe administration practices, and correct medication administration. Another component nursing professionals are accountable for is monitoring and addressing medication-related incidents and enacting strategies to prevent and reduce medication errors.

The "seven rights" refer to a set of seven guidelines for healthcare providers to follow when administering medication to patients. These standardize the medication administration process and promote a context of high-quality care. The seven rights are:

- Right medication: Providers check that the medication they are about to administer is the one that was prescribed.
- Right client: Providers check that the patient who is about to receive medication is the correct patient.
- Right dose: Providers check that the dose they are about to administer matches the prescribed dose.
- Right time: Providers check that the medication is given at the pre-determined interval.
- Right route: Providers ensure that medication is delivered in the intended method (e.g., orally).
- Right reason: Providers note that the medication is administered for a specific cause.
- Right documentation: Providers follow institutional protocol to maintain thorough recordkeeping of administered medications.

These rights work to ensure patient safety.

Patient Safety Protocols

Ensuring patient safety is one of the most important jobs for nurses. Nurses are the professionals who have the most patient contact and can best assess and prevent safety issues, such as bed sores, falls, and suicidal patients. Because nurses have the most interaction with a patient, they are able to implement measures to ensure safety and prevent common injuries from happening. Patient safety is a major area of quality improvement, which reinforces its systemic importance and the vital role nurses play in implementing it.

Rounding

Rounding is the timely process of checking on a patient's well-being, assessing their needs, and addressing any issues. Common timeframes for rounding are hourly or every two hours. While rounding, the nurse inspects the patient's room and environment looking for any potential sources of injury, such as wires that can be tripped on. They assess the patient for such aspects of care as IV lines being intact, the patient being alert or resting comfortably, and any changes in patient disposition. A systematic rounding policy reduces fall rates, call bell rings, and interruptions for the nurse. It also increases patient satisfaction because it ensures they are getting their needs met and interacting with a member of their healthcare team regularly.

As part of customer satisfaction, patients expect their call bell to be answered promptly. In many cases this is difficult for nurses, as they may be either charting or attending to another patient. Frequent rounding helps address patient needs earlier on, preventing numerous call bells later. This proactive approach addresses patients' needs faster, leading to increased satisfaction and, in the long run, better healing.

A common mnemonic to remember what to address during rounding is the Three P's, which stand for pain, potty, and position. During each rounding, the nurse should assess pain by asking the patient to rate their pain from zero to ten. If necessary, the nurse can then administer medication following provider orders and document medications given. Reassuring the patient that their pain will be rounded on and addressed at frequent time intervals is comforting to patients and families. For potty, the nurse should ask if the patient needs assistance to the restroom and provide education on not getting out of bed without assistance. Lastly, ask the patient if their position is comfortable. Remember to turn patients every two hours to prevent bed sores and skin breakdown.

Skin Integrity

Skin integrity refers to the health of a patient's skin. Skin with high integrity is free of open wounds, moisture, and infection. This is an important factor in patient health as the skin is the largest barrier between external harmful agents and internal organs, bones, and tissues. When skin integrity is low, patients become more susceptible to infection, therefore reducing recovery time and quality of care while increasing poor health outcomes (including death). When providing care to patients, nurses should ensure that surgical and recovery positioning do not compromise the skin (i.e., leaving patients in a way that would make them prone to pressure ulcers). If patients already have compromised areas, medical staff should ensure that all precautions are made to keep the wound clean, bandaged, and free of pressure or friction.

Elderly patients have an increased risk for skin injuries due to the fragility of their skin, decreased circulation, poor nutrition, decreased sensation, mental changes, and altered mobility. As the body ages, the skin becomes thinner due to decreased adipose tissue and has less elasticity. The **epidermis**, which is the outer layer of the skin, is only 0.1 millimeters thick and becomes thinner with time. Loss of collagen as the skin ages decreases the skin's elasticity, making it more vulnerable to friction and force. **Dry skin** is caused by loss of sweat and oil, and also due to a decrease in blood flow to the skin. All of these factors contribute to skin that is fragile and prone to tears. If any skin injuries are observed on a patient, the injuries must be assessed, documented, treated, and monitored for changes. Patients who require total care have the greatest risk of developing a skin tear or a pressure ulcer.

Risks for developing a skin tear or pressure ulcer include the following:

- Bedridden patient
- Wheelchair dependent
- Limited mobility
- Spinal-cord injury
- Poor nutrition
- Poor circulation to the skin, commonly due to a heart condition or diabetes
- Dependence on others for care

- Weakened immune system
- Elderly population
- Excessive pressure on the skin or on bony areas

The **Braden Scale** is used to assess the risk of patients developing pressure ulcers (commonly known as bedsores). A pressure ulcer refers to internal and/or external damage that can occur in areas of the body where areas of bone are poorly cushioned by soft or adipose tissue (such as the tailbone). This is normally the result of low mobility in a patient, resulting in constant pressure placed on the bony area and therefore resulting in bruising of or breakage in the corresponding soft tissue, blood vessels, or skin.

The Braden Scale takes into account patients' sensory perception (whether they can feel areas of pressure), moisture (how damp an area is), activity (how much patients are able to generally move on their own or with assistance), mobility (how well patients are able to generally move on their own or with assistance), nutrition (patient intake of macronutrients, vitamins, and minerals that support bodily functions), and friction (if any areas are exposed to repeated rubbing or chafing). Based on this scale, patients will be categorized as at risk, moderate risk, high risk, or very high risk of developing a pressure ulcer. Nurse monitoring and patient care should be tailored to the patient's risk category.

Bruising

Bruises or **ecchymosis** are caused by blunt force or clotting abnormalities that cause capillaries under the skin to leak blood into the tissue, causing a discolored area. Bruises can range in color from blue, brown, or purple to even green and yellow depending on the stage of healing. Bruising can occur in patients as a result of bumping into objects, multiple or failed intravenous-access attempts, medication side effects, or falling. Significant bruising that occurs without a known cause could indicate an underlying medical condition, such as a blood-clotting disorder. Bruising can also be a result of physical abuse. If suspicious bruises are noticed, it is important to ask the patient questions about the bruising. Family members should also ask staff about bruises they notice on their loved one.

Risks for bruising include the following:

- Elderly population
- Frail, thin skin
- Blood thinner medications that cause slower blood clotting times, resulting in quicker and easier bruising
- Altered mental status or disorientation (may cause a person to be unsteady or to be unaware of their surroundings)
- Environmental hazards in the patient's room, such as corners of tables, furniture, or cords that could cause tripping and bumping
- Visual or other sensory impairment (may cause falling or bumping into objects)

Restraints

Restraints can be defined as anything that is used, done, or said to intentionally limit a person's ability to move freely. Restraints, when applied properly, cannot be easily removed or controlled by the person. In addition to physical form, restraints can also be emotional, chemical, or environmental. Use of restraints is very controversial due to the ethical issue of personal freedom. These are a temporary solution to a problem and must always be used as a last resort. Restraints are used to limit a patient's movement to prevent injury to themselves or others and always require a physician's order.

Types of restraints include the following:

- Physical: vests, wrist restraints, straps, or anything that confines the body
- Emotional: verbal cues or emotions used to coerce the patient to act a certain way

- Environmental: side rails, locked doors, closed windows, or locked beds
- Chemical: any medication used to change a patient's behavior

The medical doctor or practitioner is responsible for ordering the use of restraints. Nurses are responsible for applying restraints safely and for the management of a patient with a restraint. After an order is given, the physician must visit the patient within twenty-four hours of placing the order to assess its further necessity.

The following are circumstances under which restraints are used:

- Signs of patient aggression toward self, staff, or other patients
- Interference with important medical devices, such as an IV or a catheter
- Patient movements that are potentially harmful to their health or may cause further injury
- Potential for a patient to interfere with a procedure

When applying restraints:

- Always follow the facility's restraint policy.
- Obtain an order from a physician or medical practitioner, unless it is an emergency situation.
- Obtain consent from the patient or their legal representative if the patient is not capable of understanding.
- Explain to the patient what is going to happen, even if the patient is unable to understand due to confusion or dementia.
- Always monitor the patient per facility policy, such as checking the positioning of the restraint every thirty minutes and removing every two hours for range of motion. Remember to reposition the patient and offer toileting every two hours.
- Explain the need for restraints and how long the restraints will be used.

Vests have holes for the arms and the opening crosses in the back. The straps will be secured on either side of the bed or chair, depending on the patient's location. Tie it in a quick-release knot to a lower part of the bed that does not move. Make sure that two fingers fit underneath the vest on the patient's chest so that it is not too tight.

Wrist or **ankle restraints** are cloths that wrap around each wrist or ankle. They have a strap that is tied to a lower, immovable part of the bed or chair. Tie it in a quick-release knot. Ensure the restraints aren't too tight and that the patient's arms or legs aren't in an awkward position. Usually, a pillow will be placed under the arms and/or the knees and heels.

Possible injuries from restraints can include the following:

- Broken bones
- Bruises
- Falls
- Skin tears or pressure sores
- Depression or fear due to lack of freedom
- Death from strangulation

Fall Prevention

Risk for falls is a serious consideration for all patients entering into a facility or hospital. A fall can cause injuries that worsen the patient's condition and may even lead to death. The nurse should be able to identify patients at risk for falls and implement the proper fall precautions to ensure the patient's safety.

Risk factors for falls include the following:

- Muscle weakness
- Balance and gait problems
- Dizziness related to low blood pressure, heart conditions, or medication side effects
- Slower reflexes
- Confusion or memory loss
- Foot problems and/or unsafe shoes
- Vision problems
- History of falls (Patients who have fallen before are two to three times more likely to fall again.)

A fall may occur for a number of reasons. Older adults are at risk for falls more so than younger people due to weakening muscles and bones. This weakness in the musculoskeletal system leads to an unsteady gait and poor balance. People with a weak musculoskeletal system may not be able to correct themselves as quickly or with as much agility when they lose their balance, nor can they catch themselves as well when they fall, leading to greater injury.

Fluctuations in blood pressure may cause a person to fall, especially if the blood pressure becomes too low. Blood pressure is a reflection of how well the heart is pumping oxygen-rich blood to the tissues of the body, especially the brain. If the brain is not getting enough oxygen from the blood as a result of low blood pressure, among other causes, the person may fall as a result of dizziness and/or fainting. **Orthostatic hypotension** occurs when blood pressure drops suddenly as a result of a change in position, such as from sitting to standing, and does not immediately compensate.

Low blood sugar may cause a decreased level of consciousness in an individual. The brain not only needs oxygen, but it also needs an adequate supply of blood glucose to maintain consciousness and regulate movement and coordination. When blood sugar becomes too low, the resulting altered level of consciousness may cause a person to lose balance and fall to the ground.

Patients in an unfamiliar environment may become confused when in bed or navigating themselves around their room. Confusion is common among hospitalized individuals, resulting from medication side effects and the effects of illness. A patient may suddenly attempt to get out of bed or try and walk to the bathroom, not remembering that they are attached to an intravenous pole, urinary catheter, and/or many other types of equipment, depending on their condition. This brief moment of confusion and unexpected obstacles can lead to a fall and injury.

Patients with sensory deficits may be at risk for a fall, such as those with visual and hearing impairments. Visual impairments may prevent a patient from seeing obstacles in their path. Hearing impairments may prevent a patient from hearing warning sounds or words.

There are certain measures, called **fall precautions**, which can be put in place for a patient who is at risk for a fall. The nurse can create an uncluttered, well-lit environment for the patient. Rooms that are full of clutter, equipment, and obstacles put the patient at risk for a fall. In the same way, if the lighting is not adequate for the patient, they may trip on an unseen object and fall.

Placing the call light in the patient's reach and talking to the patient about using it when needing any sort of assistance can prevent a fall. Some hospitals have a "Call Don't Fall" sign in the patient's room, indicating the patient and family should ask for help using the call light when necessary.

Patients who have displayed confusion and impulsive behavior that may put them at risk for a fall, such as suddenly attempting to get out of bed when they are not physically able or need assistance with equipment, should have special precautions put in place. A **bed alarm** is a device that sets off an alarm when the patient tries to get out of bed unassisted. It is a pad with a sensor that is placed under the patient's buttocks or under the fitted sheet of the bed; the bed itself may be equipped with an alarm device.

Some patients will be put on what is called a **low bed**, a bed that can be lowered close to the floor. This ensures that the patient will not accidentally slide or roll out of bed if they try to get out of bed before the healthcare staff can assist.

Nurses should encourage patients to use available assistive devices, such as canes, walkers, and wheelchairs. Before leaving a patient's room, make sure any assistive device that the patient can use independently is within their reach.

The use of assistive devices such as **gait belts** (also known as **transfer belts**) benefits both the nurse and the patient. When transferring or walking with a patient who needs assistance, it's advised to use a gait belt to prevent falls. When using a gait belt to assist a patient to walk, fasten the belt around their waist and hold it with both hands while standing to the side and slightly behind the patient. If the patient loses their balance and begins to fall, never attempt to catch them. Instead, continue holding the gait belt, bend at the knees, and slowly lower the patient to the floor.

Safe Transfer Techniques

When transferring a patient, the safety of the patient and the nurse are of the greatest importance. Incorrectly performed transfers can cause injury to both. Be mindful of proper transfer techniques and body mechanics, such as keeping a straight back, bending at the knees, avoiding twisting at the waist, and, most importantly, asking for additional help if needed.

When assisting a patient out of bed, always make sure that the bed is in the lowest position. Then, assist the patient to sit upright on the side of the bed with both feet on the floor. While the patient remains in this seated position, make sure they aren't lightheaded or dizzy from the position change. If the patient needs significant physical assistance other than stabilization, an assistive device should be considered. To assist the patient in standing, the nurse should stand in front of the patient, place their knees in front of the patient's knees, and hug the patient under the arms for lifting. Then instruct the patient to help as much as possible. If transferring the patient to a chair after assisting them to stand, both the nurse and the patient should take small steps, pivoting around to the chair. Make sure the backs of the patient's knees are touching the front of the seat before lowering them into the chair.

When transferring a patient, make sure that all wheels are locked on the bed and/or chair before moving the patient.

Suicide

Patients need to be interviewed regarding their life stressors and coping mechanisms. Life stressors can include losing a job, losing a loved one, divorce, chronic illnesses, and increased family obligations. The goal of risk reduction is keeping the patient safe and helping them avoid self-harm. A **suicide risk assessment** should be performed when patients verbalize suicide ideation or poor coping skills. The patient should be asked if they have a suicide plan and the means to carry it out. The SAD PERSONAS suicide risk assessment can be used to assess a patient's suicide risk. Eleven major areas (sex, age, depression, previous attempt, ethanol abuse, rational thinking loss, social supports lacking, organized plan, no spouse, availability of lethal means, sickness) are assessed and scored. The higher the score, the higher the risk.

Maintaining Records

The documentation of patient information and interventions is vitally important. A patient's chart is a legal record of assessments and care measures. Most facilities use an electronic health record, with training provided during new employee orientation. Documentation may include timing related to observations, interventions, and patient responses.

There are various charting systems used by patient care facilities to document patient data. Documentation requirements will be dictated by facility policy and regulatory guidelines. Two methods are commonly used: charting by exception and comprehensive charting.

Charting by Exception

Charting by exception requires that only vital signs and abnormal findings are documented. This charting method is somewhat controversial since a great amount of information about the patient is usually left out. It is sometimes argued that this is the safer way to chart, as only what is deviant from normal is noted, and thus, there is less room for documentation errors. The normal is assumed, unless otherwise noted. This method also saves time, as less information needs to be documented, leaving more time for patient care.

Comprehensive Charting

Some facilities prefer a **comprehensive method** of documentation, charting everything about the patient—normal and abnormal—in a very thorough manner. This way, when the patient's chart must be reviewed, especially in the case of a safety incident (e.g., a pressure sore develops or a patient falls), all details surrounding the event should be present in the medical record. This method is effective if all information is properly charted, although it can be quite time-consuming and take away from patient care time.

Documentation provides a defense for healthcare workers and patients in the case of incidents, serving as evidence of the sequence of events. There is an adage that says, "If it wasn't charted, it didn't happen." The nurse needs to be mindful that the medical record is a legal document—a complete, thorough, and accurate documentation of care, according to facility policy.

Downtime Procedures

Downtime procedures can vary from facility to facility, but the nurse should be prepared for both planned and unplanned downtime. First, what is downtime? Considering healthcare predominantly uses electronic health records, downtime is any time that an aspect of the electronic health record system is not working. Downtime can be a planned situation during which staff is informed of a certain time frame where the system will be down for updates, repairs, or a reset. It can also be unplanned in the event of an IT malfunction, cybersecurity issue, or loss of power.

During downtime, the greatest concern is patient safety, as the safeguards in place through the electronic health record are no longer accessible. The nurse's role in downtime procedures, both planned and unplanned, is to be prepared to access paper health records, understand the policy for paper documentation, and ensure no lapses in communication related to downtime. There will be minor setbacks with downtime procedures, but the goal of the nurse is to continue to provide safe, effective care to each patient.

Coaching for Documentation Performance Improvement

The nurse should become familiar with the phrase "if it wasn't documented, it didn't happen." While this may seem dramatic, it is unfortunately true in the world of the patient experience. The nurse can provide extensive care with timely intervention and implementation of all provider orders, but if that care isn't documented, the medical team will not be aware of it. Not only will the medical team be out of the loop in terms of patient care provided, so will the insurance companies, as well as the legal team in the event of a lawsuit. Proper documentation is not only the chance for the nurse to record all care provided to the patient, but also the opportunity to improve the continuum of care and quality of care.

Coaching to help improve nursing documentation should demonstrate the following:

- Document everything as soon as possible. An interval of time that is too long can lead to forgetting important details or mixing up patients.
- Follow facility protocol on times to document and any abbreviations allowed.
- Do not assume in documentation. The nurse should not say the patient "seems" a certain way—they should record only objective data or reporting from the patient.
- Be detailed enough to "paint the picture" or "tell the story."
- Follow up in a timely manner when a medical intervention is provided.

Practice Quiz

1. The professional development nurse is conducting a root cause analysis of a serious medication error. Which of the following should the nurse consider the goal of the root cause analysis?
   a. The identification and removal of the individual responsible for the error
   b. The addition of safety checks to prevent this medication error from happening again
   c. Identifying the underlying cause of the error to guide process change, which will prevent it from happening again
   d. Agreement among senior leaders on a risk-management strategy

2. Regarding ethical practice, nurses are responsible for which document?
   a. The policy and protocol of their hospital
   b. Their State Board of Nursing list of prohibited activities
   c. The AHRQ six domains for healthcare improvement
   d. The American Nurses Association Code of Ethics

3. The professional development nurse understands that HIPAA protects the confidentiality of a patient's medical information. However, she wants to know how her friend who was admitted for surgery in the morning is doing. What is the best action for the nurse to take?
   a. Look up her friend's chart.
   b. Call her colleague in surgical admissions and ask for an update.
   c. Post on social media that her friend is in surgery and ask if anyone knows how she's doing.
   d. Wait until her friend can answer the phone and tell her how it went.

4. When is root cause analysis used?
   a. When anything goes wrong in the medical setting
   b. When there are adverse events or close calls
   c. When the doctor orders one
   d. Only when a patient death or serious injury occurs

5. Nurses are responsible for which of the following elements of informed consent?
   a. Identification of alternatives to the planned procedure
   b. Description of associated risks and benefits
   c. Explanation of the planned procedure or diagnostic test
   d. Assessment of the patient's understanding of the information that is provided

Answer Explanations

1: C. The goal of a root cause analysis is to identify the underlying cause of a system failure and gather information to guide practice change aimed at preventing the error from happening again. Choice *A* is incorrect because root cause analysis is a non-punitive process and does not aim to single out an individual or assign blame. Choice *B* is incorrect because root cause analysis is a holistic, investigative process and does not start with a pre-determined solution. Choice *D* is incorrect because root cause analysis involves all levels of staff and is not a risk-management effort.

2. C. Guides for ethical decision-making for nurses include The American Nurses Association Code of Ethics, the regulations set forth by the individual's State Board of Nursing, and hospital policies and protocols, making Choices *A*, *B*, and *D* all correct. Choice *C* is incorrect because the AHRQ six domains relate to healthcare quality, not ethical decision-making.

3: D. In speaking directly with the friend, the nurse allows her friend to control their medical information. Choices *A* and *B* are HIPAA violations because the nurse does not have a treatment-related need to access the information. Choice *C* is incorrect because the fact that the patient is undergoing surgery is privileged medical information. The nurse's post on social media reveals that information to the public in violation of HIPAA.

4. B: The root cause analysis is used when there is an adverse event, a sentinel event, or a close call in the medical setting. It can also be used when there is a concern about a process due to repeated errors, when there is a possibility of serious errors, and when there are high-cost errors.

5. D: While the physician is legally responsible for satisfying all elements of informed consent, nurses are ethically responsible for assessing the patient's ability to process and understand the implications of informed consent. Nurses protect the patient's autonomy by raising these questions and concerns. The remaining elements of informed consent are required of the physician, rather than the nurses.

Evidence-Based Practice and Research

Scholarly Inquiry

Scholarly Inquiry Processes

Nursing research is a crucial component of EBP, high quality healthcare delivery, and positive patient outcomes. Effective nursing research creates and compiles bodies of knowledge relating to all clinical and non-clinical aspects of nursing. Nurses who play a role in nursing research are typically advanced-level, senior practitioners who have the necessary experience to contribute further to existing bodies of nursing knowledge through personal expertise, the ability to run or be involved in conducting research trials, and in accurately collecting and analyzing data.

Nurse researchers typically have advanced educational degrees, such as a master's or doctorate degree, and may work in specialized fields as a nurse practitioner. However, as entry-level nurses spend more time and gain more exposure to different aspects of the field, they should keep in mind that a nurse researcher is a highly skilled and rewarding career path that is critical to the development and advancement of the nursing field. High quality nursing research shapes the scope of clinical education for entry-level and experienced nurses; influences healthcare policy at the local, state, and federal levels; and enhances standard operating procedures within a healthcare organization. Together, these allow for organizations to deliver the highest level of care to patients who need them at the lowest costs.

Nurses who choose to pursue research as a career can expect to become involved in different aspects of research design and the research process. Nurse researchers will need to pass training modules that review the legalities and ethics of working with human populations in research, which is a different avenue than treating patients for disease or injury. Nurse researchers can expect to learn how to write research proposals, which serves as a large component of applying for funding, in addition to becoming familiar with seeking out viable funding sources. Depending on the end goal of the study, nurse researchers may learn how to design objective study trials, collect data through laboratory work or through sample surveys, conduct and interpret statistical data analysis, and write conclusive discussions about their findings.

Upon completion, nurse researchers can expect to be involved in the publication process, where a formal manuscript detailing the design and findings of the research study are submitted to scholarly journals. Journals often require extensive revisions and editing, so nurses should be prepared to follow up with their manuscripts. Most research projects include collaboration with doctorate-level researchers from other disciplines who share a vested interest in the topic or have skills to contribute to the project. For example, health research teams often include a biostatistician whose primary contribution is to compile, analyze, and interpret collected data. Entry-level nurses, interns, or students may choose to assist with simpler, but necessary, tasks such as survey administration or data entry. Recruiting individuals to help with these sorts of tasks can provide a great support to the research team.

The National League for Nursing (NLN) is an organization in the United States that promotes research activities through networking, support, guidelines, and funding. The NLN publishes research priorities every four years. Current priorities include further investigating evidence-based practices, promoting research exposure to student learners in order to set the foundation for health promotion and disease prevention, and evaluating best practices relating to end-of-life and other life transitional care for both patients and their families. The NLN's website, www.nln.org, is an excellent resource for current nurses to find continuing education opportunities and explore research tools to support and enhance their career paths.

Clinical inquiry is an ongoing process that evaluates and challenges clinical practice in order to propose the needed change. Clinical inquiry has several components or attributes, including critical thinking, clinical reasoning, clinical judgment, critical reasoning and judgment, and creative thinking. The process is viewed as the critical structure for the establishment of evidenced based practice and quality improvement efforts. In the Synergy Model, professional nurses employ clinical inquiry to innovate and facilitate interventions that are appropriate to patient care needs. Clinical inquiry is a rigorous process that requires attention to the rules of nursing research, such as attention to sample size, and a correct match among the data, the study design, and the statistical measures.

When used to implement evidenced based practice, clinical inquiry can result in replacing an outdated, even counter-productive nursing intervention with an intervention that effectively addresses the needs of the patient. Nurses who are involved in this form of clinical inquiry are viewed as evaluators and innovators in the Synergy Model. Matching patient needs with nursing competencies means that professional nurses are responsible for challenging all nursing interventions to be sure that they represent current best practice standards. As innovators, nurses are in the best position to research, implement, and evaluate alternative care practices.

Study Design

Simply defined, **research** involves systematically investigating an experience or observed phenomenon, either to understand what causes it, what influences it, or to develop a theory about how that experience or occurrence can cause a future event. Systematic investigation can occur through a number of different scientific methods. **Deductive research** focuses on a specific theory, and then establishes a hypothesis to methodically test the theory in order to support or discredit it. Deductive research often involves setting up experiments, trials, or data collection surveys to gather information related to the theory. **Inductive research** examines information that's already available (such as in established datasets like the U.S. Census Report) to highlight data trends and make inferences and/or projections from those patterns.

Public funds are the most common source of research funding, which means that researchers are obligated to design studies that provide valid results that are applicable to some form of patient care and to disseminate the results appropriately. Common barriers to nursing research efforts include inadequate funding, limited access to appropriate patient populations, and lack of institutional support for research initiatives. The rapid expansion of new knowledge from multiple sources can also inhibit the assimilation and application of new care interventions by expert nurses.

Research designs determine how to structure a study based on factors such as the variables being tested, the level to which the researcher is manipulating a variable in the study, the types of subjects in the study, what the study is testing or looking for, the frequency and duration of data collection, and whether the data collected is qualitative or quantitative in nature. These concepts will be examined further in the following sections.

Quantitative vs. Qualitative Research

Quantitative research utilizes logical, empirical methods of collecting information. This information is called **data** and is often analyzed using statistics. Non-experimental quantitative research includes forms of data collection where the researcher collects data that's already available in some form. They then analyze this dataset to describe the relationship between pre-determined variables. The researcher does not set up a novel system of trials to produce new data, and they can't randomize any data collected. The researcher has no part in manipulating any variables or establishing a separate control group to which they can compare collected data. The lack of a control group, researcher-controlled variable manipulation, and randomization are often seen as weaknesses in non-experimental quantitative research studies.

Qualitative research typically focuses on the analysis of a group of people (which is sometimes biased) to understand different aspects of human behavior, relationships, and social interactions. The researcher does not manipulate variables when conducting qualitative research. Qualitative research is primarily conducted without rigid structures in place.

Experimental Designs

Experimental quantitative research employs highly controlled processes, with the hope of determining a causal relationship between one or more input (**independent**) variables and one or more outcome (**dependent**) variables. It uses random sampling and assignment methods to make inferences for larger populations. Typically, it compares a control group (serving as a baseline) to a test group. Ideally, experimental studies or experiments should be able to be replicated numerous times with the same results. The ultimate goal of a well-designed experiment is to declare that a particular variable is responsible for a particular outcome and that, without that variable, the associated outcome wouldn't occur.

Quasi-experimental quantitative research employs many of these same qualities, but it often doesn't use random sampling or assignment in its studies or experiments. Consequently, quasi-experimental research produces results that often don't apply to the population at large. They do, however, often provide meaningful results for certain subgroups of the population.

Correlational Studies

These analyze the strength of the relationship between two variables in one group. One unique type of correlational design is found in **ex post facto studies**, in which the researcher examines two existing groups and analyzes the correlation between the variables of interest. Another unique type of correlational design is found in **prediction studies**, where the researcher determines a correlation between variables and then uses it to predict other correlations, related events, or future events. The strength and description of the correlation is indicated by the **correlation coefficient (r),** which falls between -1 and 1. If r = 0, it indicates there's no relationship between the two variables, while r = 1 indicates a direct, perfect correlation. If *r* equals a negative value, it indicates an inverse relationship between the two variables. If *r* equals a positive value, it indicates a direct relationship between the two variables. Regardless of how strong the correlation is between two variables, it doesn't indicate that one causes the other. It simply indicates that these two variables tend to occur (or not occur) together to some degree.

Surveys

Surveys can be conducted through telephone or face-to-face interviews. They can also be conducted through paper or electronic questionnaires (either at an external facility or at the study participant's home). Survey designs are generally used when research about a particular topic is limited, so that more information can be gathered to better shape the research question or topic. Surveys are easy (and usually cost-efficient) to administer, but they can also result in low or biased participant response rates.

Interviews are typically more personal in nature and can be conducted in person, over the telephone, or via e-mail or regular mail. The interviewer asks the individual or group a series of meaningful questions related to the research topic. The interview can be structured with the interviewer having pre-set questions to ask, or it can be unstructured with the interviewer asking questions based on the flow of conversation and the answers given by the interviewee(s).

Observational Studies

In an observation, the researcher simply watches the individual or group of interest. However, a number of additional factors usually shape the development of the observation study. The researcher can observe the participant(s) in a specific situation or highly controlled context, or the researcher can observe the participant(s) in their day-to-day routine. The participant(s) may or may not know that they are being observed for specific behaviors. The researcher can involve themselves in the context and become part of the observation study. The researcher can also freely write down data from the observations, or use a pre-made scale or data sheet to document specific behaviors.

Case Studies and Focus Groups

Case studies are detailed and documented examples of the topic of interest. They can be real or hypothetical situations. Case studies often record data over a period of time to examine a specific variable of interest. They can examine a situation involving one individual, a family, a larger community of people, or an organization. Case studies frequently look at how people relate to one another and/or to their physical or emotional environment.

Focus groups bring together a relatively small group of individuals. The group can be diverse in nature or have many similar interests. A facilitator guides a discussion within the group to discern information about individual or collective viewpoints about a specific issue.

Longitudinal Studies

A **longitudinal study** describes a research design in which information is repeatedly collected for the same research participants over an extended period of time, which can span several years or even decades. Because longitudinal studies involve observing the same individuals over the course of their lives, any differences observed in them are less likely to be due to cultural variations across generations. Longitudinal studies can be **retrospective**, which is when researchers use existing data such as medical records, or **prospective**, which entails researchers collecting new information. Though this type of research method can be structured as a randomized experiment, longitudinal studies often serve as an **observational study**.

When longitudinal studies are observational, researchers observe daily life in the real world without any efforts to control or manipulate it, as opposed to in a lab setting where more control could be exerted, thus making this research design a type of naturalistic study. Longitudinal studies are common in psychology. In social-personality and clinical psychology, longitudinal studies are typically used to observe rapid fluctuations in one's behavior, cognition, and emotions on a daily basis. And in developmental psychology, longitudinal studies observe trends pertaining to one's growth and development that occur throughout their lifespan.

Cross-Sectional Studies

Also referred to as a **transverse** or **prevalence study**, or a **cross-sectional analysis**, a **cross-sectional study** describes a research method that involves evaluating variable information gathered at a specific point in time across a sample population. This sample population includes different people with similar features being compared. Like longitudinal studies, cross-sectional studies are also **observational studies**, with researchers recording information in a population but not controlling or manipulating variables. Cross-sectional studies are also known as **descriptive research**, as opposed to being causal or relational, meaning that researchers wouldn't use this type of study to determine causality. In other words, cross-sectional studies are used to describe traits that exist within a certain group, not to determine cause-and-effect relationships between variables. This approach tends to obtain initial data and make inferences about potential relationships as a means of supporting more research.

Cross-sectional studies are often used by developmental psychologists. In developmental research, this method examines people of various age ranges at the same time, as opposed to observing individuals over many years or several decades. However, the challenge with this approach is that any differences observed in a group of people are more likely to be related to cultural differences across generations.

Data Collection

Sampling is the method of collecting participants for a study. It's a crucial component of the research design and study process. There are a number of different ways to select samples, and each method has pros, cons, and situations where it's the most appropriate one to use.

Simple Random Sampling

For this type of probability sampling, the participants are taken directly from a larger population with the characteristics of interest. Each individual in the larger population has the same chance of being selected for the sample.

Pros: closely represents the target population, thus allowing for results that are the highest in validity

Cons: obtaining the sample can be time consuming

Use When: a highly controlled experiment setting is necessary

Stratified Random Sampling

For this type of probability sampling, the researchers first examine the traits of the larger population. Traits are often demographic or social in nature like age, education status, marital status, and household income. Researchers then divide the population into groups (or strata) based on these traits. Members of the population are only included in one stratum. Researchers then randomly sample across each stratum to create the final sample set for the study.

Pros: closely represents the target population, which allows for results that are highest in validity. Since the sampling method is so specific, researchers are able to use smaller samples.

Cons: obtaining the sample can be tedious. Researchers may first need to compile and become acutely knowledgeable about the demographic characteristics of the target population before selecting a representative sample.

Use When: a highly-controlled experiment setting is necessary; demographic, social, and/or economic characteristics of the target population are of special interest in the study; or researchers are studying relationships or interactions between two subsets within the larger population

Systematic Random Sampling

For this type of probability sampling, researchers pick a random integer (n), and then select every *n*th person from the target population for the research sample.

Pros: a simple, cost-effective sampling technique that generally provides a random sample for the researchers. It ensures that sampling occurs evenly throughout an entire target population.

Cons: researchers need to ensure that their original target population (from which the sample is selected) is randomized and that every individual has an equal probability of being selected. Researchers need to be familiar with the demographics of the target population to ensure that certain trends don't appear across the selected participants and skew the results.

Use When: a highly controlled experiment setting is necessary; researchers are short on time or funding and need a quick, cost-efficient method to create a random sample.

Convenience Sampling

This is a type of non-probability sampling where researchers select participants who are easily accessible due to factors like location, expense, or volunteer recruitment.

Pros: saves time and is cost-effective since researchers can create their sample based on what permits the easiest and fastest recruiting of participants

Cons: highly prone to bias. It's difficult to generalize the results for the population at large since the sample selection is not random.

Use When: conducting initial trials of a new study, when researchers are simply looking for basic information about the larger population (i.e., to create a more detailed hypothesis for future research)

Ad Hoc Sampling

For this type of non-probability sampling, researchers must meet a set quota for a certain characteristic and can recruit any participant as long as they have the desired characteristics.

Pros: allows for greater inclusion of a population that might not otherwise be represented

Cons: results won't be indicative of the actual population in an area

Use When: it's necessary that a group within the larger population needs a set level of representation within the study

Purposive Sampling

Another non-probability sampling method used when researchers have a precise purpose or target population in mind.

Pros: helps increase recruitment numbers in otherwise hard-to-access populations

Cons: usually unable to generalize the results to larger populations beyond the sample's specific subset

Use When: researchers have a precise purpose for the study, or a specific group of participants is required that isn't easy to select through probability sampling methods

Ethical Considerations

Researchers should strive not to harm any population when conducting studies or experiments. All biomedical and behavioral research requires the approval of an independent institutional review board (IRB) to begin. In addition, the IRB monitors the research study for its duration to ensure that populations aren't experiencing any harm. Typically, IRB-approved studies require a participant consent form, the guarantee of anonymity and/or confidentiality for all participants and associated data, and strict monitoring and evaluation processes.

Researchers should also be mindful of producing, collecting, and publishing accurate, authentic, and non-biased data. Failure to collect or publish data that does not support the researchers' hypotheses or motives—or that inadvertently brings awareness to another sensitive issue—can also be grounds for ethical concern.

Accountability is an important aspect in conducting research. Researchers typically need to have a purpose for conducting their studies. This purpose should be beneficial to the target population, fair, timely, cost-efficient, and should not harm any groups in the process. Funding sources, as well as internal and external auditing groups, may regularly evaluate research operations and outcomes. This is done to ensure that the funds are used appropriately, the research process is ethical, and useful results are obtained. Typically, structured evaluation processes (such as benchmarks and reporting practices) are established and documented during the study's planning and proposal periods.

Data Interpretation

Comparing data sets within statistics can mean many things. The first way to compare data sets is by looking at the center and spread of each set. The center of a data set is measured by mean, median, and mode. These are sometimes referred to as **measures of central tendency**.

Mean

The first property that can be defined for this set of data is the **mean**. This is the same as the average. To find the mean, add up all the data points, then divide by the total number of data points. For example, suppose that in a class of 10 students, the scores on a test were 50, 60, 65, 65, 75, 80, 85, 85, 90, 100. Therefore, the average test score will be:

$$\frac{50+60+65+65+75+80+85+85+90+100}{10} = 75.5$$

The mean is a useful number if the distribution of data is normal (more on this later), which roughly means that the frequency of different outcomes has a single peak and is roughly equally distributed on both sides of that peak. However, it is less useful in some cases where the data might be split or where there are some outliers. **Outliers** are data points that are far from the rest of the data. For example, suppose there are 10 executives and 90 employees at a company. The executives make $1000 per hour, and the employees make $10 per hour.

Therefore, the average pay rate will be:

$$\frac{\$1000 \times 10 + \$10 \times 90}{100} = \$109 \text{ per hour}$$

In this case, this average is not very descriptive since it's not close to the actual pay of the executives or the employees.

Median

Another useful measurement is the **median**. In a data set arranged in numerical order, the median is the point in the middle. The middle refers to the point where half the data comes before it and half comes after, when the data is recorded in numerical order. For instance, these are the speeds of the fastball of a pitcher threw (in mph) during the last inning that he pitched (in order from least to greatest):

90, 92, 93, 93, 95, 96, 97, 97, 97

There are nine total numbers, so the middle or median number is the fifth one, which is 95.

In cases where the number of data points is an even number, then the average of the two middle points is taken. In the previous example of test scores, the two middle points are 75 and 80. Since there is no single point, the average of these two scores needs to be found. The average is:

$$\frac{75+80}{2} = 77.5\ mph$$

The median is generally a good value to use if there are a few outliers in the data. It prevents those outliers from affecting the "middle" value as much as when using the mean.

Since an outlier is a data point that is far from most of the other data points in a data set, an outlier is necessarily far from the median of the data set. The outliers can have a substantial effect on the mean of a data set, but they usually do not change the median or mode, or do not change them by a large quantity. For example, consider the data set (3, 5, 6, 6, 6, 8), which has a median of 6 and a mode of 6, and a mean of $\frac{34}{6} \approx 5.67$. Now, suppose a new data point of 1000 is added so that the data set is now (3, 5, 6, 6, 6, 8, 1000). The median and mode, which are both still 6, remain unchanged. However, the average is now $\frac{1034}{7}$, which is approximately 147.7. In this case, the median and mode will be better descriptors for most of the data points.

Outliers in a given data set are sometimes the result of an error by the experimenter, but oftentimes, they are perfectly valid data points that must be taken into consideration.

Mode

One additional measure to define for X is the **mode**. This is the data point that appears most frequently. If two or more data points all tie for the most frequent appearance, then each of them is considered a mode. In the case of the test scores, where the numbers were 50, 60, 65, 65, 75, 80, 85, 85, 90, 100, there are two modes: 65 and 85.

Correlation Coefficient

As mentioned previously, the **correlation coefficient (r)** measures the association between two variables. Its value is between -1 and 1, where -1 represents a perfect negative linear relationship, 0 represents no relationship, and 1 represents a perfect positive linear relationship. A **negative linear relationship** means that as x values increase, y values decrease. A **positive linear relationship** means that as x values increase, y values increase.

Frequency Distribution

A set of data can be described in terms of its center, spread, shape and any unusual features. The center of a data set can be measured by its mean, median, or mode. The spread of a data set refers to how far the data points are from the center (mean or median). A data set with all its data points clustered around the center will have a small spread. A data set covering a wide range of values will have a large spread.

When a data set is displayed as a graph like the one below, the shape indicates if a sample is normally distributed, symmetrical, or has measures of skewness. When graphed, a data set with a normal distribution will resemble a bell curve.

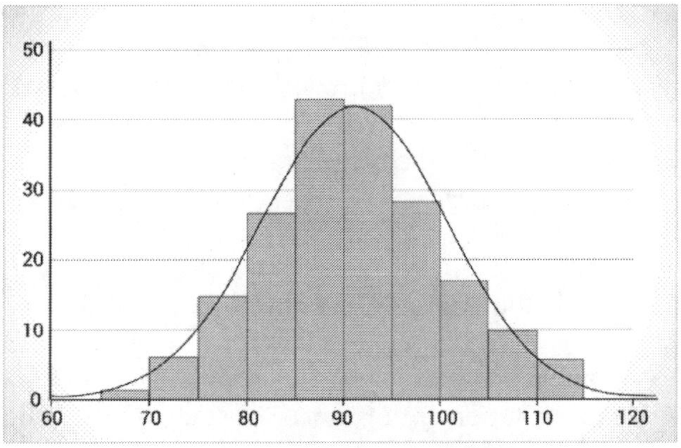

If the data set is **symmetrical**, each half of the graph when divided at the center is a mirror image of the other. If the graph has fewer data points to the right, the data is **skewed right**. If it has fewer data points to the left, the data is **skewed left**.

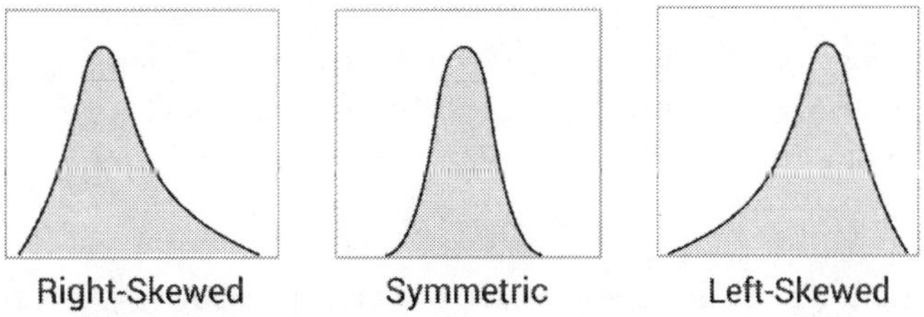

A description of a data set should include any unusual features such as gaps or outliers. A **gap** is a span within the range of the data set containing no data points. An **outlier** is a data point with a value either extremely large or extremely small when compared to the other values in the set.

The previous graphs can be referred to as **unimodal** since they all have a single peak. In contrast, a bimodal graph has two peaks.

Descriptive and Inferential Statistics

The field of statistics describes relationships between quantities that are related, but not necessarily in a deterministic manner. For example, a graduating student's salary will often be higher when the student graduates with a higher GPA, but this is not always the case. Likewise, people who smoke tobacco are more likely to develop lung cancer, but, in fact, it is possible for non-smokers to develop the disease as well. **Statistics** describes these kinds of situations, where the likelihood of some outcome depends on the starting data.

Descriptive statistics involves analyzing a collection of data to describe its broad properties such average (or mean), what percent of the data falls within a given range, and other such properties. An example of this would be taking all of the test scores from a given class and calculating the average test score. **Inferential statistics** attempts to use data about a subset of some population to make inferences about the rest of the population. An example of this would be taking a collection of students who received tutoring and comparing their results to a collection of students who did not receive tutoring, then using that comparison to try to predict whether the tutoring program in question is beneficial.

Processes, Translation, and Dissemination of Research

Research Process

The research process in nursing is similar to the research process in any workplace, with the goal of finding and accumulating information in attempts to further knowledge. The importance of routine research within healthcare cannot be overstated. With evolving technology and improvements in care processes, protocols are almost constantly changing. For the nurse to stay up to date in the constantly evolving healthcare system, using the proper form of research is essential. Just as important as the concept of research itself is the correct practice and use of the research. Credibility is of utmost importance in clinical research. The following is a review of the procedural process of nursing research:

1. Select the specific topic: While this step sounds relatively straightforward, the research team will need to understand the importance of selecting an appropriate topic. While there are plenty of issues that warrant discussion, not all issues are appropriate for a research topic. The research team needs to be sure that the topic selected has an attainable solution or outcome. The topic will also need to be specific enough to be measurable.

2. Find additional background information on the specific topic and formulate hypotheses: This stage can be known as the pre-planning phase, as the research team will be looking for general background information to formulate hypotheses. The point of this phase is to further assess the quality of the topic selected for a research project.

3. Design framework for research: This stage can be known as the planning phase. The research team will focus on finding the appropriate forms of data collection and establishing specific roles for the extraction of the data. The goal is to find data specific enough to answer the research topic/question while maintaining practical and ethical values.

4. Utilize approved resources for detailed data collection: Data collection is the meat and potatoes of the research process. It is the unrefined collection of data that is related to the research topic. The importance of data collection is to obtain unbiased information from credible sources. Most facilities/agencies will have a resource library that can be freely used, but access to multiple credible sources is the best research practice.

5. Organize data collected and evaluate findings: Separating the data into quantitative and qualitative sections can help with the organization and evaluation of data. Using visuals for the quantitative data (based on numbers/measurable) and using direct quotes for the qualitative data (interpretive/subjective) can help the research team organize the information to closely assess the general findings.

6. Analyze and interpret data collected: Analyzing the data and interpreting the results is rarely the form of closure to the research topic. This stage usually brings clarity on the need for further research on the topic, research on an additional topic, or revision of the entire research plan. This stage allows the research team to review the interpreted data with the hypotheses.

7. Properly cite any sources: Properly citing sources is not only giving credit to the original author but also avoiding plagiarism. Giving credit to the original source—whether it's a demonstration of the research or written literature—also allows the audience to follow the research.

Literature Review

A **literature review** is an analysis of publications related to a specific topic. It is a way to investigate and study work that has already been developed, gain understanding of a topic, and learn how the topic can be progressed through future work. The literature review is an essential component to researching disease because it gives those involved an idea of the current understanding of the disease and prevents conducting experiments that have already been performed and published. Conflicting theories can also be examined to determine the best course of action in disease prevention strategies. Literature surveyed can include books, published articles from journals, theses from universities, and past medical surveillance data to help form a full understanding of the disease or situation as it currently stands. The literature review then organizes this data and presents an analysis of how it may relate to the situation that needs to be addressed.

The first step in developing a complete literature review is to define a set of goals or objectives that need to be accomplished. This will provide insight on where to look for relevant literature and the type of information that will be most useful when conducting research. The next step is to complete the proper research, including selection of the articles or information that are the most relevant and useful to accomplish the goals. It is important to read as much information on the topic as possible to obtain an understanding of the type of data that is the most useful. Also, vetting sources for authenticity and credibility will guide which ones are known to be used frequently and are the most reliable. Once the best sources have been selected, a summary of each source that examines its credibility and suggestions to further the research should be written. Then, it will be possible to select the sources that are the most helpful to the current problem and document this reasoning to formulate the literature review.

Critically Appraising Literature

When performing a literature review, it is important to be able to identify what sources have the most useful information related to a current problem. Not all sources are trustworthy, and not all trustworthy sources are relevant. It is up to the researcher conducting the literature review to determine which sources contain the most useful, credible data. When critically appraising literature related to healthcare and disease prevention, it is important for each source to be free of errors that might steer the course of further research in the wrong direction. Literature should be appraised based on credibility, relevance, and date of publication.

The most **credible literature** comes from academic sources that have been peer reviewed by professionals before publication. For disease prevention, scientific and healthcare-related medical journals are the best source for finding data and articles that have been well researched and cross-examined by multiple parties. Information that has already been confirmed by those in the same industry will have the least chance of containing misleading errors or too much unrelated or opinionated information. The relevance of the literature also needs to be compared with the problem that is being researched. Before conducting research, it is important to set goals and write questions that need to be solved to help the situation. The most relevant data is the data that directly solves these goals and answers the questions that have been laid out in relation to the current problem.

Literature that includes too little or too much data that may be hard to interpret should be avoided. Also, it is important to pay attention to when the literature was published to avoid using data that may be out of date or proven to be ineffective. The most recent articles are the most helpful because they contain the most up-to-date data collection methods and pertain to more modern health problems than those published before newer advancements in modern science were made.

Dissemination of Research Findings

The final step of the clinical inquiry process, knowledge translation or dissemination, may be the most important step. Knowledge translation refers to the complex process of synthesizing the research findings, disseminating those findings to others, and integrating the findings into clinical practice. Barriers to this process include lack of rigor in the original research design with respect to sample size, data interpretation, and the applicability of the research findings. The failure of nursing researchers to access all possible modes of the dissemination of study results has also been identified as a significant barrier to the application of new interventions. All of these system-wide and individual barriers potentially limit the use of innovative patient care interventions.

Evidence-Based Practice

Evidence-based practice (**EBP**) is a research-driven and facts-based methodology that allows healthcare providers to make scientifically supported, reliable, and validated decisions in delivering care. EBP takes into account rigorously tested, peer-reviewed, and published research relating to the case; the knowledge and experience of the healthcare provider; and clinical guidelines established by reputable governing bodies. This framework allows healthcare providers to reach case resolutions that result in positive patient outcomes in the most efficient manner. This, in turn, allows the organization to provide the best care using the least resources.

There are seven steps to successfully utilizing EBP as a methodology in the nursing field. First, the work culture should be one of a "spirit of inquiry." This culture allows staff to ask questions to promote continuous improvement and positive process change to workflow, clinical routines, and non-clinical duties. Second, the PICOT framework should be utilized when searching for an effective intervention, or working with a specific interest, in a case. The **PICOT framework** encourages nurses to develop a specific, measurable, goal-oriented research question that accounts for the patient population and demographics (P) involved in the case, the proposed intervention or issue of interest (I), a relevant comparison (C) group in which a defined outcome (O) has been positive, and the amount of time (T) needed to implement the intervention or address the issue. Once this question has been developed, staff can move onto the third step, which is to research. In this step, staff will explore reputable sources of literature to find studies and narratives with evidence that supports a resolution for their question.

Once all research has been compiled, it must be thoroughly analyzed as part of the fourth step in the process. This step ensures that the staff is using unbiased research with stringent methodology, statistically significant outcomes, and reliable and valid research designs. Furthermore, it includes verification that all information collected is applicable to their patient. For example, if a certain treatment worked with statistical significance in a longitudinal study of pediatric patients with a large sample size, and all other influencing variables were controlled for, this treatment may not necessarily work in a middle-aged adult. Therefore, though the research collected is scientifically backed and evidence-based for a pediatric population, it does not support EBP for an older population. The fifth step is to integrate the evidence to create a treatment or intervention plan for the patient. The sixth step is to monitor the implementation of the treatment or intervention and evaluate whether it was associated with positive health outcomes in the patient. Finally, practitioners have a moral obligation to share the results with colleagues at the organization and across the field, so that it may be best utilized (or not) for other patients.

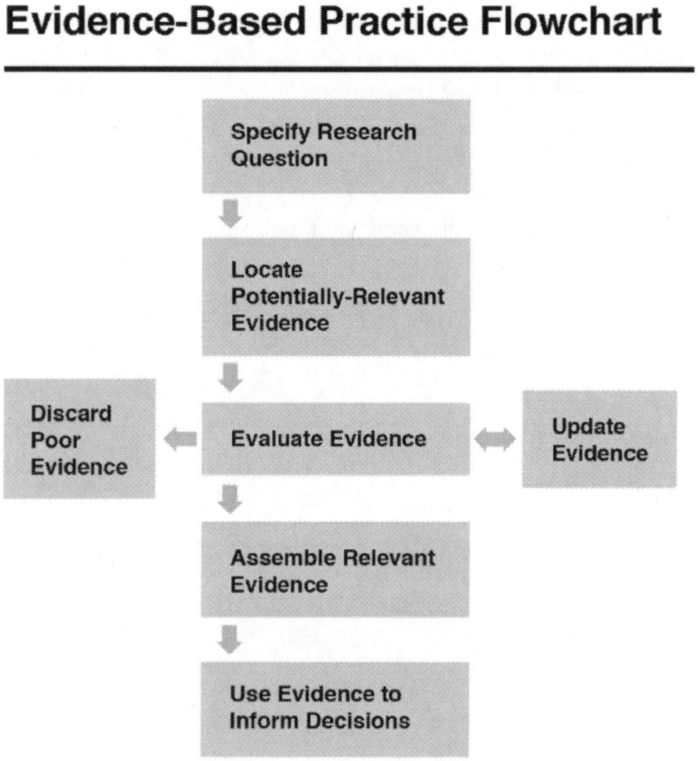

Legislative and Licensure Requirements

Similar to the procedural scope of practice for nurses, there are legislative and licensure requirements for the use of evidence-based practice (EBP) and research. As with the procedural scope of practice, each state board of nursing will have specific guidelines for EBP and research practices. The nurse must understand the similarities and differences between EBP and clinical research. While both serve as pivotal tools in the improvement of safe, effective patient care, the actual processes and end results are different.

Evidence-based practice looks towards evidence seen in clinical practice to make informed decisions on patient care. Evidence-based practice puts the gathered information into practice. Research focuses more on validating the current nursing practice and gathering information that is already in practice.

Quality Improvement

Quality improvement is influenced by the collection and analysis of data. **Data** can be collected on a grand scale or on a more specific level. For example, HAIs in hospitals produce high morbidity and mortality. Acute care facilities track data on HAIs to determine areas of improvement. On a grand scale, the data is captured from the hospital as a whole, meaning all areas of patient care are included. Typically, critical care areas contain the highest risk for HAIs due to the acuity of patients and the complexity of treatment. However, the data may be offset by lower-risk patient care units, such as labor and delivery. When identifying opportunities to improve performance and avoid negative outcomes, it is important to research the data from independent levels.

For example, the infection control department of a hospital is tasked with researching an increasing rate of *Clostridium difficile* (*C. diff*) infections in patients. The first step would be to analyze the data and determine the problem areas. Should the data reveal that most *C. diff* infections are occurring in a specific patient care area, such as the intensive care unit, the infection control team would primarily focus their implementation strategies there. As part of the research, the team would identify the current infection control practices, such as hand washing, antibiotic use, cleaning practices, and staff education. Any deficiencies identified for any of the factors would prompt the infection control team to establish an implementation strategy. For example, further research revealed that the patient care rooms were being cleaned with a disinfectant not specifically approved to eliminate the bacterial spores associated with *C. diff.* Improper cleaning practices increase the risk of illness transmission. Should another patient be placed in the same room, the risk of acquiring *C. diff* would be increased. The infection control team may use this data to introduce a new cleaning product. Ongoing research would include the impact of the new product on the HAI rates within the hospital.

Practice Quiz

1. When developing evidence-based practice protocols for a perioperative unit, the professional development nurse should rely primarily on which type of source?
    a. Up-to-date patient satisfaction data
    b. Opinions of surgeons and senior medical officers at the organization
    c. The bedside practice of veteran staff nurses
    d. Peer-reviewed research and published guidelines from reputable governing bodies

2. Which of the following is cited as the MOST common source of funding for nursing research?
    a. Pharmaceutical companies
    b. Public funds
    c. Non-profit organizations
    d. Private institutions

3. Which of the following is a characteristic of high-quality research evidence?
    a. Results obtained from observational studies
    b. Variable estimates of effect size
    c. RCT study design
    d. Case controlled analytics

4. Placebos may be used at which level of research?
    a. Level I
    b. Level II
    c. Level III
    d. Level IV

5. Which of the following may be necessary to treat the Hawthorne effect?
    a. Random selection
    b. Random assignment
    c. Blinding of the researcher
    d. Placebo control group

See answers on the next page.

Answer Explanations

1: D. Evidence-based practice refers to a methodology based on peer-reviewed research, clinical practice statements, and guidelines published in reputable medical, nursing, and allied health publications, as well as other scientific sources. It does not rely on consumer or practitioner opinion or defer to traditional practice. While Choices *A*, *B*, and *C* are important factors to consider in creating protocols, they are not the primary source for evidence-based practice.

2. B: Research indicates that public funds are the most common source of funding, which means that researchers are obligated to design studies that provide valid results that are applicable to some form of patient care and to disseminate the results appropriately. The remaining sources listed in Choices *A*, *C*, and *D* also provide funding; however, public funds are noted to be the common source.

3. C: The randomized controlled trial (RCT) is regarded as the research design that best controls researcher bias. RCTs tend to be expensive and large-scale; however, the number of subjects often corresponds with the quality of the results. The level of confidence in observational studies is proportional to the control of bias in the specific design, but the evidence is generally considered to be of low quality; therefore, Choice *A* is incorrect. Variable or imprecise estimates of effect size that require additional investigation before the results of the research can be directly applicable are considered as only moderate-quality evidence; therefore, Choice *B* is incorrect. Case controlled analytics are also considered to be moderate-quality evidence; therefore, Choice *D* is incorrect.

4. D: Placebos are used in level IV randomized clinical trials to combat the Hawthorne effect. This phenomenon occurs when test subjects give false replies to test items to please the researcher. If the study participants understand that they may have received no treatment at all, they are more likely to provide true answers to the test items. Placebos are not used at levels I, II, or III; therefore, Choices *A*, *B*, and *C* are incorrect.

5. D: The Hawthorne effect occurs when research participants tell researchers what they want to hear instead of providing accurate answers. Adding an additional section of subjects who receive an inactive substance that resembles the research treatment means that the researcher can have greater confidence in the results. The remaining choices are elements of the RCT study design, but none of these choices treats the Hawthorne effect; therefore, Choices *A*, *B*, and *C* are incorrect.

Technology

Information Systems and Management

Business Tools

Document Production

When producing educational documents, organizational restrictions may require logos, dates, or clearance from public relations or another department. The type of document required should fit the purpose. Anything that is patient related must adhere to HIPAA guidelines and regulations. Nurses must have expertise on technology usage to produce documents that are able to convey the message in the right forum. Documents may be used as posters for public or widespread information sharing, as memos sent via email or shared using online platforms, or in ways that share critical information needed for patient acuity and staffing schedules. When producing documents, it is important that the information is presented utilizing the business rules of the organization. Accuracy and clarity are essential; therefore, having a trusted colleague proofread prior to submission can be beneficial. Documents posted on an open forum must be regularly updated to provide records of progress and reflect any changes that have been made since they were originally produced.

Spreadsheets

Spreadsheets are valuable tools for nurses to employ to display, explain, and organize information in a structured and cohesive way. Spreadsheets can be used to track continuing education credits, certifications, and skills development, ensuring compliance with licensing requirements. These applications can also record participation in workshops, conferences, and training sessions, helping to identify areas for growth. Personal and professional goal setting and progress tracking can be mapped out for academic and career advancement. Nurses may elect to use this type of tool to build a professional portfolio, which may include sections for reflective quips on clinical experiences or mentorship activities. Within healthcare organizations and application to clinical care, spreadsheets offer a method of data analysis, tracking trends of quality improvement projects or research initiatives, and evaluating evidence-based practices. Working use of spreadsheet applications is imperative to be able to interpret large amounts of data for meaningful use. Nurses must be able to aptly present this data in a way that is understandable to other professionals across the healthcare domain.

Presentation Software

Nurses seeking advancement into leadership or educational roles must have expertise in the use of presentation software. This skill facilitates effective communication, education, and collaboration. Tools such as Microsoft PowerPoint, Prezi, and Google Slides provide a medium to create engaging presentations for training sessions, workshops, and conferences. These platforms help convey complex medical information clearly while supporting continuous learning and skill enhancement. Presentation software allows nurses to share research findings, best practices, and case studies with colleagues, fostering a culture of evidence-based practice. Visual aids such as charts, images, and videos improve understanding and retention of information. Creating effective presentations bolsters remote learning, expanding access to professional development opportunities regardless of location. Presentation software provides an opportunity to add interest to educational offerings with graphics, animation, and video, resulting in improved audience engagement and knowledge retention.

Virtual Meetings

Since the COVID-19 pandemic, virtual meetings have become a mainstay in organizations across healthcare and other industries. Meeting in a virtual environment has expanded opportunities in education, professional development, and lifelong learning by increasing the accessibility to attend events and training that may not have been previously attainable. This method has also allowed for the recording of events so that participants may attend at their own pace or time.

Through these virtual platforms, nurses can attend webinars, workshops, and case discussions that enhance their clinical skills and keep them informed on current healthcare trends and practices. Virtual meetings can also promote interdisciplinary communication, encouraging teamwork and comprehensive patient-focused care. As virtual meetings provide additional flexibility, this allows nurses to participate without the need for travel expenses or time away from work, thus supporting improved work-life balance. Virtual meetings are an efficient, cost-effective way to ensure that nurses remain competent, informed, and engaged in their ongoing professional development. This increases opportunities to build community and professional networking connections, which can improve job satisfaction and reduce burnout.

Utilization of Information Technology Systems

Information technology (**IT**) is a field of nursing that continues to evolve with the rest of healthcare. Nurses must not only understand the science that is associated with nursing, but they must also be able to navigate various forms of technology. While there are nurses still in the workplace who can recall what it was like to physically fill out forms and track vitals on paper, there are also nurses who have no concept of having documented their activities in these systems. All nurses must be able to function within today's technologically advanced world.

IT is important for many reasons including:

- Cost savings
- Decreased medication errors
- Improved documentation efficiency by removing paper charting
- Enhanced accessibility to quality health care

Medical technology needs to be fully integrated in a larger system within an institution to support the continuum of patient care. This connection provides information sharing throughout each stage of the treatment period and eventually allows for the collection of statistical data in the future.

Next, medical technology must support the user's ability to navigate without difficulty. The goal here is not to slow down the pace of the medical environment, but to increase efficiency so that technology is seamless. These qualities then allow for real-time data and real-time decision-making capabilities, while reducing the risk of errors or redundancy.

There are a few gaps that remain on the IT front of the medical environment that have their roots in the computerized physician order entry (CPOE) arena. In some instances, CPOE software is not able to meet the needs of various interdisciplinary roles, such as in the OR. The reason for this is that it tends to favor the inpatient setting.

Health care IT (**HIT**) has characteristics that are steeped in supporting broad processes or functions. HIT is software that can perform operations associated with:

- Admissions
- Scheduling
- Clinical documentation
- Pharmacy
- Laboratory
- Clinical Information Technology

Clinical IT (**CIT**) concentrates on a particular set of clinical tasks, instruments, equipment, and imaging.

Radio frequency identification (**RFID**) provides support for real-time surgery scheduling. This technology has been shown to drastically enhance the structure and functions within medical software. RFID functions on wireless networks, helps to "tag" items, and tracks their movement as they remain on or leave a particular unit. This may be especially important when tracking equipment or supplies that are used to care for the patient or during a surgical procedure.

Technology Trends in Healthcare

Nurses will need to stay current with IT trends and engage in ongoing education and exposure to technology. Continuing education and training can be accomplished through independent reading, e-learning, and live classroom instruction.

Nurses may encounter a broad range of technologies including:

- Robots
- Medication delivery devices
- Instruments
- Biotechnology and nanotechnology
- Digital tracking
- Mobile and wireless devices
- Nurse Informatics

Nurses may assist in the development of standards for EHR (electronic health records) or other clinically based IT systems that nurses utilize for their sphere of health care. In today's landscape, many nursing applications fall into a variety of categories including:

- Internet-based patient education systems
- EHR
- Telemedicine and telenursing

These systems have the capacity to exchange information and enable the decision-making process to progress along the continuum.

Some nurses possess a master's degree in **informatics** and work in a variety of roles to assist with development of clinical systems designed to support nurse activities including:

- Business or clinical analyst
- Project management
- Software developer

These systems are designed to accommodate patient education resources, nursing procedures, and critical pathways, to name a few.

Nurses may also serve in the role of perioperative **robotics nurse specialist**. As robotic surgery utilization continues to evolve into standard practice, the robotics nurse specialist supports a variety of tasks, ranging from scheduling maintenance to assisting during surgery.

Security Measures

The role of information technology (IT) in nursing professional development is growing, with a strong focus on enhancing patient care and safeguarding sensitive data. As nurses increasingly use electronic health records (EHRs), telehealth platforms, and clinical decision support tools, a firm understanding of cybersecurity is essential to maintain patient privacy and comply with regulations such as HIPAA. To prevent unauthorized access, healthcare systems must implement strong security measures, including complex password policies, multi-factor authentication, and routine system updates. Encryption protects data in both transmission and storage, while user access controls ensure that only authorized individuals can view or modify patient information. Educating nurses on cybersecurity practice, such as spotting phishing attempts and understanding digital threats, further reinforces data protection efforts. Ongoing professional development in IT security with the input of nursing informatics mitigates risks and promotes industry best practices through creating a culture of safety and accountability. Embedding robust cybersecurity measures into nursing practice not only protects patient information but also strengthens the integrity and trustworthiness of digital healthcare delivery.

Databases

Professional development in nursing increasingly depends on the effective use of research databases to strengthen knowledge, enhance skills, and support evidence-based practice. Resources such as CINAHL, PubMed, and the Cochrane Library offer access to up-to-date research, clinical guidelines, and peer-reviewed literature, enabling continuous learning and the delivery of high-quality patient care. By regularly consulting these databases, nurses can stay informed about emerging healthcare trends, sharpen critical-thinking abilities, and improve clinical decision making. These tools are essential for integrating evidence into practice and ensuring safe, effective care. In addition to informing practice, databases support participation in research initiatives, involvement in clinical studies, and the pursuit of advanced education or certifications. As the healthcare landscape evolves, proficiency in accessing and applying information from professional databases is vital for lifelong learning and professional growth. Ultimately, this competency leads to better patient outcomes and advances the nursing profession.

Learning Management Systems

Utilizing learning management systems (LMS) for nursing professional development provides a flexible and effective approach to enhancing knowledge and skills. LMS platforms offer access to a diverse array of courses, tutorials, and resources designed to support various specialties and clinical competencies. This technology enables ongoing education, keeps nurses current with evidence-based practices, and helps meet licensure or certification requirements. Interactive elements such as quizzes, discussion boards, and multimedia content promote engagement and enhance knowledge retention. LMS platforms also support progress tracking and performance monitoring, allowing for the development of personalized learning pathways. Integrating LMS into nursing professional development encourages lifelong learning, elevates the quality of patient care, and nurtures a culture of continuous improvement across healthcare settings.

Electronic Health Records

One way of improving patient outcomes is with the use of **electronic health records** (**EHRs**). EHRs help health care providers to access complete and accurate health information in a timely fashion. EHRs have also been shown to reduce (and even prevent) medical errors due to misinterpretation of handwriting. EHRs also allow built-in systems designed to prevent treatment errors. All documentation is typically added to an electronic health record (EHR), due to the need to maintain patient privacy and confidentiality. Anyone who accesses this information will be tracked and monitored. Most institutions will conduct routine audits to see who has been accessing which records and if they were authorized to do so. The use of paper records continues, but due to the sheer volume of information collected and the need to ensure the security of this record, this practice will soon be phased out. Basic standards of care require the EHR contains all pertinent information and that it is updated frequently as the plan of care changes. Basic demographic information, along with treatment protocols and correspondence, is readily available to be accessed by the necessary practitioners associated with the case. Further, the meaningful use of file sharing is expected. Meaning, one of the main stipulations of the use of the EHR is that the client and provider benefit from the use of the EHR in quantifiable and qualitative ways. For this reason, it is imperative that all healthcare providers periodically document in the EHR, addressing the client's progress throughout the treatment plan.

Technology Tools and Strategies

Learning Technology Principles

With the ever-changing and improving world of technology, it is more crucial than ever to evaluate and integrate technology within the healthcare industry. **Technology** allows healthcare organizations to enhance patient care, improve operations, and create better outcomes. Some common areas that nurse administrators need to consider include telehealth, predictive analysis, and remote monitoring since these can affect technology evaluation and integration. **Telehealth** can affect technology evaluation and integration because administrators must assess the available technology, evaluate workflows, train staff, optimize infrastructure, and ensure compliance with regulatory requirements to successfully implement telehealth in their healthcare organization. **Remote monitoring** is a form of telehealth that allows healthcare providers to monitor patient data outside of healthcare settings, such as their homes. Nurse administrators must assess these technologies and their integration with electronic health records to successfully utilize remote monitoring in patient care. **Predictive analysis** allows nurse administrators to make data-driven decisions regarding technology evaluation and integration. By utilizing predictive analysis, nurse administrators can make informed choices that will improve patient care measures and operational efficiency.

Technology Evaluation

In simple terms, **technology evaluation** is the systematic assessment of technological solutions being utilized by an organization to determine their effectiveness and suitability for the needs of an organization. The purpose of evaluating technology is to confirm that the investment is worthwhile, align with organizational goals, and delivers the promised benefits.

Steps in Technology Evaluation

The first step in evaluation of technology is for the nurse administrator to identify the needs of the organization. The goal is to identify areas where technology can remedy organizational challenges or enhance processes.

The next step in the process is to establish criteria. For the technology evaluation to be effective, the nurse administrator must define specific measurements of focus. For example, they may choose to focus on cost, functionality, or security.

Once criteria are established, the nurse administrator must research the technology and develop a shortlist of preferred options. This can help identify potential technological solutions that fall within the chosen criteria.

When the shortlist is generated, it is time to assess the options available by interviewing vendors, participating in site visits, and having demonstrations of such technology.

The nurse administrator must decide which to choose by comparing the strengths and weaknesses of each option. They should choose the option that is the most appropriate for their organization and its needs.

Once the technology option has been chosen, it is important to test such technology in a controlled environment to determine its functionality and feasibility to the needs of the organization. This is called **pilot testing**.

A plan needs to be implemented to run pilot testing. The nurse administrator will create a detailed plan to implement the technology, which can include training modalities, stakeholder roles and support, and requirements of the organizational infrastructure.

Once pilot testing is implemented, there should be continuous evaluation. This includes monitoring the technology's performance and gathering feedback from those using the technology to determine areas for improvement.

Best Practices in Technology Evaluation

There are several best practices that nurse administrators should follow when it comes to technology evaluation. They need to engage stakeholders, involving them in the evaluation process. **Stakeholders** can include nurses, IT staff, and other administrators.

Another important consideration for best practice is **interoperability**. The nurse administrator should ensure that chosen technology can integrate seamlessly with existing systems that are in place; furthermore, the communication between these technological platforms must be viable.

Evaluating the long-term costs of technology improvements is another important factor in the decision-making process. It is the responsibility of the nurse administrator to consider the financial burden of implementation, maintenance, and upgrades of the implemented technology.

Since medical information is protected by laws such as HIPAA, assessment of security measures is a vital component of best practice. It is important to evaluate the technology's security features and how they comply with regulations set forth by not only the hospital, but also national laws and regulations.

Finally, the nurse administrator should ensure that the technology aligns with the goals of the organization. This includes the organization's overall vision and strategic objectives.

Teaching Strategies Using Technology

Simulations

Hands-on training in a safe, controlled environment is essential for effective learning, allowing nursing students and professionals to build knowledge and gain practical experience. Simulation-based education is a powerful method for professional development, offering opportunities to enhance clinical skills, critical thinking, and decision making without endangering patient safety. Through realistic scenarios involving medical equipment, supplies, and clinical applications, nurses can practice complex procedures, respond to emergencies, and improve communication techniques. This immersive, experiential learning builds confidence, sharpens problem-solving abilities, and reinforces technical proficiency in a safe and supportive environment.

Simulation experiences also promote teamwork and interprofessional collaboration, which are key elements in delivering high-quality healthcare. By replicating real-world challenges, nurses can practice alongside other disciplines to collaborate on current best practices and technological innovations. As a component of ongoing professional development, simulation supports licensure maintenance, career advancement, and the cultivation of a lifelong learning mindset. This approach improves clinical competence and contributes to safer, more effective patient care through enhancing performance in real-world situations.

Gaming

Game-based learning offers a dynamic and interactive approach to nursing professional development, supporting both skill acquisition and knowledge reinforcement. Through simulated scenarios, nurses can safely practice clinical decision making, critical thinking, and problem solving, leading to increased confidence and competence in real-world situations. This method encourages active engagement, enhances motivation, and improves knowledge retention by providing immediate feedback and rewarding progress.

Game-based activities also foster collaboration and effective communication among participants, reinforcing the interdisciplinary teamwork that is essential within healthcare environments. These simulations create an engaging environment that encourages active participation, reinforces knowledge through repetition, and improves retention by offering instant feedback and achievement-based rewards. The game-like structure enhances motivation while reducing the fear of making mistakes, allowing nurses to build confidence in a risk-free setting. Integrating gaming into ongoing education helps nurses stay current with evolving clinical protocols and best practices. As healthcare technology continues to advance, the use of gaming in nursing education offers an innovative approach to lifelong learning, ensuring that nurses are well-prepared for complex clinical challenges.

Computer-Based Learning

Computer-based learning (CBL) provides a flexible, accessible approach to nursing professional development, supporting the ongoing enhancement of clinical skills and knowledge. This method enables nurses to update competencies, stay informed about medical advancements, and fulfill licensure requirements at a self-directed pace.

CBL comprises a variety of formats, including online courses, simulations, webinars, and interactive modules. These are aimed at increasing learner engagement and improving information retention. This delivery method keeps up with the rigors of advancing medical knowledge and clinical skill development through reiteration and challenging critical thinking, incorporation of evidence-based practice, and continuous improvement in practice. With personalized learning pathways, CBL allows content to be tailored to meet individual learning needs and competency deficits. Healthcare organizations also benefit from this model, gaining a more competent workforce, improved patient care outcomes, and cost-effective training solutions. As digital tools continue to advance, CBL remains an essential component of nursing education, empowering nurses to meet emerging healthcare challenges and maintain high standards of care. Computer-based learning aligns with the dynamic demands of the nursing profession by offering efficient, current, and adaptable educational resources.

Virtual Reality

Virtual reality (VR) is transforming nursing professional development by offering innovative, immersive training experiences that strengthen clinical skills and elevate patient care. Through realistic simulations, nurses can safely practice complex procedures, sharpen critical thinking, and enhance decision making in a controlled environment that incorporates psychological safety. VR enables hands-on learning for tasks such as IV insertions, emergency interventions, and patient communication without jeopardizing patient safety. This technology supports continuous education by helping nurses stay updated with the latest clinical practices and evolving protocols.

Using advanced technology to deliver education is appealing and easily adopted by the younger generation of nursing staff who have grown up in a digital age. In addition, VR fosters collaboration through interactive scenarios that encourage teamwork and interdisciplinary communication, which are key elements in the current healthcare delivery model. Its flexibility and cost-effectiveness make VR an accessible training tool, available anytime and anywhere to support ongoing professional growth. By integrating VR into nursing education, healthcare organizations can build a confident, competent workforce equipped to meet today's complex clinical demands. Ultimately, VR contributes to improved patient outcomes and advances the quality of care across healthcare settings.

Virtual Education

Virtual education plays a vital role in nursing professional development by offering flexible and accessible learning opportunities. Through online platforms, nurses can engage in a variety of courses, webinars, and certification programs that accommodate demanding schedules while supporting up-to-date knowledge of current healthcare practices. This mode of learning promotes lifelong education and allows nurses to develop new competencies in areas such as patient safety, healthcare technology, and specialized clinical skills. Virtual education also fosters collaboration through discussion forums, virtual workshops, and online conferences, encouraging knowledge exchange and peer interaction.

Access to expert instructors and diverse global perspectives further enriches the learning experience and supports broader professional growth. As the healthcare landscape continues to evolve, virtual education remains a key resource for nurses striving to improve patient care, maintain certifications, and advance within the profession. By integrating virtual learning opportunities into nursing professional development, nurses gain skills to be adaptable, technologically savvy, and prepared to meet the dynamic needs of modern healthcare.

Clinical Technologies

While it is easy to assume technology in healthcare revolves around electronic health records, the nurse will be able to use other types of technology including complex equipment. The nurse should be prepared to use and troubleshoot the equipment in their field of practice, including but not limited to IV pumps, mechanical ventilators, bladder scanners, and/or smart beds. To review, listed below are a few of the more common types of equipment the nurse should feel comfortable using and troubleshooting.

Smart Pumps

IV Pump

IV pumps are used in a wide variety of medical settings. Every manufacturer provides a slightly different set of instructions, but there are a few basic steps in using any IV pump. The IV pump is in place to help the nurse provide a consistent administration of ordered medication or fluids, but it is the nurse's responsibility to ensure the correct flow rate, medication, and compatibility with other medications (if applicable). IV pumps need to be inspected routinely for accuracy, but there are still some alarms that the nurse will need to troubleshoot. The two alarms that the nurse should be prepared to troubleshoot are the presence of air in the tubing and a distal occlusion. In the event of air in the IV line, the pump should be stopped, and the air should be removed from the line prior to administration of any further infusions. Regarding a distal occlusion, the catheter is either in a place that allows the patient's movement to affect flow (e.g., flow can be obstructed by bending an elbow with an AC catheter) or there is a kink in the IV line.

Feeding Tube Pump

Like IV pump alarms, enteral feeding pumps sound an alarm in the event of a blockage or air present in the tubing. A blockage can be the result of a few things and will require the nurse to use nursing judgement. The blockage could be the result of administering a medication that was not intended to be crushed or was not adequately crushed, not flushing the line after administering medications and food, or a kink in the tubing. Nursing interventions include removing any formula present in the tubing and attempting to flush with warm water. Using a feeding tube syringe, a pull-push method can be used gently to try and clear the tubing. Air in the tubing may alarm as "NO FOOD," as the device does not detect the enteral formula, but detects the air bubble instead. Adequately priming the tubing and removing air bubbles will resolve this issue.

Bedside ECG Monitor

Depending on the clinical setting, the patient may be set up on a continuous bedside monitor or telemetry. For these monitoring tools to be effective, the nurse must be prepared to recognize arrhythmias and respond accordingly. Common issues with the use of continuous bedside monitoring include misplacement of electrodes, not replacing electrodes routinely, and faulty wiring or a faulty monitor that requires maintenance or new batteries.

Mechanical Ventilator

Mechanical ventilators are seen in the critical care environment and in the home health environment for long-term usage. The nurse should be prepared to recognize and respond to vent alarms, as a ventilator is a life-sustaining piece of equipment. The main alarms the nurse must be prepared to respond to are high-pressure alarms and low-pressure alarms. High-pressure alarms sound in response to high amounts of pressure fighting back on the ventilator. The causes can include the patient coughing, the patient fighting the vent, the presence of a mucus plug or thick secretions, or a kink in the tubing. Low-pressure alarms sound when there is not enough pressure detected and are most often the result of the patient not receiving adequate amounts of ventilation. The causes include disconnected tubing, a dislodged trach tube or ET tube, or an air leak in a cuffed ET tube. For both ventilator alarms, the nurse's first step is to assess whether the patient is in any distress. Interventions can be provided when the airway is patent and respirations are being provided.

Patient Barcode Scanners

Failing to identify patients correctly can cause mistakes and miscalculations regarding medication, transfusions, test procedures and results, procedures involving the wrong person, and discharging infants to the wrong families. It is essential to utilize two **patient identifiers**, which allows for the patient to be involved in the identification process and ensures dependability and consistency in the process. Using two identifiers also helps guarantee an accurate match between the service or treatment and the patient, helping to prevent mistakes and improve patient care.

There are a number of patient identifiers depending on the healthcare facility. Some examples include patient name, birthdate, address, phone number, Social Security Number (SSN), photograph, or their medical record number.

The nursing team must make sure that two of these above identifiers are assigned to each patient according to the facility's policy. Additionally, these same two identifiers must be linked to the patient's medication, blood product, treatment, procedure, or specimen container via an attached label. It is imperative to always check a client's ID band to verify it matches the name on the chart and the orders being performed. These identifiers must be used to verify a patient's identity when admitted or transferred to another hospital or care location and prior to caring for the patient. It is important to avoid using the patient's room number, which could result in a patient misidentification. The nursing team also needs to be aware of how to integrate automated systems into the patient identification process if used in their facility. These are utilized in order to decrease the likelihood of identification inaccuracies and reduce **medication errors**. Some examples include the following:

- **Computerized provider order entry** (**CPOE**): A system that allows healthcare personnel to enter and send treatment orders electronically.
- **Barcoding**: Computerized reference numbers that contain descriptive and other essential data.
- **Radio Frequency Identification** (**RFID**): Wireless technology utilizing radio waves and signals to communicate data.
- **Biometric identification**: The measurement and statistical analysis of a patient's individual features for the purpose of identification.

Smartphones/Tablets

Healthcare providers utilize a variety of resources to meet patient and family needs, exchange health information, and promote better health outcomes. In the hospital setting, these resources can begin with specialized counseling services (e.g., lactation consultants, diabetic educators). Hospitals may also collaborate with case management and insurance providers to coordinate the provision of medical equipment (e.g., medical beds, assistive devices, continuous oxygen, etc.) to meet a variety of patients' needs. In the outpatient care setting, providers are increasingly using at-home testing to help identify and treat issues such as cardiac dysrhythmia or sleep apnea.

Smartphone technology has also opened a massive database of potential resources for patients and families. There are applications that allow users to track nutrition intake, which can be used for health promotion activities. Other applications provide access to resources and exercises to help reduce stress and anxiety or offer the ability to track health data, such as weight, blood pressure, or menstrual cycles, for health promotion. Additionally, there are applications which provide a means to track caregiving tasks more effectively. Those patients and family members who do not have access, the desire, or the ability to utilize smartphone apps can also benefit from the use of printed or written materials to track health data.

Device Integration

Integration of advanced clinical technology devices into healthcare practice enhances patient care and safety. These devices, such as electronic health records (EHRs), infusion pumps, and bedside monitoring systems, work to streamline data collection and facilitate real-time decision making. For nurses, proficiency in operating these technologies is essential for accurate documentation, medication administration, and monitoring of patient status. Ongoing education and training ensure that nurses stay current with evolving device functionalities and safety protocols. Effective integration of clinical technology not only improves workflow efficiency but also reduces errors and promotes evidence-based practices. As healthcare continues to evolve, nurses must embrace technological advancements through continuous professional development, fostering a culture of innovation and excellence in patient care. Emphasizing technology competency within nursing education and training programs is vital for preparing a skilled workforce capable of navigating modern healthcare environments.

Networking Tools

Nurses seeking advancement in professional development and career promotion must be skilled at navigating clinical technology and networking tools to increase their circle of influence. Communication tools may be used within the workplace for sharing patient and professional information. Many organizations offer networking opportunities through forums and learning events. Nurses are encouraged to participate in education, training, and seminars that provide opportunities for interacting with other disciples. This practice leads to improvement in communication, collaboration, and understanding among healthcare teams.

Online learning platforms and webinars also enable nurses to stay current with the latest evidence-based practices and certifications. Networking tools, such as professional social media platforms and nursing associations, facilitate connections with peers, mentors, and industry leaders while championing knowledge sharing and collaboration. These tools collectively support continuous education, skill development, and professional growth, ensuring that nurses are well-equipped to meet evolving healthcare demands. While networking may occur in structured or casual environments, it is important to note that nurses should always present themselves in a courteous and professional manner while representing their respective cohorts.

Practice Quiz

1. An elderly patient is receiving teaching about the use of a home blood pressure monitoring device. Which statement made by the nurse would be the LEAST effective for assessing patient comprehension?
   a. "Show me how you will measure your blood pressure."
   b. "Where does the cuff go?"
   c. "Tell me which button you will press to see previous results."
   d. "Do you have any questions?"

2. Which of the following is a potential barrier to electronic care innovations?
   a. Identity theft
   b. Patient costs
   c. Age
   d. All of these are potential barriers

3. Clinical information technology is associated with which of the following?
   a. Clinical tasks
   b. Admissions
   c. Pharmacy
   d. Laboratory

4. Which of the following can be a barrier to communication?
   a. Quiet environment
   b. New computer technology and applications
   c. Low turnover productivity standards
   d. Prioritizing during documentation

5. Which is an example of how an electronic health record (EHR) improves patient outcomes?
   a. By reducing medical errors due to misinterpretation of handwriting
   b. By increasing the time a nurse spends researching the patient's disease process
   c. By decreasing the interdisciplinary team's access to patient information
   d. By discouraging the use of built-in systems in preventing treatment errors

See answers on the next page.

Answer Explanations

1. D: Choice *D* is the least effective statement to assess for patient comprehension, as this is a closed-statement question that does not require the patient to demonstrate or verbalize proof of comprehension. Choice *A* would be incorrect, as this statement would be the best way to assess a patient's overall understanding of the process. Choice *B* is incorrect because the patient is able to demonstrate whether they understand appropriate blood pressure cuff placement. Choice *C* is also incorrect because the patient is required to verbalize or point to the appropriate button to access previous measurements, which assesses understanding of how to access that feature.

2. D: All the choices have been identified as barriers to the use of electronic healthcare innovations.

3. A: Clinical information technology centers on a set of clinical tasks, instruments, equipment, and imaging. The other options listed are mainly associated with healthcare information technology, which has a broader base of processes and functions such as laboratory, pharmacy, and admissions.

4. B: New technology and limited understanding of the new technology can prove to be a barrier to communication for staff who are unable to access information, document patient data, or share results with fellow staff. Disruptive surroundings may also prove to be a detriment to effective communication (e.g., alarms, high volume, and rapid turnover). Nurses should prioritize the appropriate time to document and which information to document; this allows for smoother workflow and allocates time for communication.

5. A: EHRs have been shown to reduce (and even prevent) medical errors due to misinterpretation of handwriting. EHRs also allow built-in systems designed to prevent treatment errors. EHRs do not relate to the time spent researching a disease process.

Performance Improvement and Project Management Methodologies

Continuous process improvement applies broadly to operations across healthcare, business, the public sector, nonprofits and beyond. Process improvement can occur incrementally over time or happen in a discrete breakthrough; however, continuous process improvement is the paradigm of viewing such improvements as part of a repeating cycle for the development of better work processes. Three central concepts to continuous process improvement are the Plan-Do-Study-Act (PDSA) cycle, "Lean Leadership" business planning, and responding to system failures through systems thinking and root cause analysis.

PDSA Cycle

Fundamental to the paradigm of continuous process improvement is the **Plan-Do-Study-Act cycle**, sometimes also referred to as Plan-Do-Check-Act (**PDCA**). Healthcare leaders can use this method to implement change in a systematic way. It allows for testing, assessing, and adjusting changes on a limited scale to maximize the chance of success once the change is rolled out broadly.

Plan

Healthcare leaders assess the need for change, the conditions surrounding the process, and the desired outcomes. They may interview staff, collect data, and reach out to peers at other organizations to learn from their experiences and methods. They may also observe the different systems within the healthcare environment (e.g., nursing, pharmacy, respiratory therapy, and environmental services) to learn the way they interact, contribute to, or hinder the process in question. Then, leaders begin to form a plan for improvement, usually targeted to an initially limited scope that will be implemented in the "Do" step.

Do

Healthcare leaders then implement the plan in the "Do" stage of the PDSA cycle. In this phase, it is important to stay in communication with stakeholders, staff, and other allied health colleagues to monitor for any safety issues and to check on participation and staff buy-in.

Study (or Check)

This is the phase during which healthcare leaders step back and assess the results of the process change. Was it a success? Were the desired outcomes achieved? Again, this may involve data collection, discussions with staff, and considerations of any safety implications. In this step, healthcare leaders can make adjustments and may consider issues involved in scaling up the change.

Act

Actions taken in this last step depend on what was learned in the "Study" step. If the change was unsuccessful, the cycle begins again with an adjusted or even entirely new plan. If the attempted change was successful, the "Act" step allows healthcare leaders to make minor adjustments and consider issues involved in scaling up the change. If the change was successful, this is the step during which the change is rolled out to a larger audience. Additionally, measures are taken toward permanent implementation and ongoing assessment of outcomes.

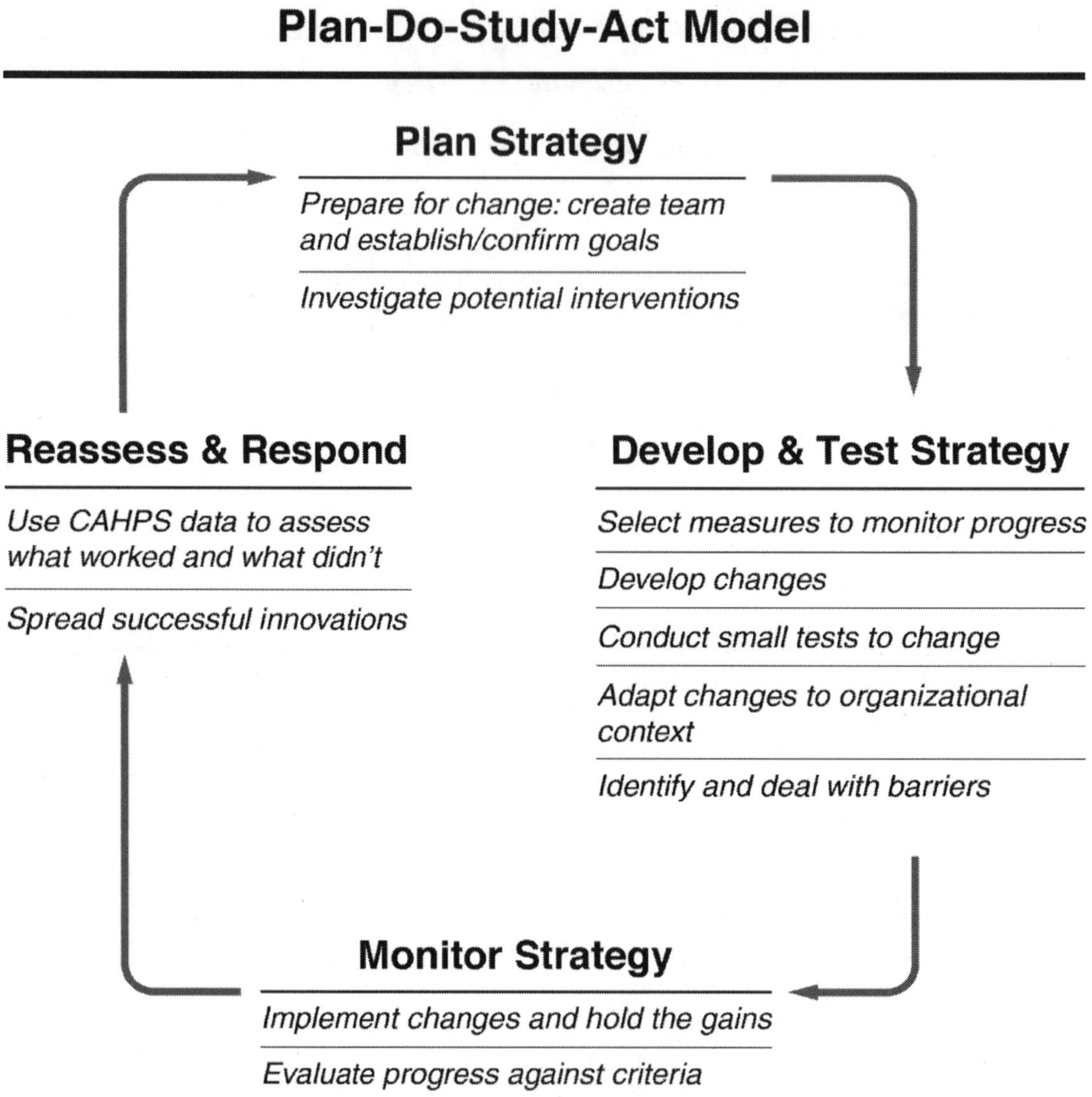

Lean Leadership

"**Lean**" is a system of thinking and practicing that originated with the Toyota car company. It aims to produce maximum value with minimum waste. "**Lean leadership**" relies on respect for the people who carry out the daily operations of the organization and employs a continuous learning cycle to deliver process improvement. The "**lean approach**" in healthcare focuses on the patient and what is of value to them, such as reduced wait times, a quiet sleep environment, reduced readmission rate, and on-time discharge. However, the lean approach can be targeted toward any group, such as frontline nurses or physicians, and attempt to deliver value to that group in the most resource-efficient manner possible.

The lean approach pursues continuous process improvement on a granular and incremental level, aiming for ever increasing efficiency, flow, and elimination of waste. It does this by first determining a valuable measure, such as a reduction in medication errors or increased patient satisfaction. The next steps involve identification of a purpose or problem to be solved, the work necessary to solve that problem, and the capabilities required for the desired solution. These capabilities can include management and leadership actions, both material and human resource needs, and developing awareness and buy-in among staff. The lean approach attempts to remove barriers or workflow steps that do not contribute to producing the maximum value.

Standard work is an example of a lean-based practice that has been widely adopted in hospitals and healthcare systems. Standard work protocols aim to add value to the patient experience by training staff in best practices to reduce many healthcare-related risks, such as infection, transfusion reaction, and falls. The lean approach identifies the value being delivered (e.g., reduced healthcare risks), a problem to be solved (e.g., inconsistent use of best practices), and what capabilities are required in the effort to produce maximum value with minimum waste (e.g., standardization, ease of use, and ease of access). The result is that best practices for many different procedures are available for use in front-line practice, and are easy to update, disseminate, and access.

Systems Thinking

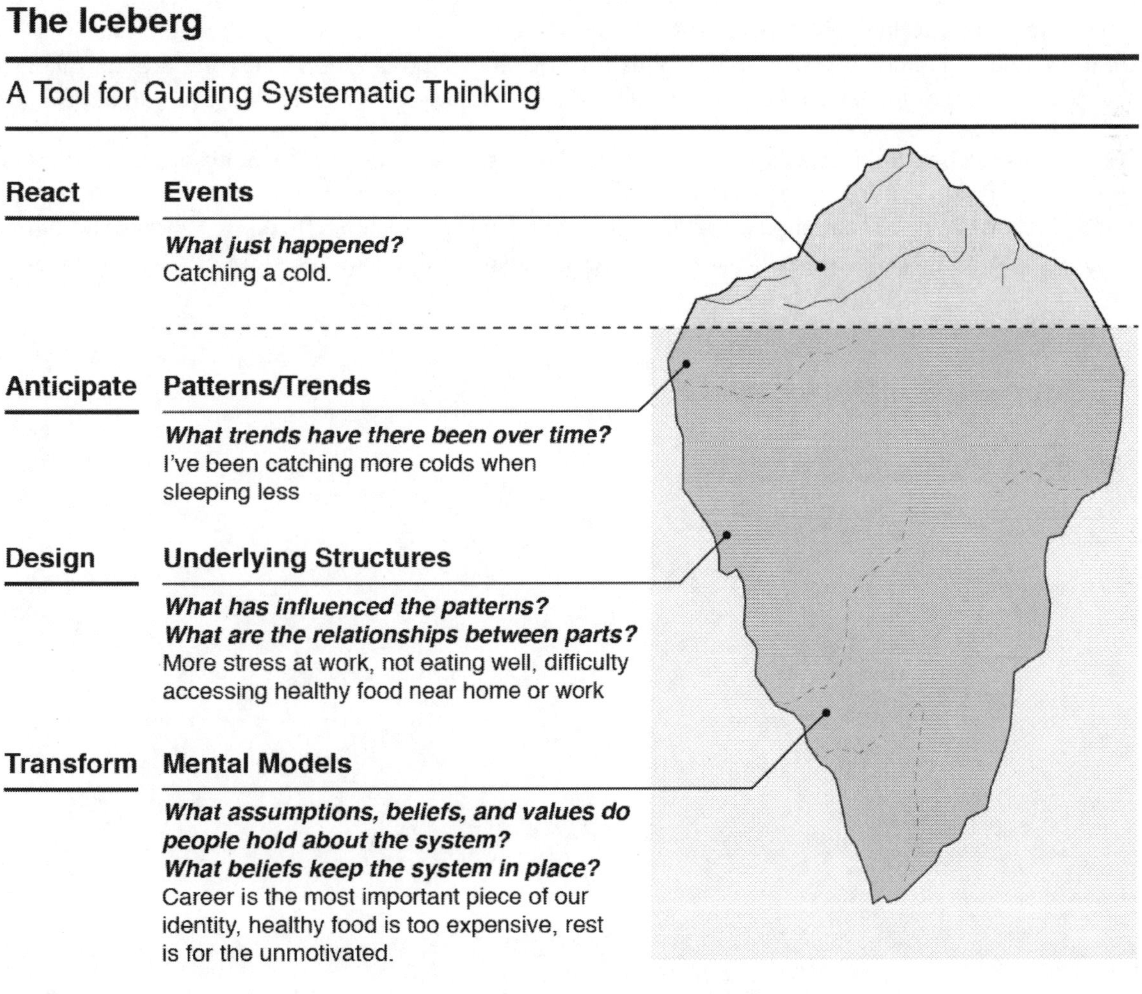

Systems thinking is defined as a link between individuals and their environment. For nurses, this refers to their ability to understand the influence of the healthcare environment on patient outcomes. Systems thinking is identified as the goal of all of the Quality and Safety Education for Nurses (QESN) competencies, which are acquired by nurses on a continuum that ranges from the care of the individual patient to the care of the entire patient population. The QESN competencies were originally identified to improve patient outcomes in response to extensive research that identified a significant difference between the care of patients and the improvement in patient outcomes resulting from that care. The nursing competencies include patient-centered care, evidence-based practice, teamwork and collaboration, safety, quality and improvement, and informatics. Successful interventions associated with each of these criteria for professional nursing practice require the ability to apply the systems thinking approach to care.

Competency related to systems thinking requires appropriate education and clinical experience, and is also identified as one of the nursing competencies in the Synergy Model. In that model, novice nurses view the patient and family as isolated in the nursing unit rather than being influenced by the healthcare system, while experienced nurses are able to integrate all of the resources in the healthcare system to improve patient outcomes. Several of the learning activities designed to improve nurses' ability to acquire systems thinking include creation of a grid that identifies the nursing competencies across the continuum from isolated, individual care to the level of care associated with systems thinking. There are assessment models that apply this exercise to specialty care units such as emergency care, long-term care, and outpatient care, which identify specific systems needs for these areas. Other exercises include tracking unit statistics for the QESN competencies followed by the creation, implementation, and evaluation of a plan that applies systems thinking to address that competency. All of these activities help nurses integrate patient needs with all available resources in order to improve outcomes.

Root cause analysis can also be used as a learning exercise for systems theory because this process, which is commonly used to investigate errors, looks at all elements of an institution's relationship with the error. Case studies and reflection are also recommended as useful learning aids for systems thinking. In addition, there are valid assessment instruments that can be used to assess systems thinking skills acquired through these learning activities.

A cause-and-effect diagram can show relationships between factors and can organize potential causes into smaller categories in order to find out why something happened or how it could happen. It is also known as an Ishikawa diagram, named after the man who designed it, Kaoru Ishikawa. Although it was originally developed as a quality control tool, in the healthcare setting the diagram is used to discover the root cause of a problem, uncover bottlenecks in a process or identify where and why a process isn't working. This is called a **root cause analysis** or a **cause-and-effect analysis**.

Example of a Root Cause Analysis

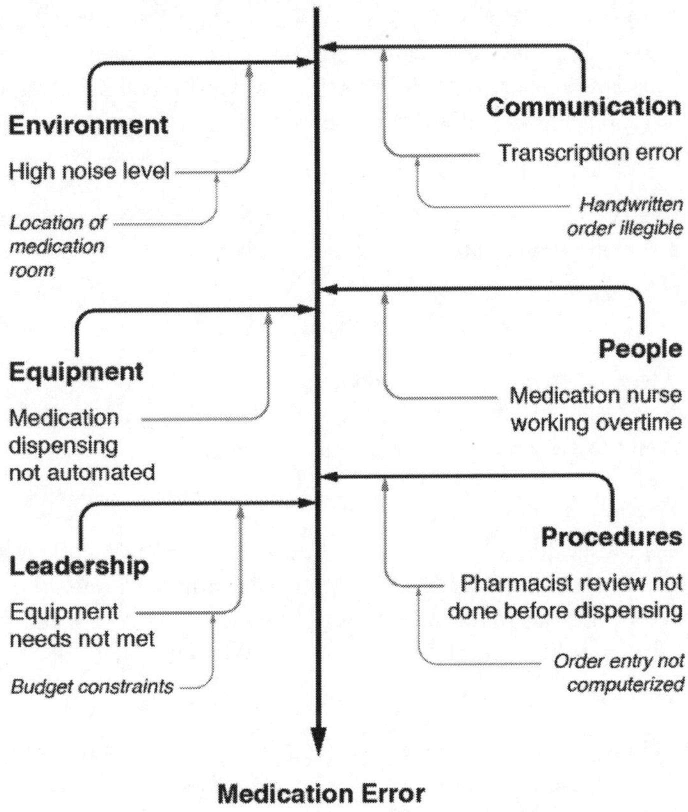

The root cause analysis (RCA) is used when there is an adverse event, a sentinel event, or close call in the medical setting. It can also be used when there is a concern about a process due to repeated errors, when there is a possibility of serious errors, and when there are high-cost errors. The RCA answers the following critical questions:

- What happened or is still happening?
- How did it happen?
- Why did it happen?
- How can we prevent it from happening again?
- What can we learn from this?

Organizational Performance Indicators, Priorities, and Trends

Patient Experience Facilitation

Patient experience is a concept that reflects the goal of healthcare systems to provide patient-centered care. **Patient experience** encompasses the entire scope of the patient's interaction with those that provide their inpatient, outpatient, and at-home care. It includes fundamental healthcare behaviors, such as communication, information sharing, coordination, cultural awareness, and support for self-management. Understanding patient experience requires healthcare staff and leaders to see things from the patient's point of view.

The focus on patient satisfaction has received criticism in recent years. While patient experience differs represents a neutral view of a patient's interaction with the healthcare system, **patient satisfaction** focuses on whether the patient's expectations for the interaction were met.

The **Consumer Assessment of Healthcare Providers and Systems** (**CAHPS**) arm of the Agency for Healthcare Research and Quality (AHRQ) provides patient experience surveys tailored to a wide variety of different service lines and care delivery systems. The CAHPS patient experience survey assesses patient experience with questions that address if and how often specific actions occurred. For example, a patient will be asked if they experienced emotional difficulties related to their illness and, if so, whether their healthcare team gave them advice or assistance with coping mechanisms.

Experience of care is one of three points in the **Institute for Healthcare Improvement**'s (**IHI**) Triple Aims for improving the U.S. healthcare system, along with population health and reducing per-capita cost. Patient experience comprises the six domains of healthcare quality: safety, effectiveness, patient-centeredness, timeliness, efficiency, and equity. Research supports the link between positive patient experience and improved healthcare outcomes.

Patient experience data should be approached as an **indicator**, not an outcome. This data can be used to identify areas for improvement and target system-level process improvements, such as shortening wait times in outpatient clinics or improving response time to call bells in the inpatient setting.

Five C's of Patient Experience

Patient experience is essentially the patient's cumulative exposure to the healthcare system. From primary care offices and clinics, to hospitals and acute care facilities, to telehealth and home health services, the patient's healthcare experience can become very disjointed without the assistance of a devoted healthcare team. To improve the patient experience, the nurse should remember the five Cs (consistency, coordination, continuity, caring, and correction):

- Consistency: Consistent patient care is consistency across the entire healthcare experience. From varying nurses to varying shifts, there is vast potential for a lapse in consistency. Effective communication and routine training are key to a consistent nursing practice.
- Coordination: Coordination is the teamwork and communication of the interdisciplinary team. An example of poor coordination would be the nurse educating the patient on a medication that the medical provider just discontinued. Effective communication is essential for coordination of the patient's healthcare experience.
- Continuity: While similar to consistency, continuity of care is the smooth transition of care. Continuity of care can be seen in the nursing shift change. The patient would experience continuity of care if there were no lapse in quality of care during the change of staff at regular shift changes.
- Caring: Caring in nursing can drastically affect the patient experience. Empathy, respect, and the practice of active listening are all key practices involved in being a caring nurse.
- Correction: Lastly, correction can improve an issue a patient experiences in the course of their care. Human error is inevitable, but the patient experience can be improved with the recognition of the issue and measures put into place for resolving the issue or preventing a recurrence.

Patient Experience Strategies

Patient experience facilitation is a collaborative process that involves understanding patient goals and desires and setting patient expectations. Some healthcare systems employ designated patient facilitators who work as multidisciplinary coordinators and advocates to individualize interventions and improve patient experience. Patient experience facilitators are sometimes called patient experience managers, liaisons, or directors. While these roles are fairly new, many existing roles in the hospital contribute directly to facilitating patient experience, such as bedside nurses, social workers, care coordinators, and discharge coordinators.

All members of the healthcare team and support staff contribute to patient experience, even those who are not directly involved in patient care. For example, an understaffed pharmacy team can impact patient experience if there are delays in the delivery of needed medications, even if the patient never meets the pharmacy staff.

The patient's physical environment plays a large role in their experience. Pay attention to accessibility needs, comfort, and ease of use for the patient and family. Dietary and environmental service teams have a direct impact on patient experience and should not be overlooked.

Facilitating patient experience requires flexibility and creative thinking. Many strategies and tools are available to healthcare staff and leaders as part of the process.

In the inpatient setting, it is important to ask open-ended questions on admission to give the patient a voice in their plan of care and to understand what unique issues and priorities the patient has for their stay. These may include dietary needs, communication needs, or cultural concerns related to their care.

The nurse's **bedside shift report** involves the patient and family in the handoff of care between nurses. This allows the patient and family to meet their new caregivers face-to-face, communicate their goals and desires for their care, update their caregivers on their status, and prevent incorrect information from being passed on.

Multidisciplinary rounding contributes to a positive patient experience by improving communication between the patient and different disciplines, such as physicians, nurses, and pharmacists. As a result, the negative effects of lapses and breakdown in communication are avoided.

Dry-erase boards with updated information on the patient's care team, goals, and plans for the shift help patients and families understand what to expect. Providing a notepad and pen to write down questions and concerns to share during rounds also helps patients and families communicate with their healthcare team.

Discharge is an exciting but vulnerable time for patients. Family and/or care partners should be included in the **discharge process**. Using strategies such as **teach-back**, where the nurse teaches the learner, then has the learner demonstrate or "teach" the skill back to the nurse, helps patients and families feel more confident in managing their care at home. Including home-health liaisons and social workers in the discharge process helps promote a seamless transition from hospital to home. Even the trip from bedside to car can have an outstanding impact on patient experience.

In the outpatient setting, the friendliness and efficiency of front desk staff contributes to the beginning of a positive patient experience. Consider the cleanliness and comfort of the waiting area as well.

A great deal of outpatient care is managed by phone and, increasingly, by **secure messaging** on online portals. Methods for communicating with the care team from home should be easy to understand and access, and responses from the care team should be timely.

The more data that healthcare leaders have regarding the actual events of the patient experience, the better they can target improvements. Surveys should be provided frequently and should be easy to complete and return.

Patient experience is a primary driver of where patients go for their medical care. Ongoing positive patient experiences will not only improve safety and health-related outcomes, but they will also improve the reputation of the healthcare provider or system in the community.

Patient Satisfaction

Patient satisfaction is a term used in healthcare to describe an organization's ability to meet patient expectations. Hospitals have a duty to provide safe and effective care while also maintaining a favorable patient experience. This can be challenging to achieve, and the implications are significant. Not only does patient satisfaction have an impact on health outcomes, but it also impacts organizational business and financial success.

Patient satisfaction is a highly valued benchmark of healthcare quality. Data relating to patient satisfaction can be collected internally by a healthcare organization or through external institutions that focus on healthcare quality. In the business of healthcare, patient satisfaction often serves as the "demand" in a supply and demand economy. Higher patient satisfaction scores are associated with better patient health outcomes, and consequently associated with happier patients, patients who are more likely to return to and recommend a particular healthcare organization, higher quality of medical staff that the healthcare organization retains, increased level of outside funding that the healthcare organization receives, and fewer medical malpractice suits. Patients report higher satisfaction when they receive care that they find to be tailored to their needs, care that is safe yet efficient, and care that is accessible. In this regard, healthcare delivery requires a nuanced level of customer service; however, rather than delivering a tangible manufactured product, medical staff deliver a product that affects the patient's ability to live well and their long-term physical, mental, and emotional state.

Business and Financial Impact

Patient perception of experience is increasingly being used to measure hospital performance and reimbursement eligibility. The *Hospital Consumer Assessment of Healthcare Providers and Systems* (HCAHPS) survey, for instance, nationally collects and reports how patients perceive their healthcare experiences. The results, which are available to the public, can impact a hospital's image, marketability, and opportunities. Other federal initiatives, like the *Value-Based Purchasing* (VBP) *Program*, seek to put quality controls in place for hospitals receiving funding from the Centers for Medicare and Medicaid Services (CMS). A quality score—significantly tied to patient experience—is assigned to healthcare organizations and used to determine a small percentage of reimbursement as well as the provision of bonuses or penalties.

Management of Patient Satisfaction

Hospitals are extremely complex systems that handle a high volume of potentially sensitive and stressful patient interactions. Despite their best efforts at maintaining quality and patient satisfaction, hospitals inevitably will receive complaints and grievances. These concerns can be raised by anyone within or outside of an organization and can be received as an informal comment or a formal grievance filed with the organization or a regulatory body.

Nurses are in a unique position to intervene to recognize and possibly mitigate concerns raised within the care setting. When recognized and addressed early, development of serious grievances can sometimes be avoided altogether, and patient experiences can be improved. Nurses often directly and indirectly assist with the service recovery process (i.e., make things right) by being empathetic, helping to problem solve, escalating as required, or providing comfort and additional customer service measures to improve the experience of a disgruntled patient or family member. Nurses can also advocate for patient rights, such as the right to a second opinion, by providing information and discussing available resources.

Additionally, nurses are called—both professionally and ethically—to speak up when they identify an issue related to practice. A concern with an individual, ideally, would be addressed with the individual in a professional manner.

However, nurses may also be required to escalate or report via additional channels, including supervisors, ethics committees, Human Resources departments, regulatory agencies, or even lawmakers.

Service Recovery

As previously discussed, the skill of recognizing an issue and working towards correction is crucial for the nurse. With a lapse in care quality, trust can be compromised, and the patient may lose confidence in the ability of the healthcare team to provide care. The goal with service recovery is restoring trust and restoring confidence in the healthcare team.

Restoring Trust

Restoring trust will require the nurse to acknowledge the issue with honesty. Allowing the patient time to ask questions while maintaining an apologetic attitude can restore respect, which can be an initial step to restoring trust. Making any amends necessary/appropriate can also assist in restoring trust.

Restoring Confidence

Simply put, restoring confidence will include resolving the issue. Fix the issue, follow up, and follow through:

- Fix the issue with the assistance of the entire interdisciplinary team to ensure adequate coordination.
- Follow up by checking with the patient after the issue has been fixed, both to ensure that the issue is in fact fixed and that the patient does not require additional assistance.
- Follow through by ensuring that any promises or plans made are effectively in place.

Care Delivery Evaluation

Evaluating the delivery of patient care is an essential part of nursing practice. By evaluating the care that is being implemented, professional development nurses can identify areas of improvement, guarantee quality patient care, and help strengthen overall healthcare outcomes for patients.

Importance of Care Delivery Evaluation

Care delivery evaluation is important because it helps enhance patient outcomes. When nurse leaders identify and fix gaps in patient care, this leads to fewer adverse events and higher patient satisfaction. Evaluating care delivery helps identify areas for improvement. This allows for delivery processes to be enhanced, specifically with the incorporation of evidence-based guidelines and best practices in nursing care. Moreover, evaluation allows for quality improvement initiatives to be created and implemented. When quality improvement initiatives are implemented, they improve the overall safety, success, and productivity of the healthcare services provided.

Key Concepts

There are four **core measures** in care delivery evaluation: performance measurement, outcome evaluation, process evaluation, and structure evaluation. **Performance measurement** involves evaluating the quality and effectiveness of healthcare delivery through a variety of performance metrics. Such metrics include patient outcomes, adherence to protocols, and resource utilization. **Outcome evaluation** is when the impact of care delivery is assessed based on several indicators, including, but not limited to, morbidity, mortality, and patient satisfaction. **Process evaluation** occurs when the individual processes involved in care delivery are assessed. Some examples include clinical guideline adherence, interdisciplinary collaboration, and the efficiency of workflow on a daily basis. Finally, **structure evaluation** is the assessment of the overall organizational structure and the available resources to help facilitate care delivery. Some factors that are assessed include staffing levels, equipment, and infrastructure of facilities.

Methodologies

Professional development nurses can use several methods, including qualitative, quantitative, mixed-methods, and benchmarking, to obtain data that can be analyzed. **Qualitative methods** involve the use of interviews, focus groups, or observations to collect descriptive data regarding the care delivery process, patient experiences, and the workflow of nurses. **Quantitative methods** incorporate data collection tools, conduct surveys, and utilize statistical analyses to measure specific variables to assess care delivery outcomes. Factors in the healthcare setting that can be measured using quantitative methods include infection rates, medication errors, and patient satisfaction scores. A **mixed-method approach** incorporates both qualitative and quantitative data collection methods. This allows for a more comprehensive understanding of care delivery and provides validation of data. Lastly, **benchmarking** is a method that utilizes the comparison of delivery performance metrics with established standards to help determine areas of improvement. This allows for goal setting and quality improvement overall.

Quality Indicators

There are several indicators that nurse administrators should assess during care delivery evaluation. These include structure, process, outcome, safety, and nurse indicators. When looking at **structure indicators**, the nurse administrator focuses on assessing the organizational resources, policies, staffing levels, education, and training opportunities. This is a non-exhaustive list, however. Some of the process indicators that nurse administrators assess to ensure that they are adhering to evidence-based practices can include interdisciplinary communication, documentation practices, and the use of standardized protocols. In terms of outcome indicators, nurse administrators evaluate mortality rates, readmission rates, infection rates, and patient satisfaction ratings. **Safety indicators** that nurse administrators utilize in the evaluation process include medication errors, falls, hospital-acquired infections, adverse events, and similar measures.

Nurse-sensitive indicators are indicators that reflect the quality and effectiveness of nursing care. Nurse administrators should consider the following common nurse-sensitive indicators: patient satisfaction, patient falls, pressure ulcers, hospital-acquired infections, medication errors, nursing staffing levels, patient readmissions, nurse turnover, and job satisfaction.

Below is an example of the care delivery evaluation process in action:

Sarah is the nurse administrator in a busy surgical unit. She understands the significance of medication safety in achieving positive patient outcomes, having fewer adverse events, and increasing patient satisfaction. She has a goal to improve the medication administration process on her unit—specifically reducing medication errors related to high-alert medications. She knows that if medication administration practices are improved on her unit, overall patient safety and surgical unit productivity will be improved.

The first action Sarah takes is to determine the objectives for the care delivery evaluation plan. The main objective she decides to address is to decrease medication errors related to high-alert medications by 50% within six months. This is a SMART goal—one that is specific, measurable, achievable, relevant, and time-bound.

Next, Sarah collects baseline data on medication errors with high-alert medications over the past fiscal year using both quantitative and qualitative methods. She looks at documented medication errors, reviews staff surveys, and observes daily medication administration. Once data is collected, she analyzes the data to identify what types of errors are occurring, any contributing factors, and any patterns. The purpose of this baseline data is to allow for comparison of future outcomes. Sarah determines that errors are mainly occurring with drugs that have similar names.

After data collection, Sarah looks inward to the facility and unit itself, focusing on its infrastructure, available resources, and compliance with evidence-based practices and guidelines regarding medication safety. Some of the important concepts she identifies are effective communication, double-checking procedures, barcode scanning, clear labeling, and staff education and training. These concepts will help her develop an interventional plan. Sarah notices that the two main issues found were nurses not double-checking medications and the fact that labels from the pharmacy were very similar, making it difficult to differentiate certain medications. There were also a few incidences of mislabeling from the pharmacy, which the barcode cannot detect.

To develop an intervention plan, Sarah works closely with the interdisciplinary team. This includes her nursing staff, hospital pharmacists, physicians, and other relevant stakeholders. Together, they come up with a plan to implement several strategies. First, they will implement a new standardized medication administration process. Next, they will improve communication channels, highlighting the importance of closed-loop communication. They will also conduct regular and unannounced competency assessments. Ongoing education and training for staff will be implemented. Sarah and her team find it important to implement a **double-checking system** with another nurse when administering high-alert medications.

Sarah implements the intervention plan with the help of her nursing staff and the rest of the interdisciplinary team. They ensure clear protocols and guidelines are developed for medication administration, monitor the distribution of appropriate supplies and resources (such as labeling and barcode systems), and facilitate educational workshops for staff.

To monitor the interventional plan and evaluate its effectiveness, Sarah creates a **reporting system** for medication errors. Nurses are instructed to report incidents in a prompt and thorough manner. Periodic medication safety audits and observations are also conducted to identify any gaps or areas for improvement.

Sarah will retrieve all collected data that has been reported through the new reporting system, safety audits, and observations to provide a thorough analysis. She compares this data to the baseline data that was obtained prior to the implementation of the interventional plan. Data is analyzed to identify medication errors, contributing factors, and recurring patterns and issues. This will allow her to identify gaps in the interventional plan that require further improvement or alteration. After the six months is over, Sarah determines that errors have decreased by 40%—not the 50% that she was hoping for.

Sarah decides to meet with the interdisciplinary team to create additional changes and implement them accordingly. They decide to revisit the **"look-alike drug" policy** by coordinating with the pharmacy and **electronic medication administration record** (**eMAR**) systems to utilize capitalization in several look-alike drug names. This will help reduce errors with mislabeling. They also decide to provide training modules, including mock scenarios and situations for the staff to practice, to determine areas that still need improvement. To ensure that high-alert medications being administered are accurately confirmed before administration, a mandatory double-check system with the charge nurse is implemented on the unit.

Since care delivery evaluation is an ongoing process, Sarah ensures that she maintains an environment of monitoring and evaluation within the surgical unit. She continues to have randomized and unannounced observations, audits, and staff discussions, so she can monitor medication safety practices. This allows her to identify any shortfalls with adherence to established protocols and guidelines, which she addresses immediately.

Care delivery evaluation is not a one-time process. It is an ongoing and lengthy process that needs to be thorough. Even if new interventional practices are implemented that meet set SMART goals, there are always additional factors that may arise and cause issues within the system. An example of this would be new staff members joining the nursing or pharmacy team. Although additional safety measures have been put in place, new staff members have the potential to make medication errors due to inexperience or lack of knowledge. This factor could be something that the nurse administrator can create an interventional plan for—to help onboard new hires through extensive training programs in this area.

Patient Outcome Measures

Professional development nurses should understand that the patient outcomes rely on a complex combination of the patient's individual biological pharmacotherapeutic profile, degree of adherence with the plan, socioeconomic factors, and existing comorbidities. Much of the research on patient adherence focuses on economic factors, while many providers believe that the patient outcomes should be the top priority. Quality improvement activities at the administration level can address many of these issues by standardizing the provider approach to the development of the therapeutic plan. Some of the issues addressed can include methods of education, monitoring procedures for drugs with known or high-risk for the development of adverse drug reactions, and examination of hospital readmissions following the administration of the target drug.

Nurses promote best patient outcomes by providing education to patients and families by utilizing best practice guidelines and using these in the nursing process. Ultimately, the purpose of education, care bundles, core measures, and guidelines is to promote the best possible **patient outcomes**. Patient outcomes are identified as high priority by nurses, physicians, patients, families, professional organizations, and governing bodies. One of the quality objectives of the **Affordable Care Act (ACA)**, enacted in 2010, is fewer avoidable hospital readmissions. Avoidable hospital readmissions are considered negative outcomes for all parties involved, but especially for the patients. The **Institute for Healthcare Improvement (IHI)** is a worldwide driver of healthcare improvement and best patient outcomes. The IHI's work focuses on improvement capability, person- and family-centered care; patient safety; and quality, cost, and value. These focus groups are all aimed to improve patient outcomes.

The **Centers for Medicare and Medicaid Services (CMS)** was formed in 1977. CMS provides value-based incentives to providers and institutions by tying reimbursement to better patient outcomes. Conversely, CMS withholds reimbursement to institutions and providers if a patient is readmitted to the hospital within thirty days of discharge if the readmission is related to the same problem causing the initial hospitalization. For instance, a patient is admitted to the hospital with CHF exacerbation, treated, and released. Two weeks later, the patient is readmitted with CHF exacerbation. Neither the hospital nor the physician is reimbursed for care related to the readmission.

TJC created the Surgical Care Improvement Project (SCIP) with the goal of substantially reducing negative patient outcomes (surgical mortality and morbidity), specifically **surgical site infection (SSI)** and venous thromboembolism (VTE).

Project Management

Understanding the project management process is extremely practical and beneficial for the professional development nurse. Basic steps in project development include the following:

Initiation

- Understanding the root issue
- Defining measurable goals and outcomes
- Recognizing any limitations or restrictions
- Example: The root issue is a poor documentation system. The goal is to implement a new electronic documentation system. Limitations include potential lapses in documentation during the shift of documentation systems and barriers with technology among staff

Planning

- Establishing the "how" of obtaining the measurable goals and outcomes
    - Once defined, educating staff on the steps/procedures in place to obtain the goals/outcomes
- Establish all equipment, supplies, manpower, and education needed for the next phase

- Example: The project management team will need to plan for potential downtime for documentation, an expert documentation team, and education in-services on the new electronic documentation system

Execution

- Implementing the plan
- Example: The new electronic documentation system will be implemented with the planned resources in place

Monitoring/Controlling

- Closely monitoring the implementation
- Measuring the actual outcome with the planned goals and outcomes
- Monitoring will occur continuously or at regular intervals
- Example: The project management team will monitor documentation standards and staff understanding/compliance

Closing

- Closing out the process once the implementation process is sustainable
- Example: The project management team will close the project when the documentation system is successfully in use with the routine quality assurance checks in place for documentation standards

Quality Improvement

Quality is an integral component of healthcare, including in nursing. High quality care is linked with improved patient satisfaction, improved patient health outcomes, and a significant reduction in medical errors. In recent decades, **quality improvement** in healthcare has focused on eliminating paper charting and replacing it with electronic medical records. This improvement has standardized patient records, reduced human input error, and allowed multiple providers across disciplines to easily access and update patient charts. Other example of quality improvement measures include the following: establishing training protocols, standardizing patient hand-off and transitions between staff members (as studies have found this period to be most vulnerable to medical errors), using benchmarking reports to standardize operating procedures and set performance goals, conducting regular internal and external audits and evaluations, and encouraging healthcare organizations to develop a culture of continuous quality improvement.

Quality improvement is a systematic, data-driven approach to reducing inefficiencies and improving value provided by operational processes. Inefficiencies may be discovered by regularly conducting **gap analyses** that examine workflow processes individually to determine whether any critical steps are missing that might lead to errors. Additionally, **value stream mapping** examines workflow processes to ensure that each step provides irrefutable value; if they do not, the process may need to be rewritten in order to remove unnecessary steps. Poor quality procedures may also be discovered during audits or reporting periods if steps come back non-compliant or organizational data appear to fall below acceptable benchmarks.

Models that can be used to improve quality include the **Plan-Do-Study-Act** (**PDSA**) framework, which encourages examining a process for a gap and inefficiency, planning a test of change, implementing the change for an experimental period of time, studying the results, and making positive changes a permanent part of the workflow.

Lean Six Sigma is another type of quality improvement approach, which uses the **Define-Measure-Analyze-Improve-Control** (**DMAIC**) process on existing procedures to improve their outputs while keeping inputs and costs as low as possible.

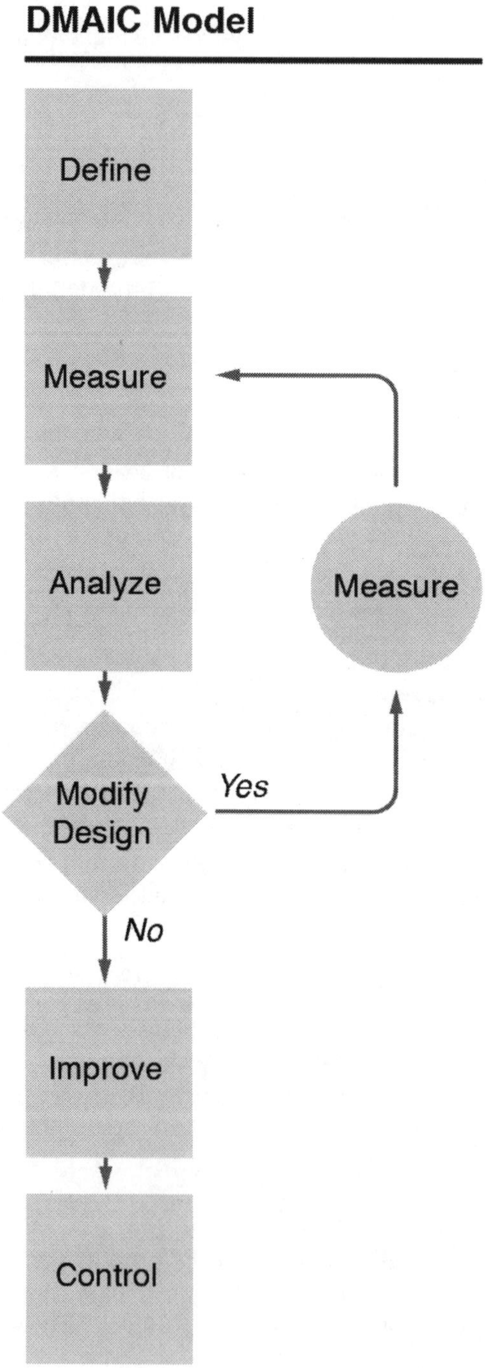

Best Practice

Best practices refer to a set of procedures that are generally accepted to be the most effective method of accomplishing a specific goal. These are shaped by evidence-based practice, professional expertise, and patient or client input. Organizations should follow established best practices in an industry in order to maintain high-quality standards. If an organization is underperforming in an area, researching established best practices for that area and implementing change to reflect best practices is likely to result in improved quality.

Quality Measures

Quality measures are used to determine how effective a quality process is. These can be classified into three categories: structural, process, and outcome measures. Structural measures refer to tools available within an organization that support high-quality processes, such as software or highly credentialed personnel. Process measures refer to the assessment of actual steps in a procedure, such as determining if nurses are verifying identity before administering a medical procedure. Outcome measures refer to whether structures or processes in place make a difference, such as the number of patients with bedsores in inpatient settings.

Quality Assurance

Quality assurance refers to an established system within an organization that has the function of ensuring that processes and outcomes are free of error. Quality assurance practices use administrative and process controls to ensure that variation from the start of the process to the end of the process is limited, therefore creating relatively standardized inputs that lead to an expected output. These factors are associated with efficiency, cost and resource reduction, and reduced product and service defects. Examples of quality assurance practices in the healthcare setting include electronic medical records, which reduce documentation error within and between different healthcare facilities, sanitation checklists, standardized training protocols for staff, and identity verification before medical procedures.

Quality Improvement Activities

The nursing team should participate in, and initiate, quality improvement activities in an effort to improve patient care and the overall profession. There are constant opportunities for practice improvement, and ideally, the team should foster an environment that is open to exploring these opportunities.

One of the best opportunities to learn about quality improvement activities is at trade shows and poster presentations. It is very beneficial to review what other institutions have researched or implemented in order to improve patient safety and patient care. These projects can range from changes to workflow and process to introducing tools to improve the hand-off of care in between care areas. After learning about these projects, the team can determine if implementing a similar project may be beneficial at their own facility while ensuring there are not overwhelming changes that may be a distraction to the team.

With the adoption of electronic medical records and electronic documentation, another great opportunity for research and improvement is using analytic tools to analyze and interpret the data at the facility. There are many examples of nursing teams using their own data for initiatives such as decreasing postoperative nausea and vomiting (PONV) using premedication or decreasing unnecessary overtime.

Performance Improvement

Performance improvement is a mechanism to continuously review and improve processes in a system, ensure that work is completed in the most cost-effective manner, and produce the best possible outcomes. Healthcare facilities are constantly aiming to drive down cost and increase reimbursements while delivering the highest quality of healthcare and utilizing analytical methods to achieve this. These analyses and implementations may be done by top administrative employees at the organization and be executed across the healthcare system, or within a particular department. Leadership support is always crucial for positive change to occur and sustain itself.

All processes should be regularly monitored for opportunities for improvement. Common opportunities include areas of reported patient dissatisfaction; federal, state, or internal benchmarks that are not being met; areas of financial loss; and common complaints among staff. While multiple opportunities for improvement may exist, focusing on one at a time usually produces the greatest outcome. When choosing a process to improve, it is important to select one that has the potential to be changed by the members involved (e.g., medical staff often do not have control over external funding sources). Processes where minimal resources are required for change, but that can produce positive end results, are also preferable to more costly improvements. Once the process has been selected, a group of stakeholders that are regularly involved in the process should map out each step while noting areas of wasted resource or process variation. From here, stakeholders can develop a change to test.

The **PDCA cycle** provides a framework for implementing tests of change. *Plan*, the first step, involves planning the change. This will include accounting for all workflow changes, the staff members involved, and logistics of implementation. It should also include baseline data relating to the problem. *Do*, the second step, involves implementing the change. During this step, data collection is crucial. For example, if a department believes that implementing mobile work stations will decrease nurses' wait time between patients, the department should keep a detailed record of the time spent with and between each patient. *Check*, the third step, involves checking data relating to the change with the baseline data and determining if the change improved the process. *Act*, the final step, involves making the change permanent and monitoring it for sustainability.

New Product/Technology Implementation

It is important to ensure that **technology integration** in healthcare is seamless with the current workflows and processes of an organization. When effective technology integration occurs, there is enhanced communication, increased efficiency, and improved patient outcomes.

There are several strategies that a nurse administrator can utilize to help integrate technology into their organization. The first step is to assess how implementing technology will impact current workflows and determine what adjustments are needed. The nurse administrator should also consider offering training programs and additional support to help staff members become familiar and comfortable with newly implemented technology. When it comes to choosing technology to utilize in an organization, it is important to consider usability. In other words, choosing user-friendly technology that is easy to navigate will help make the transition easier for staff. The use of "**super-users**", or staff members with advanced training in the new technology, can be a great resource to aid those with questions during the implementation process. Another strategy the nurse administrator can utilize is to facilitate collaboration between hospital IT staff and healthcare providers to identify areas where technology can be integrated or improved. Finally, the nurse administrator should continuously monitor the integration of technology, gather feedback, and determine areas that need improvement.

The following is a real-world example of a nurse administrator who is planning to integrate technology in his hospital after evaluating existing methods.

Mark is a nurse administrator working for a hospital that is looking to implement a new **electronic health record (EHR)** system to improve patient care and make documentation easier and more efficient. Currently, nurses are using manual charting methods and keeping paper records. Mark's role is to evaluate the technology and oversee its integration throughout the hospital.

The first thing Mark will do is participate in a technology evaluation.

Mark begins to identify the current issues and challenges in documentation at the hospital. He determines that there are issues in manual charting and insufficient communication between nursing staff and healthcare providers. These are the main areas that the EHR system can help fix.

Next, Mark identifies specific criteria on how to evaluate the EHR systems available. He chooses to focus on ease of use, data security, interoperability, and functionality. Mark works closely with the nurses, physicians, and hospital IT staff to obtain input and ensure that the selected criteria align with the goals of the hospital organization.

Once criteria are established, Mark conducts research on current EHR systems available and generates a shortlist of preferred options. Some important factors that he evaluates include user reviews and overall features. He decides on three potential vendors that meet the established criteria.

Now Mark is tasked with evaluating the options. He does so by arranging vendor demonstrations and site visits for EHR system to understand their functionality and capabilities. He pays close attention to overall user experience, ease of navigation, and interoperability capabilities.

Once all vendor demonstrations and site visits are complete, Mark composes lists of strengths and weaknesses of each EHR system. He considers the cost, user feedback, implementation timeline, and reputation of the vendors. After consulting with the executive leadership of the hospital and the IT department, they come to an informed decision and select the most suitable EHR system for their organization that helps them meet their strategic goals.

Finally, it is time for pilot testing. Mark chooses to implement the new EHR system within the neurology department. He works closely with IT and nursing staff to help customize the system according to the needs of their workflow. Mark closely monitors the performance of the system, its usability, and its impact on patient care and overall documentation processes. He regularly obtains feedback from the nursing staff and IT via surveys and interviews to identify areas of improvement before implementing the system in the entire hospital.

Once the evaluation piece has been completed, Mark decides to integrate the new EHR system within the rest of the hospital.

Mark assesses how the EHR system can impact **workflows**. He collaborates with frontline staff and nursing managers on each unit, adjusting workflows to align more closely with the capabilities of the new EHR system. This allows for an easier, more seamless integration.

Mark develops a comprehensive training program with the help of the IT department, vendor, and nursing managers to ensure that healthcare providers are proficient in using the new EHR system. Initial training is provided for all staff, but there is ongoing support through the vendor and IT department. Super-users are assigned in each unit who can help provide guidance and support to their coworkers.

Mark wants to ensure that the system is **user-friendly**. He works closely with nurses, physicians, and other healthcare providers to obtain input on the layout of screens and the organization of patient information. This allows him to work with IT and the vendor to customize the system, preventing duplicate data entry and ultimately optimizing data retrieval.

Mark also utilizes change management strategies that can help address any resistance from staff members regarding the new EHR system and facilitate the transition. He communicates the benefits of the new system to the staff and helps address their concerns. Highlighting the fact that there will be continuous support and communication throughout the implementation process will help provide successful integration overall.

Finally, Mark continuously monitors the integration process. He obtains feedback from all end-users to help determine staff satisfaction. He also assesses data to determine the impact on patient care, its efficiency, and documentation accuracy. By reviewing key performance indicators regularly, Mark can determine the success of the EHR system and work with IT to adjust if warranted.

Strategies for Sustaining and Maximizing Outcomes

Process improvement and quality initiatives require measurement, analysis, improvement, and sustainability to be effective. The first component, measurement, involves process mapping as well as data collection and analysis. Both qualitative and qualitative research used in the process must have statistical significance to support change. Nurse leaders must be experts in both interpreting the data and producing quality data visuals that can be easily understood by a broad audience.

Next, analysis tools must be employed to identify the involved processes and failure points. There are a variety of approaches and improvement models that can be utilized to manage a process improvement project. Common models include Plan Do Study Act (PDSA), Just Do It, Rapid Process Improvement Workshop, and Root Cause Analysis. One methodology often used in healthcare and nursing settings is continuous improvement. This model aims to reduce wastes that consume resources but do not add value, eliminate overuse of unneeded items, and lessen burden on resources. Selection of an analysis tool depends on the type of project. For projects in which the problem is not well defined, a deeper analytical tool such as a fishbone diagram or the 5 Whys may be used to disseminate an issue into respective components until the root cause is discovered.

Once the root cause is determined, actions and initiatives should be aimed at directly addressing the identified underlying reasons for the specific issue. When developing actions, it is important to ensure that they target the root cause, are measurable, have defined timeframes, and are feasible and current to the needs of the organization or individuals involved. Outcomes measurement should be planned once the action is developed to support effective measurement of the goal and improve success of the project.

While managing a process improvement project, it is vital to seek feedback and contributions from those individuals who will be most affected. Having these members on the project improvement team can decrease unforeseen complications with implementation ahead of time. Assessing the feasibility of change prior to implementation and gaining buy-in from the start can greatly enhance the probability of adoption and prevent resistance.

Practice Quiz

1. The professional development nurse is discussing process changes with their team based on the lean approach. Which statement should the nurse use to best explain the goal of lean management?
    a. Lean management aims to deliver maximum value to the patient with minimum waste and wait.
    b. Lean management helps reduce staffing and spending as much as possible.
    c. Lean management ensures that every step in a workflow is covered by a policy or protocol.
    d. Lean management addresses the healthcare system's legal and financial exposure to risk.

2. The professional development nurse is reviewing several surveys to assess patient experience. The nurse expects a patient experience survey to focus mainly on which type of questions?
    a. Questions that measure the patient's satisfaction and if their expectations were met for their care on a scale of one to ten.
    b. Questions that ask which behaviors and events occurred during the patient's stay, usually in a yes/no format.
    c. Short-answer questions that ask the patient to reflect on what went well or didn't go well with their care.
    d. Questions related to demographic and health history information.

3. Which action is the cornerstone of providing a positive patient experience?
    a. Maintaining a clean and comfortable physical environment
    b. Preventing errors
    c. Talking with the patient about their own goals, fears, concerns, and priorities
    d. Using plain language to discuss medical care so that the patient and family can understand

4. Which of the following is NOT an example of a nurse-sensitive indicator on an inpatient obstetric unit?
    a. Catheter-associated urinary tract infection (CAUTI) rates
    b. Patient falls
    c. Primary C-section rate
    d. Patient satisfaction scores

5. Regulatory bodies such as TJC and CMS clearly identify which need as one that must be fulfilled in order to promote optimal patient outcomes?
    a. Holistic care model
    b. Discharge planning
    c. Culturally-based care
    d. Patient education

See answers on the next page.

Answer Explanations

1: A. Lean management aims to deliver maximum value to the patient with minimum waste and wait. All other choices are incorrect because they do not represent the goals of lean management. It doesn't aim to reduce staffing or spending as much as possible, Choice *B*. While it is important to know if a workflow is covered by a policy or protocol, Choice *C*, that is not the goal of lean management. Being aware of exposure to risk is not part of lean management, making Choice *D* incorrect.

2: B. Patient experience refers to what did or did not happen in the patient's course of care. Patient satisfaction is distinct from patient experience in that it gauges whether their expectations were met, which makes Choice *A* incorrect. Choice *C* is incorrect because patient experience data does not focus on the patient's opinion about what happened. Choice *D* is incorrect because demographic and health history information is not a primary focus of patient experience.

3: C. While Choices *A*, *B*, and *D* are all contributors, placing the patient at the center of conversation, listening to their concerns, and making them feel included and respected is the fundamental basis of a positive patient experience.

4: C. C-section rates are not a nurse-sensitive indicator because they reflect physician decision-making, not the quality and effectiveness of nursing care. Choice *A*, CAUTI rates, are a nurse-sensitive indicator because they are directly related to activities such as catheter placement and care, which nurses perform. Choice *B*, patient falls, are a nurse-sensitive indicator because they are directly related to nursing activities during patient transfer and ambulation. Choice *D*, patient satisfaction scores, are a nurse-sensitive indicator because they reflect the nurse's interactions with the patient.

5. D: Regulatory bodies such as TJC and CMS clearly identify patient education as a need that must be fulfilled in order to promote optimal patient outcomes. While holistic care, discharge planning, and culturally-based care are important aspects of nursing, these are not identified by TJC and CMS as ones that must be fulfilled in order to promote optimal patient outcomes.

Practice Test #1

1. What would be the best way to evaluate the effectiveness of a training program for new nurse hires on the critical steps of the cleaning process?
   a. Wait until the training course is over to see if they implement their education in the correct way.
   b. Test them on the subject matter before they start working.
   c. Allow them to create their own cleaning solution.
   d. Hold one-on-one meetings with each new hire to receive feedback on their opinions of the cleaning process.

2. Which of the following statements best identifies the meaningful use initiative?
   a. The meaningful use initiative provides financial rewards to providers for better patient outcomes.
   b. The meaningful use initiative is focused on decreasing medication errors.
   c. The meaningful use initiative requires the use of the SOMR for compliance.
   d. The development and use of the electronic health record is the focus of the meaningful use initiative.

3. Which of the following nursing models refers to the patient-focused care that centers around the integration of patient characteristics and nurse competencies within the healthcare environment?
   a. Nursing Leadership Model
   b. Professional Practice Model
   c. Synergy Model
   d. Modular Nursing Model

4. The professional development nurse is providing guidance on the use of a new central line dressing kit. The nurse is implementing which educational concept?
   a. Competency
   b. Knowledge
   c. Training
   d. Evaluation

5. Which of the following is an example of a healthcare provider showing cultural consideration to a patient?
   a. A healthcare provider does not allow a patient's same-sex spouse to visit in the recovery room due to the healthcare provider's religious beliefs.
   b. A healthcare provider allows a patient of the Islamic faith to keep her headscarf on during a physical exam.
   c. A healthcare provider tells a person who identifies as Asian on his intake form that she does not like Chinese food.
   d. A healthcare provider tells an older patient that unless he or she enrolls in the online patient portal, the provider will not provide treatment.

6. When attempting to lift something heavy, which of the following should NOT be done?
   a. Keep the legs straight and bend over to use back muscles.
   b. Spread legs apart and bend at the knees.
   c. Stand close to the object.
   d. Use only feet and legs to turn.

7. A nurse is concerned about the current nursing care delivery system, which relies on traditional task-oriented nursing care. The nurse believes that this system does not provide optimal care for patients, particularly those with complex medical needs. They are considering advocating for a different nursing care delivery system. What is the most appropriate nursing care delivery system for a patient with complex medical needs?

a. Task-oriented nursing care
b. Functional nursing care
c. Team nursing care
d. Patient-centered nursing care

8. The nurse involved in a research study wants to ensure that data was properly analyzed and collected. This nurse is ensuring what aspect of study design?

a. External validity
b. Generalizability
c. Internal validity
d. Replicability

9. Studies have shown that which of the following practices has the most positive impact on patients?

a. Personalized comfort measures in their post-operation room, such as a favorite snack or book
b. Internet and television access during their clinical stay
c. An attentive communication style between their nurses and physicians
d. Visible operation and safety checklists that staff members regularly check and notate

10. The nurse is caring for a patient who is one day post-op from a lung resection and chest tube placement. The patient has been receiving acetaminophen (Ofirmev) 1000mg every 6hrs and requests to have something additional for pain management. The nurse understands that recovering from this surgery with a chest tube can be extremely painful and contacts the surgeon to request an additional PRN medication for pain. This nurse is exhibiting which level of advocacy and moral agency?

a. Level 1
b. Level 2
c. Level 3
d. Level 5

11. At minimum, which sets of standards and guidelines should all nurses familiarize themselves with?

a. FDA and EPA standards and guidelines
b. OSHA and ANA standards and guidelines, in addition to the guidelines of the state in which they work
c. HHS and DPH standards and guidelines for the country and state in which they work
d. CDC standards and guidelines

12. What is the e-prescribing process?

a. The patient electronically contacts their healthcare provider to request new prescriptions.
b. The healthcare provider sends the patient's prescriptions electronically to their pharmacy.
c. The pharmacy accesses the patient's EHR to determine when to automatically refill a prescription.
d. The healthcare provider integrates their EHR system with a partner pharmacy's EHR system.

13. How can the professional development nurse best communicate appropriate and acceptable behaviors within the workplace?

a. Specifically communicate this information to employees during orientation.
b. Hang posters with federal and state regulations in break rooms and lunchrooms.
c. Consistently display ethical, reliable, and acceptable behaviors.
d. Communicate the required behaviors via email and newsletters on a regular basis.

14. A healthcare facility maintains a database that tracks immunization and health screening details required for employees that reduce their risk of healthcare-associated infections. It is designed to flag those individuals in need of updates. The professional development nurse notes that five employees show flags for an update on TB screening. What is the next step?
   a. A group email is sent to these five individuals with locations where the screening may be conducted.
   b. At the next staff meeting, the five individuals are asked to stay behind and are verbally informed of this requirement as a small group.
   c. Each individual is sent a memo making them aware of this situation and a deadline by which the screening should be completed.
   d. Nothing is done; it is assumed that the individuals know what to do and when to do it.

15. In the AACN Synergy Model of nursing practice, which of the following is one of the eight types of client characteristics?
   a. Medical knowledge
   b. Predictability
   c. Insurance coverage
   d. Positivity

16. The professional development nurse is working to create a research project on nosocomial infection. The nurse understands that the PICOT question format refers to which elements?
   a. Population, introduction, cost, outcome, test group
   b. Practice, intervention, change, options, time
   c. Participation, inquiry, cooperation, organization, teaching
   d. Population, intervention, control, outcome, time

17. Which of the following is the best option for erasing confidential digital records?
   a. Hire a certified digital sanitization service.
   b. Delete the files, and empty the computer's recycle bin.
   c. Utilize an open-source disk cleaning software.
   d. Transfer the files to an external storage unit and destroy that storage device.

18. Which of the following is NOT an outcome of the performance management process?
   a. Salary increases and promotions
   b. Growth and development opportunities
   c. Employee satisfaction and morale rate
   d. Disciplinary actions and training needs

19. Which of the following statements is consistent with the concept of moral agency?
   a. The patient's decisions will always be honored.
   b. Nurses assume accountability for their decisions.
   c. Institutions rarely act as moral agents.
   d. Advocacy and moral agency are interchangeable concepts.

20. A nurse is completing a history and physical on a newly admitted patient. How should the nurse communicate with a Spanish-speaking patient?
   a. Speak loud and slowly.
   b. Use a monotone voice to avoid inflection.
   c. Phone the interpreter line for assistance.
   d. Request that a family member translate the discussion.

21. Any deviation from the standard process typically results in higher risk, according to which methodology?
   a. 5 S Methodology
   b. Six Sigma
   c. Lean
   d. National Safety Standards

22. Susan is preparing her team's department objectives that will be used to create individual goals and accomplishments for her employees' performance reviews. What should Susan ensure that each of these objectives includes?
   a. Well-written, clear, concise, and specific language to ensure understanding
   b. Specific, measurable, achievable, relevant, and time-bound aspects
   c. Professional growth, development, training, and learning opportunities
   d. Recognition and appreciation for previous performance and accomplishments

23. In performance management, what is a principal function of rating?
   a. Rating allows management to identify their most productive workers and provide them incentives to retain them.
   b. Because of its narrow statistical application, rating is generally an infrequent practice by management.
   c. Rating provides a way for management to designate their most favored employees.
   d. By having employees rate management, they can more accurately decide for whom and under which conditions they wish to work.

24. What are the two most common workplace safety risks?
   a. Bloodborne pathogens and tripping hazards
   b. Lockout/tagout and confined space hazards
   c. Noise exposure and bloodborne pathogens
   d. Lockout/tagout and tripping hazards

25. A small group of clinical nurses is choosing to improve an existing process related to patient discharge. They have identified that patients have a high re-admittance rate during the summer months. After mapping the current process, they note that patients leave the printout of discharge instructions that they are provided in their hospital room approximately 65% of the time. The nurses set up a meeting to review potential solutions. In which part of the PDCA cycle is this performance improvement plan?
   a. Plan
   b. Do
   c. Check
   d. Act

26. Which of the following nursing interventions is most consistent with the competencies of caring practices, advocacy, and moral agency?
   a. Developing cultural awareness of care team members
   b. Mentoring novice nurses in the use of research findings
   c. Facilitating the patient's transition from one level of care to another on the health continuum
   d. Refining educational programs for patients and families

27. Which statement best describes the Lean Six Sigma approach to process improvement?
    a. The continual and collaborative discipline of measuring and comparing the results of key work processes
    b. A plan to eliminate or lower the likelihood of an error, or to make the occurrence of an error so obvious that any possibility of that error impacting the consumer is practically impossible
    c. To produce more effective processes, policies, and procedures that reduce variation and significantly lower the chances of negative outcomes
    d. A specific methodology that calculates the true costs of a potential solution compared to the actual benefits

28. A nurse follows up with a patient after their treatment has finished, ensuring that the patient is familiar with low-cost outpatient treatment options. Which of the following principles of proper healthcare management is that nurse using?
    a. Idealized influence
    b. Resource utilization
    c. Overprovision
    d. Permanent care maintenance

29. Under HIPAA, when can a patient request an amendment of their health information?
    a. When they disagree with the physician's diagnosis
    b. When the EHR has a factual inaccuracy
    c. When a second provider has provided an alternative diagnosis
    d. When the patient is transferring to the care of a new healthcare provider

30. Which of the following ethical principles is MOST closely related to advocacy?
    a. Distributive justice
    b. Beneficence
    c. Nonmaleficence
    d. Fidelity

31. Which of the following is NOT included in the post-exposure care of a healthcare worker following occupational exposure to the HIV virus?
    a. Post-exposure anti-viral therapy is contraindicated if the exposed person is pregnant.
    b. HIV testing will be repeated at 6 weeks, 12 weeks, and 6 months at a minimum.
    c. The exposed person should avoid blood or tissue donation, breastfeeding, or pregnancy for 6 to 12 weeks after exposure.
    d. Renal and hepatic studies and a CBC will be done at baseline and repeated frequently.

32. Which of the following is NOT one of the domains of the Siebens Domain Management Model for geriatric patients?
    a. Medication management
    b. Medical and surgical diseases
    c. Environmental safety
    d. Physical function

33. Which statement best describes the evaluation phase of the nursing process?
    a. Subjective, objective, and psychosocial data are gathered in this phase.
    b. Nursing diagnoses are formulated during this phase.
    c. Evaluation happens across the continuum of the nursing process.
    d. This phase often begins with educating the patient on expected outcomes.

34. Which of the following is NOT a performance domain designated by CMS for participation in a VBP program?
   a. Clinical outcomes
   b. Patient volume
   c. Safety
   d. Efficiency and cost reduction

35. Which of the following is an example of a short-term strategy to develop workforce competencies?
   a. Increase the academic and professional qualifications in job postings.
   b. Enroll targeted employees in a high-potential development program.
   c. Reassign underperforming employees to positions that better fit their skills.
   d. Organize a week-long training class focused on development of the desired skill.

36. A 60-year-old patient who recently immigrated to the United States and does not speak English fluently has been admitted to the hospital with chest pain and is experiencing significant anxiety due to their inability to communicate effectively with their healthcare providers. What is the best way to provide patient and family-centered care in this situation?
   a. Assigning a nurse to their care who speaks the patient's native language
   b. Providing a professional medical interpreter during all healthcare encounters
   c. Utilizing family members as interpreters during healthcare encounters
   d. Providing written materials in their native language for the patient and family to read

37. Which communication technique hinders the discussion between the nurse and the patient?
   a. Empathetic engagement
   b. Open-ended questions
   c. Nurse-focused answers
   d. Restating

38. Which of the following is NOT one of the measures involved in regulatory compliance to maintain accreditation?
   a. Patient satisfaction
   b. Infection control
   c. Staff qualifications
   d. Emergency preparedness

39. When the nurse is communicating with patients and family members to give education and instruction, which communication approach should they use?
   a. Assertive
   b. Aggressive
   c. Passive
   d. Submissive

40. Which of the following is NOT a benefit of using SBAR?
   a. Nurses spend an excessive amount of time writing, but they are able to draw attention to adverse events using this process.
   b. Nurses are able to focus on patient care.
   c. The SBAR process increases communication among members of the nursing staff.
   d. SBAR eliminates the need for face-to-face communication.

41. Which of the following choices is most consistent with nurses' responsibilities for advocacy?
    a. Notify the nursing supervisor of any conflict to assure resolution of the patient issue.
    b. Consider the patient's point of view and support and explain the point of view as needed.
    c. Provide comprehensive documentation of the patient's care in the EHR.
    d. Understand all relevant laws associated with the nursing care of the patient.

42. Which of the following is an example of the assessment stage of nursing practice?
    a. A newly written policy is reviewed to ensure that it aligns with current accreditation standards.
    b. After the cause of several falls is identified, patient rounds are increased to every 15 minutes for high-risk patients.
    c. A root cause analysis is completed on a unit that demonstrates chronically late medication administration times.
    d. After implementation of an intervention, data is gathered on the metrics related to new wounds acquired on a palliative care unit.

43. To what extent is a medical practice able to guarantee the security of patient information when delivered to the patient electronically?
    a. All digital communications are secure if encrypted.
    b. All digital communications are secure if a patient password is required for access.
    c. Digital communications are mostly secure but can be compromised by human error.
    d. Digital communications are not secure, and physical access to patient information is preferred.

44. Resiliency and stability are examples of traits in which aspect of the Synergy Model?
    a. Nursing competencies
    b. Quality outcomes
    c. Client characteristics
    d. Healthcare environment

45. What is one benefit of electronic health records?
    a. They can be accessed across multiple medical facilities.
    b. They can be accessed internationally, as many countries have adopted the same system.
    c. They require minimal training to adopt.
    d. They can be easily accessed in areas with limited internet service, such as rural areas.

46. Which of the following would be the quickest way to correct a lapse in the practice of wearing gloves while working with patients who may be carriers of infectious disease?
    a. Schedule several training seminars throughout the month so each worker has a chance to attend and learn about the importance of wearing gloves.
    b. Retrain the entire staff on the procedures of caring for patients with a possible infectious disease.
    c. Create a notice that reminds and educates workers on the importance of wearing gloves while working and post the notice around the hospital in areas where it can be clearly read.
    d. Develop a system where workers can provide feedback regarding why they sometimes do not wear gloves.

47. What is the best general definition of a patient portal?
    a. A website that gives patients access to their personal health information
    b. A website that allows patients to send direct messages to their doctors
    c. A website from which patients can download medical-related forms
    d. A website on which patients can make payments for medical services

48. What is the main federal government agency that is responsible for ensuring the health of Americans in their places of employment through the enforcement of regulations and laws?
   a. Department of Labor
   b. Department of Health and Human Services
   c. Centers for Disease Control and Prevention
   d. Occupational Safety and Health Administration

49. Which of the following is true of competitive benchmarking?
   a. It is not advised by TJC.
   b. It can be done by reviewing a competitor's public summary.
   c. It helps improve internal quality processes.
   d. It involves comparison of functions within an organization to each other.

50. Risk managers are trained to evaluate which of the following?
   a. Potential for harm
   b. Outcomes of events
   c. Patient safety
   d. All of the above

51. Which of the OARS communication tools can potentially enhance the patient's self-efficacy?
   a. "Tell me more about that experience."
   b. "Are you saying that ...?"
   c. "I understand your concerns."
   d. "Is there anything else that you would like to say?"

52. When working with adult learners, it is important for the nurse to incorporate which concept into their lesson plan and teachings?
   a. Relate teachings to real-life experiences.
   b. Assume the patient has no prior knowledge of the topic.
   c. Maintain authority and control of the patient during education.
   d. Keep objectives fluid and subjective.

53. Which ethical principle guides the nurse's actions while guaranteeing that the patient with the most critical condition receives priority treatment?
   a. Hedonism
   b. Virtue ethics
   c. Act deontology
   d. Utilitarianism

54. Susan is a professional development nurse in an emergency department. Each morning, she asks her entire staff to convene in the break room for fifteen minutes. During this time, she gives everyone the opportunity to share any concerns for the day. She also goes around the room and asks everyone to briefly share, in one sentence, the biggest event occurring in their personal lives. She closes this session with a minute-long group meditation. Each morning, she also provides a card that has a relaxation exercise to each of her staff members to try during the day. In which stage of the CISM model is Susan engaging her staff?
   a. Pre-Crisis
   b. Acute
   c. Post
   d. Recovery

55. Which of the following is the most important consideration in remote monitoring?
   a. Patient safety and confidentiality
   b. Patient education on the remote monitoring system
   c. Access of data by the patient's PCP
   d. Provider training on remote monitoring

56. Which of the following benefits is associated with a diverse workplace?
   a. Higher employee retention
   b. Higher employee complaints
   c. Increased training needs
   d. Higher employee turnover

57. Which of the following would be the most effective way to present information about workplace misconduct to employees?
   a. Give employees a checklist of workplace DON'Ts based on EEOC guidance.
   b. Show news stories of the recent high-profile cases, along with commentary from legal experts about corporate liability and other worst-case scenarios concerning violations of workplace conduct policies.
   c. Set up a self-paced, remote training session to allow for greater flexibility so the information can reach as many employees as possible.
   d. Schedule mandatory in-person training with employee involvement, such as skits, role plays, and mock juries, to encourage engagement and focus on real-world implications.

58. The professional development nurse has appointed a committee to conduct an audit of its infection prevention program. Although three of the members have done an audit previously, the audits involved acute care facilities and a hemodialysis facility. What should the committee do first?
   a. Review facility policies and procedures to create a checklist.
   b. Collaborate on past experience to create audit tools and timelines.
   c. Visit the CDC website for facility-specific checklists and resources.
   d. Conduct a gap analysis of existing data to prepare a checklist.

59. Which of the following policies encourages openness and transparency with employees?
   a. Communications policy
   b. Social media policy
   c. Open-door policy
   d. Code of conduct policy

60. Which statement correctly identifies the distinction between equitable healthcare and equality of healthcare?
   a. Equitable healthcare means that everyone in a population receives all the care that they require.
   b. Equality of healthcare means that scarce resources are managed appropriately.
   c. There is no distinction between the two kinds of healthcare.
   d. Equality of healthcare means that all people are treated equally.

61. A healthcare provider scores in the 75th percentile for their achievement score for a certain VBP performance domain and in the 97th percentile for their improvement score in the same domain. How many points will they receive, and for what score?
   a. They will receive the maximum number of points due to their achievement score.
   b. They will receive the maximum number of points due to their improvement score.
   c. They will receive less than the maximum number of points due to their achievement score.
   d. They will receive less than the maximum number of points due to their improvement score.

62. Which of the following is a tool from the Six Sigma approach?
  a. Value stream mapping
  b. HRIS
  c. SMART
  d. Flow state diagram

63. Regarding the documentation of care, which choice best reflects the types of items that should be included in the patient's social history on the EHR?
  a. Number and health of friends and relatives; types of regular social activities
  b. Alcohol, smoking, and drug use; living arrangements; marital status; occupation
  c. Chief complaint; review of symptoms; past medical history; family history
  d. Occupation history; compliance with treatment; test and examination results

64. When healthcare providers see patients who are unconscious or not of a sound state of mind, what principle is utilized in order to provide treatment?
  a. Assumption
  b. Risky consent
  c. Informed consent
  d. Implied consent

65. While explaining discharge instructions, the nurse finds that the Japanese American patient frequently nods their head. How should the nurse understand this behavior?
  a. The patient agrees to the discharge plan.
  b. The patient is nervous and unsure of the plan.
  c. The patient is producing normal cultural conduct.
  d. The patient is encouraging the nurse to finish their sentence.

66. Explaining which of the following is NOT a required component in informed consent?
  a. Medical team members involved in treatment or procedure
  b. Risks and benefits of alternative options
  c. Reason for the treatment or procedure
  d. Alternative treatment options

67. The nurse is planning to teach a newly diagnosed diabetic patient, their mother, and their spouse how to draw up and inject insulin before the patient is discharged from the hospital. Which teaching style would be most effective for this group and learning objective?
  a. Lecture
  b. Discussion group
  c. Online module
  d. Hands-on workshop

68. What is one of the main differences between the POMR and the SOMR?
  a. Only nurses can add data to the SOMR.
  b. The POMR facilitates the assessment of patient outcomes.
  c. The SOMR generates less paper.
  d. The POMR separates the notes from each discipline.

69. A healthcare organization is implementing a new electronic medical record (EMR) system, and the nursing staff is expected to complete training and begin using the new system within the next month. However, one nurse is resistant to change and expresses frustration with having to learn a new system, stating that they have always used paper charts and do not see the need for an electronic system. The nurse is a seasoned staff member who has been with the organization for over 20 years. Which stage of the change management process is the nurse in, based on the ADKAR model?

a. Awareness
b. Desire
c. Knowledge
d. Ability

70. According to the nursing theories of culturally sensitive practice, which of the following is the FIRST step?

a. Cultural self-awareness
b. Cultural skill development
c. Cultural knowledge acquisition
d. Cultural implementation training

71. The following are the federally protected classes of the Equal Employment Opportunity Commission EXCEPT?

a. Pregnancy status
b. Genetic information
c. Disability
d. Employees/applicants between eighteen and twenty-six years old

72. The nurse is caring for a patient who comes from a different cultural background than themselves. The nurse respectfully asks the patient about different foods they prefer to eat in their culture so those foods can be discussed with the dietician. This nurse is at which level of responding to diversity in the Synergy Model?

a. Level 1
b. Level 2
c. Level 3
d. Level 5

73. An influx of patients with a known or suspected communicable disease may indicate an act of bioterrorism or an outbreak of a particular disease that is unrelated to bioterror. How do medical personnel and public health officials monitor data in order to identify a situation that may require response protocols?

a. Reference the CDC database for reported cases
b. Use a syndromic surveillance system
c. Receive Federal Emergency Management Agency (FEMA) notification
d. Review electronic medical records

74. A novice nurse is caring for a patient who requires a blood transfusion. The patient, however, has refused the transfusion due to a religious objection. The nurse says, "I don't understand why the patient's sister can't donate the blood. No one should object to receiving blood from a family member when you need it." Which of the following statements correctly identifies the critical issue in this situation?

a. The nurse is displaying an ethnocentric attitude.
b. The nurse thinks that the patient is concerned about contracting an infectious disease.
c. The nurse thinks that the patient doesn't understand the necessity of the blood transfusion.
d. The nurse believes that blood donation from family members is safe.

75. A nurse who is completely engaged in client care and can help anticipate the needs of the patient and family members is said to be at which level of caring practice?
   a. Level 1
   b. Level 3
   c. Level 4
   d. Level 5

76. How does each state board of nursing set the standards a nurse is expected to maintain in practice?
   a. Through its Nursing Practice Act
   b. By mandating a minimum number of continuing education units (CEUs) by nurses in all 50 states
   c. By defaulting to each institution's policies and procedures
   d. Individual states do not set these standards; federal guidelines govern these standards.

77. What is the correct order of the steps for a nurse to create and implement new evidence-based practice guidelines?
   a. Evaluate, appraise, ask, gather, act
   b. Ask, gather, appraise, act, evaluate
   c. Gather, ask, act, appraise, evaluate
   d. Ask, act, evaluate, gather, appraise

78. Which action ensures the successful integration of remote monitoring?
   a. Training nursing staff on the proper use of remote monitoring equipment and software
   b. Establishing partnerships with remote monitoring device manufacturers
   c. Expanding telehealth services to new patient populations
   d. Conducting market research on the latest remote monitoring technologies

79. What should the professional development nurse educate perioperative staff to do during a postoperative follow-up call?
   a. Assess for any changes in health status, address patient and family concerns, validate medication regimen, and provide additional education.
   b. Conduct patient satisfaction surveys.
   c. Assess for changes in health status, but avoid excessive reinforcement education activities.
   d. Focus on positive postoperative outcomes instead of highlighting discrepancies in the patient's recovery.

80. The nurse is delegating the task of getting a set of vital signs to the certified nursing assistant (CNA). The nurse tells the CNA the task to complete, the CNA repeats the task instructions back to the nurse, and the nurse verifies that the message is correct. This is an example of what kind of communication?
   a. Closed-loop communication
   b. Call-out communication
   c. Feedback communication
   d. Open-loop communication

81. What type of programs are used to promote organizational culture by identifying and rewarding individual employees for the work done?
   a. Special event programs
   b. Recognition programs
   c. Inclusion programs
   d. Incentive programs

82. Two nurses get into an argument during their shift about restocking the supply room and go to the professional development nurse to intervene. What is the first step of conflict resolution the nurse should instruct them to take?

a. Present their sides of the argument.
b. Come to a compromise.
c. Discuss options for resolution in detail.
d. Dismiss their argument as non-productive.

83. What is a Lean way of communicating HR programs, policies, and practices, including real-time updates?

a. An employee handbook that is reprinted and redistributed with each new version
b. In-person conferences that regularly review protocols
c. An online employee handbook that is accessible to every employee and is updated online
d. Social media

84. A 72-year-old patient who is postoperative day one after undergoing hip replacement surgery has a patient-controlled analgesia (PCA) device to manage their pain, which they are instructed to use as needed. The nurse is alerted that the PCA device is not functioning properly, and the medication is not being delivered. Which of the following is the appropriate initial action by the nurse when troubleshooting the PCA device for this patient?

a. Discontinuing use of the PCA device
b. Assessing the patient's pain level and providing alternative pain management
c. Checking the connections of the PCA device and repositioning as needed
d. Contacting the healthcare provider for an order to change the medication

85. Which of the following information is NOT included in a literature review?

a. Opinions about the usefulness of each source
b. An analysis of the credibility of each source
c. A summary of each source
d. Test data performed by the researcher

86. A nurse who is at a level 3 of team collaboration according to the Synergy Model has which of the following characteristics?

a. Participates in collaborative efforts
b. Initiates collaborative efforts
c. Mentors others in collaborative efforts
d. Teaches collaboration techniques to others

87. An 80-year-old patient with hearing aids is scheduled to start a new antibiotic regimen with their morning medications. As the nurse is hanging the new medications, they verbally explain what the new medications do and their possible side effects. This nurse is at which level of facilitation of nursing according to the Synergy Model?

a. Level 1
b. Level 2
c. Level 3
d. Level 5

88. What ethical principle sets forth that the nurse must maintain truthful engagements with their patient?

a. Justice
b. Veracity
c. Nonmaleficence
d. Beneficence

89. In reading through annual performance reviews, a leader at a healthcare provider notices that many employees report feeling dissatisfied with their job and unmotivated by the work they do on a regular basis. What style of leadership might the leader find most helpful in amending such an issue?
  a. Democratic leadership style
  b. Laissez-faire leadership style
  c. Situational leadership style
  d. Transformational leadership style

90. Which of the following patients is LEAST likely to experience suboptimal patient care related to implicit bias?
  a. A 45-year-old Caucasian male receiving treatment for congestive heart failure
  b. A 23-year-old Hispanic female receiving treatment for pneumonia
  c. A 78-year-old Caucasian male receiving treatment for urinary tract infection
  d. A 50-year-old African American female receiving treatment for breast cancer

91. Which of the following is the best way to prevent the spread of infection?
  a. Keeping the mouth covered when coughing or sneezing
  b. Disinfecting shared patient equipment
  c. Practicing proper hand hygiene
  d. Avoiding contact with infectious patients

92. Which of the following word pairs identifies the C's of caring practices that demonstrate a commitment to lifelong learning?
  a. Compassion and curiosity
  b. Confidence and collaboration
  c. Conscience and creativity
  d. Commitment and competence

93. Which of the following details are necessary in order for checklists to be effective standardization tools?
  a. Checklists need to be aesthetically pleasing to the practitioner's eye so that he or she is more likely to use it.
  b. Interdisciplinary team members must commit to using the checklist and all members must use the checklist in the same context.
  c. Checklists need to be varied enough so that a diverse group of staff members has appropriate tasks (pertaining to their job role) to check off.
  d. A checklist must have a global presence in order to be considered a standardization tool.

94. A healthcare provider receives additional reimbursement from a private insurance company for meeting certain standards of care against certain populations. This is an example of which of the following?
  a. Shared-risk reimbursement
  b. Capitation
  c. Quality incentives
  d. Bundled payments

95. Which choice provides the most accurate description of MedWatch?
   a. The Food and Drug Administration's system for the public to report drug reactions and drug failures; providers use a different system for medical errors.
   b. The Food and Drug Administration's system for providers and the public to report medical errors, drug reactions, product quality problems, and drug failures
   c. The National Institutes of Health's online system for providers to access the latest publications in medical research and archives of medical news
   d. The National Institutes of Health's online system for the public to access the latest regulations, reports, and other updates concerning healthcare

96. Which action should the nurse delegate to the unlicensed assistive personnel (UAP)?
   a. Obtain sterile equipment
   b. Document early detection education
   c. Provide discharge teaching
   d. Prepare an incident report

97. HR wants to organize a training program on cultural differences in the workplace. Whom should this training target?
   a. Managers and other employees in leadership positions, so they can communicate key practices to their subordinates
   b. Employees who have had problems with cultural misunderstandings in the past
   c. New employees because they are more likely to come from diverse backgrounds
   d. Employees from all levels of the organization

98. Which of the following is NOT one of the eight indicators of nursing competencies?
   a. Systems thinking
   b. Facilitation of learning
   c. Clinical inquiry
   d. Adherence to discharge plans

99. The professional development nurse is gathering a team to conduct a root cause analysis after a sentinel event. Which statement should the nurse use to best describe the overall goal of the team?
   a. "We will be looking to identify the person most responsible for the sentinel event so that we can take appropriate action to either remediate or discipline their behavior."
   b. "We will try to identify the greatest risks to our organization created by this sentinel event and mitigate them."
   c. "We will be looking for the system, human, and cultural failings in the organization that led most directly to this sentinel event so that we can change them."
   d. "We will be conducting a literature search on the best ways to prevent this kind of event from happening in the future."

100. Which of the following sources would contain the most credible information related to sexually transmitted infections (STIs) in college students?
   a. Student publications
   b. Personal anecdotes of those who have been tested for an STI
   c. A hospital report about the types of STIs that are prevalent in an area
   d. A campus survey

101. Which of the following culturally and linguistically appropriate services (CLAS) criteria requires mandatory compliance and reporting for all federally assisted healthcare institutions?

a. Provide effective, equitable, understandable, and respectful quality care and services.
b. Recruit, promote, and support a culturally and linguistically diverse governance, leadership, and workforce.
c. Conduct ongoing assessments of the organization's CLAS-related activities.
d. Ensure the competence of the individuals who provide language assistance.

102. Which of the following is the best example of a patient-centered health goal statement?

a. Patient will demonstrate safe and effective self-administration of insulin.
b. Patient will complete IV antibiotic therapy in two days.
c. Patient will be able to walk for ten minutes, twice daily, before discharge.
d. Patient will verbalize pain level of five out of ten or less throughout day shift.

103. The problem list generated in a POMR is most often displayed as a database. Which of the categories is an essential element of that database?

a. The patient's age
b. The date of onset of the problem
c. The list of the patient's previous medications
d. The patient's weight

104. Evelyn is a professional development nurse who is having trouble with supervisors not submitting their employee evaluations on time. What should Evelyn immediately do to engage the management and supervisory staff in the performance management process?

a. Provide training, forms, required timeline (including due dates), and coaching on delivering employee evaluations.
b. Suggest implementation of a new policy that requires evaluations be conducted by the annual due date or disciplinary actions will be taken.
c. Discuss the situation with the HR director and CEO and request their immediate attention to the issue.
d. Continue to send out emails and communications requesting the documents within the time frame needed.

105. Which process administers, manages, and supports significant transitions related to resource allocation, operations, business processes, and other large-scale changes?

a. Risk management
b. Strategic planning
c. Critical evaluation
d. Change management

106. "The protection, promotion, and optimization of health and abilities, prevention of illness and injury, alleviation of suffering through the diagnosis and treatment of human response, and advocacy in the care of individuals, families, communities, and populations." This statement is best described as which of the following?

a. The ANA Code of Ethics
b. The AACN definition of clinical care
c. The ANA definition of nursing practice
d. The five assumptions of the Synergy Model

107. Which of the following correctly identifies a critical distinction between the two concepts of advocacy and moral agency?

a. Advocacy is legally binding.
b. Moral agency requires accountability for right and wrong decisions.
c. Advocacy is implied in the paternalistic view of patient care.
d. Moral agency only refers to support for at-risk populations.

108. When creating a lesson plan to teach a new topic to a patient and their family, which of the following components would NOT help create and foster a comprehensive lesson plan?

a. Set goals.
b. Create open-ended objectives.
c. Focus on one or two topics.
d. Assess the patient's understanding.

109. Which of the following would be the best source of information related to the way patients were treated to handle the symptoms of hepatitis B in the past?

a. Medical libraries
b. Web browsing
c. Old television hospital dramas
d. Recent medical journals

110. A quality improvement tool is being used to determine the most frequently occurring factors related to increased respiratory infection rates in a healthcare facility. The tool uses a bar graph to determine the frequency of occurrence. This quality improvement tool is known as a:

a. Fishbone diagram
b. Pareto chart
c. Flow chart
d. Gap analysis

111. The professional development nurse is seeking information to improve quality practices related to electronic health record safety. Which organization is most likely to provide information specific to this query?

a. Centers for Disease Control and Prevention (CDC)
b. National Committee for Quality Assurance (NCQA)
c. Centers for Medicare and Medicaid Services (CMS)
d. World Health Organization (WHO)

112. Which of the following agencies ensures safe working conditions for employees by establishing process safety management standards?

a. ADA
b. OSHA
c. HIPAA
d. SOX

113. Which of the following statements most accurately describes the difference between how achievement scores and improvement scores are calculated?
   a. Achievement scores are calculated by determining how effective a patient's particular treatment course was, whereas improvement scores are calculated by determining how cost-efficient a patient's particular treatment course was.
   b. Achievement scores are calculated by comparing a healthcare provider's performance to that of other healthcare providers, whereas improvement scores are calculated by comparing a healthcare provider's current performance to their previously calculated performances.
   c. Achievement scores are calculated by assessing the effectiveness and efficiency of healthcare leaders, whereas improvement scores are used to calculate and assess care effectiveness and efficiency for all healthcare employees.
   d. Achievement scores are used to calculate quality of performance for healthcare providers already considered to be in the top 50% for patient outcomes and experiences, whereas improvement scores are used to calculate quality of performance for healthcare providers ranked in the bottom 50% for patient outcomes and experiences.

114. In the cognitive domain of Bloom's Taxonomy, which of the following is the highest level of cognitive complexity?
   a. Understanding
   b. Analyzing
   c. Applying
   d. Evaluating

115. What does the HCAHPS survey purport to do?
   a. Calculate and publicize data on the likelihood of various medical complications at different healthcare providers.
   b. Estimate how much a healthcare provider spends on each of its patients.
   c. Calculate and show medical team leaders the unique strengths and weaknesses of each of their team members.
   d. Collect and publicize patients' perspectives on healthcare providers and the quality of care they received.

116. A nurse is reading a research article on new treatments for patients with COPD. In order to critically read, the nurse should actively try to determine all of the following aspects of the article EXCEPT:
   a. Thesis
   b. Process
   c. Outcomes
   d. Funding

117. What is the suggested preparatory schedule for accreditation?
   a. Six months of current-process analysis in advance of survey
   b. One year of current-process analysis prior to survey
   c. At least one year of current-process analysis, followed by status updates every three months
   d. One should begin preparing for the next survey immediately after the current one ends.

118. The nurse is completing discharge teaching for a 35-year-old patient who is a lawyer at a local law firm. This patient was admitted following a new breast cancer diagnosis and initiation of chemotherapy. This patient's readiness to learn is most likely to be impacted by which barrier?
   a. Physical restriction
   b. Literacy barrier
   c. Emotional lability
   d. The patient will not be impacted by any barriers.

119. Innovation in healthcare can best be described as which of the following?
   a. Spreading of a new process in a passive manner or unplanned fashion
   b. A form of predictive technology that will enhance physicians' ability to provide medical care
   c. Developing a new process, policy, or standard that improves upon the quality outcomes of previous processes
   d. Providing a format to create uniformity of practice across other departments within the organization

120. Patient rights related to confidentiality and release of medical information are protected by which of the following?
   a. Patient's Bill of Rights
   b. The WHO Surgical Safety Checklist
   c. The Health Insurance Portability and Accountability Act (HIPAA)
   d. TJC National Patient Safety Goals (NPSG)

121. A professional development nurse is evaluating potential education options for teaching in the community about healthy food choices and preventative diabetes care. What type of role would this advocacy fall under?
   a. Public health
   b. Legal
   c. Home health
   d. Patient rights

122. Amy is a nurse practitioner that has begun her shift. Using her designated log-in, she signs into a mobile clinical workstation and reviews how many patients are scheduled for appointments with her during this shift. She notices that her first patient has already been checked in by the front desk staff, so she logs out of the workstation and greets her patient. Once roomed, Amy logs back into the room's clinical workstation and pulls up the patient's medical history and chief complaint to review with him. The patient mentions he has a new allergy to NSAIDs, which Amy documents in his electronic medical record. Later, the patient goes to the clinic's pharmacy to pick up a prescription that Amy ordered. The pharmacist is able to note the patient's updated allergy information and double-checks that the patient's prescription won't cause any issues. He also provides the patient with a patient portal log-in so that the patient can order a refill when he's out of his current medication. What primary tool is the medical organization effectively utilizing to streamline processes, improve documentation, and enhance accessibility to care?
   a. Healthcare information technology
   b. Paper-charting documentation
   c. A nearby pharmacy
   d. A customer-service oriented pharmacist

123. What is a benefit of providing a digital patient portal for a practice's EHR?
   a. Patients can renew prescriptions online.
   b. Patients can digitally sign an ROI.
   c. Patients can check the process of an insurance claim.
   d. Patients can schedule appointments online.

124. Which Lean Six Sigma format targets current processes?
   a. Define, measure, analyze, improve, and control
   b. Define, maintain, analyze, improve, and control
   c. Define, measure, analyze, design, and verify
   d. Define, measure, analyze, investigate, and contain

125. Which piece of federal legislation guarantees 12 weeks of protected, unpaid time off from work for certain employees?
   a. The Americans with Disabilities Act
   b. The Affordable Care Act
   c. The Consolidated Omnibus Budget Reconciliation Act
   d. The Family and Medical Leave Act

Answer Explanations #1

1. B: Regular testing should be done before new hires are considered able to begin work to ensure they fully understand the most critical cleaning procedures taught in training. Waiting until they start working, Choice *A*, or allowing them to try creating their own cleaning solutions, Choice *C*, could result in harmful mistakes. Simply asking for feedback, Choice *D*, may not provide enough quantitative data as to whether or not the educational program is effective because individuals may overestimate their level of confidence in the material.

2. D: The meaningful use initiative is a government-funded incentive program that requires the development and implementation of the EHR. It is based on the assumption that the use of the EHR will positively impact the quality of patient care. The meaningful use initiative rewards are determined by the implementation of the EHR, rather than by patient outcomes. The nurse should be aware that there are other government-funded programs that reward providers for improved outcomes and that this is why medical record models that facilitate outcomes assessment are commonly used by providers. However, Choice *A* is incorrect. The implementation of the EHR may improve patient care error rates; however, that is not the basis for the meaningful use initiative; therefore, Choice *B* is incorrect. The meaningful use plan does not require a specific medical record model, but the literature seems to suggest that the POMR is superior to the SOMR regarding outcomes measurement; therefore, Choice *C* is incorrect.

3. C: The model of nursing that shows the interactions and interconnectivity of a patient's health, the nurses' knowledge and clinical expertise, and the healthcare environment describes the Synergy Model of nursing practice. The Synergy Model encompasses eight client characteristics, eight nursing competencies, and six indicators of quality outcomes in the healthcare environment. Choice *A* is incorrect because the Nursing Leadership Model describes collaborative nursing environments that encourage teamwork and motivation. Choice *B* is incorrect because the Professional Practice Model refers to the overarching model of nursing practice that describes general values and beliefs in the nursing profession. Choice *D* is incorrect because the Modular Nursing Model describes the hierarchy and separate care units involved in patient care.

4. C: Choice *C*, training, is the correct educational concept being used by the professional development nurse. Training involves hands-on experiences, whether simulated or actual, to ensure competency with a new process. Choice *A* is not correct because competency is the term used to describe the efficacy of performing an action. Providing guidance does not guarantee competency. Choice *B* is not correct because knowledge is a broad concept that can be obtained through theory or experiences. Providing hands-on guidance goes beyond a knowledge base. Choice *D* is not correct because evaluation is a tool used to determine whether the implementation is successful.

5. B: In this case, the healthcare provider considered religious and cultural beliefs of the patient to make her feel comfortable during the exam. Effective cultural considerations improve patient satisfaction scores. In the other options listed, the healthcare providers act inconsiderately, insultingly, and make assumptions about the patient's culture.

6. A: When lifting a heavy object, the lower back should not be strained; therefore, bending over and using the back muscles should be avoided. Choices *B*, *C*, and *D* should be done when lifting. Stand close to the object, bend at the knees with legs apart, and use feet and legs to turn if needed.

7. D: Patient-centered nursing care is an approach to care delivery that prioritizes the patient's needs and preferences. This model focuses on individualized care, shared decision-making, and collaborative communication among patients, families, and healthcare providers. Patient-centered care is particularly important for patients with complex medical needs who require individualized attention and comprehensive care plans. Choices *A* and *B* are less comprehensive approaches to care that may not meet the needs of patients with complex medical needs. Choice *C* is a collaborative approach to care delivery but may not provide the level of individualized care needed for patients with complex medical needs.

8. C: Checking that data is properly collected, analyzed, and from an unbiased source ensures that data for a study is internally valid. Choice *A* is incorrect because external validity is ensuring that results in the study participants can be applied to other outside populations. Choice *B* is incorrect because generalizability is a type of external validity where the study results can be useful to larger groups of the population. Choice *D* is incorrect because replicability is the ability for a study to be reproduced and generate outcomes similar to the original study.

9. C: Patients respond favorably to positive intrapersonal communication between their attending nurses and physicians. The other options may be nice for patients, but studies indicate that nurse and physician relationships have the most impact on a patient's overall experience.

10. A: The nurse who is easily able to advocate for a patient and agrees morally with the decision the patient is making is exhibiting Level 1 advocacy and moral agency, the most basic level that emphasizes the work of the nurse. There are three levels of nurse advocacy and moral agency: Levels 1, 3, and 5. Choice *B* is incorrect because Level 2 is not a level of advocacy and moral agency. Choice *C* is incorrect because Level 3 advocacy and moral agency has the nurse advocate for the patient even if what they are advocating for does not directly align with their own personal values. Choice *D* is incorrect because Level 5 advocacy and moral agency is when the nurse uses their position and power to empower clients to request the care and resources that are within their best interests, even if it goes against their personal values.

11. B: Nurses across disciplines are held accountable to the standards and guidelines established by the Occupational Safety and Health Administration, the American Nursing Association, and the specific state where they are licensed and employed. They aren't held accountable individually to any guidelines of the Food and Drug Administration, the Environmental Protection Agency, the Department of Health and Human Services, or the Centers for Disease Control, making Choices *A*, *C*, and *D* incorrect.

12. B: E-prescribing is the process by which a healthcare provider uses electronic communication to send prescriptions directly to the pharmacy. Choice *B* is correct. Choice *A* is incorrect because most prescription refills require an in-person appointment to determine if the medication has an appropriate effect on the illness. Choices *C* and *D* are incorrect because pharmacies and healthcare providers do not operate at that level of electronic integration.

13. C: The best way for HR leadership to communicate appropriate and acceptable behaviors within the workplace is to consistently behave in an ethical, reliable, and acceptable manner. Choices *A, B,* and *D* are all acceptable best practices to ensure that the message of what is appropriate behavior is communicated frequently; however, the best way to communicate this is to model the behavior daily.

14. C: All medical data are private, even for employees, so private notification of required immunizations and screenings is necessary. A deadline encourages compliance in a reasonable time frame. The memo may also include locations where the screening is available. A friendly reminder of required immunizations or screenings is generally appreciated and highly recommended to protect employees and patients from healthcare-associated infections. Choices *A* and *B* are incorrect because both email and small group notification violate Health Insurance Portability and Accountability Act (HIPAA) regulations—they are not private. Choice *D* is incorrect. Although some employees may keep careful track of their own information, many lose track.

15. B: Predictability is one of the eight types of client characteristics in the AACN Synergy Model. The other client characteristics are resiliency, stability, vulnerability, complexity, resource availability, participation in care, and decision-making ability. Choices *A, C,* and *D* are incorrect because these are not characteristics or factors that affect the patient aspect of the Synergy Model.

16. D. The PICOT acronym in research refers to population, intervention, control, outcome, and time.

17. A: Hiring a certified service provider gives the strongest guarantee that the files will be deleted and no remnant of them will remain on the server or storage device. Choices *B* and *D* do not address the possibility that the files could be recovered after deletion. Choice *C* is inappropriate because open-source software—while cost efficient—is generally not certified for use with confidential material.

18. C: The rate of employee satisfaction and morale (Choice *C*) is not an outcome of the performance management process. This rate is determined by an employee survey to establish what the organization does well and what needs to be improved. Standard outcomes of the performance management process are salary increases and promotions, growth and development opportunities, and disciplinary actions and training needs (Choices *A, B,* and *D*).

19. B: When nurses act as moral agents, they are required to also assume responsibility for their decisions. The patient's opinions will be identified and accommodated whenever possible; however, there may be conflict between the patient's opinions and the recommended plan of care, making Choice *A* incorrect. The institution may act as the moral agent for patients without any social support, making Choice *C* incorrect. The difference between moral agency and advocacy is the element of accountability. Moral agents are required to take responsibility for their decisions, making Choice *D* incorrect.

20. C: Choice *C* indicates the appropriate professional response by the nurse to address the present language barrier. Choices *A* and *B* would not directly support communication that is free from misunderstanding and should be omitted. Choice *D* would not rely on a professional, non-biased party for translation and should be avoided if possible.

21. B: According to Six Sigma, any deviation from the standard process typically results in higher risk. Choice *A*, the 5 S method, is incorrect because it is an organization tool used in Lean. Choice *C*, Lean, is incorrect because it focuses specifically on reducing waste, not variety. The National Safety Standards are not a methodology in process improvement, so Choice *D* is incorrect.

22. B: Susan should ensure that each objective includes the SMART aspects: specific, measurable, achievable, relevant, and time-based. Without these aspects, an objective may not be met, or the status could be unknown. By including the SMART aspects, there can be a clear understanding of performance expectations. Choice *A* is incorrect because all language should be well written, clear, concise, and specific, but without SMART aspects, there could still be misunderstandings as to what is to be accomplished. Choices *C* and *D* are inaccurate because professional development and recognition are items within a performance review that are separate from performance objectives. If a training opportunity is to be an objective for an employee, the item should be written as an objective, containing the SMART aspects.

23. A: There are multiple functions of rating in performance management. The first purpose of rating is to give management the opportunity to identify the best performing employees. Once this is done, these employees can be rewarded in various ways, making Choice *A* correct. Conversely, rating is a technique used by management to distinguish poorly performing employees. Underperforming employees can be dealt with in many ways: they can receive a decrease in pay, be forced to attend additional training programs, or ultimately have their employment terminated. Choices *B, C,* and *D* do not accurately reflect functions of rating in performance management, since rating is used frequently and not for the purpose of designating favorites or employees rating management.

24. A: Although all of the hazards listed can occur in a workplace and employers should have a plan to address each, the most common workplace safety risks are bloodborne pathogens and tripping hazards, making Choice *A* correct.

25. A: The nurses are in the planning stage. When they develop a change to implement, they'll be in the Do stage. Once the change has been implemented, they'll check the results and compare them to their baseline re-admittance and printout retention rates. Finally, they'll act to sustain any positive changes.

26. C: Facilitating a patient's transition from one point on the health continuum to another requires caring practices in addition to advocacy and moral agency. Moral agency may be employed to ensure that the patient's wishes are considered, especially those wishes associated with end-of-life concerns. Developing cultural awareness is an example of a response to diversity, and the remaining two choices refer to the facilitation of learning.

27. C: The primary goal of Lean Six Sigma is to produce more effective processes, policies, and procedures that reduce variation and significantly lower the chances of negative outcomes.

28. B: By following up with a patient after their treatment has ended and suggesting further outpatient treatment options, the nurse is ensuring that that patient is offered the most effective and cost-efficient care available. Such efforts are an example of proper resource utilization. Consequently, the correct answer is Choice *B*. Choice *A* is incorrect because such a method can only be practiced between a leader and their team member, not between patient and provider. Choice *C* is incorrect because by offering the patient low-cost treatments, the nurse is in no way contributing to the phenomenon of overprovision. Choice *D* is incorrect because it is not a widely used or known term in the healthcare industry.

29. B: HIPAA provides patients with the right to request a change to their health records if the patient believes the record is based on incorrect facts. HIPAA does not give patients the right to request amendment of a physician's diagnosis; therefore, Choice *A* is incorrect. Choices *C* and *D* are incorrect because these changes do not require the physician to alter their own records.

30. A: Distributive justice refers to the allocation of scarce resources, and advocacy is support for policies that protect at-risk populations. The nurse understands that scarce resource allocation may be sub-standard in certain populations. In nursing, nonmaleficence refers to the act of inflicting the least amount of harm possible in order to reach a favorable result. Fidelity refers to faithfulness but does not specifically address resources or the patient population.

31. A: Anti-viral therapy will be started immediately after exposure, without waiting for further specialty consultation if the exposed person is pregnant due to the risk of the unborn fetus. HIV testing will be conducted at frequent intervals to monitor for the presence of evidence of infection; therefore, Choice *B* is incorrect. The precautions listed in Choice *C* are necessary to prevent possible contamination in the event that the exposure has resulted in infection of the exposed individual by the HIV virus; therefore, Choice *C* is incorrect. Renal, hepatic, and hematology studies are monitored to assess any effects of the HIV virus and/or the effects of anti-viral medications if ordered; therefore, Choice *D* is incorrect.

32. A: Medication management is not included in the Siebens Domain Management Model. The missing domain is mental status, which also includes emotions and coping. The remaining choices are consistent with the model that was developed to plan the care for elderly patients by consideration of the limitations imposed by the subcategories of each domain. Therefore, Choices *B, C,* and *D* are incorrect.

33. C: The final phase of the nursing process is evaluation; however, evaluation happens across the continuum of the nursing process, not just at the end. The nurse frequently evaluates the effectiveness of care plans, adjusts as necessary, and reevaluates. Data is collected during the assessment phase. Nursing diagnoses are formulated in the diagnosis phase. The implementation phase often begins with educating the patient on expected outcomes.

34. B: In order for a healthcare provider to be allowed to participate in a VBP program, there are four distinct performance domains for which they need to demonstrate quality of care. These domains are clinical outcomes, person and community engagement, safety, and efficiency and cost reduction. Therefore, the correct answer is Choice *B* because no considerations are made depending on the overall number of patients a healthcare provider sees and treats. All of the other answer choices accurately reflect the various performance domains designated by CMS for participation in a VBP program.

35. D: Organizing a week-long training class focused on desired skill development, Choice *D*, is the best strategy. Although building the skills, knowledge, and competencies of the workforce is an ongoing responsibility of the HR department, sometimes there are short-term skills gaps that need to be closed. In this case, organizing a class or workshop to directly target the missing skill is a practical and effective approach. For example, if many employees are struggling with adopting new workplace software, a few training courses can help them get up to speed. Choice *A* is not the best choice because interviewing and onboarding new employees is very time-consuming and not the best short-term strategy. Choice *B* is also not the best choice because a high-potential development program should carry employees throughout the time at an organization until they are positioned to become leaders; again, this is a long-term rather than short-term development strategy. Finally, Choice *C* is not the best choice because, while internal reassignment can help employees to find positions that best fit their competencies, this choice does not solve the problem because it removes underperforming employees without replacing them or building the skills of remaining workers.

36. B: Providing a professional medical interpreter will ensure that the patient is able to communicate their needs effectively and receive appropriate care, while also alleviating the anxiety that they are feeling in this difficult situation. Choice *A* is not always a possible solution. Choice *C* can lead to inaccurate communication, as they may not be trained in medical terminology and may have difficulty remaining objective. Choice *D* may be helpful but does not give the patient or their family the opportunity to communicate their needs.

37. C: Choice *C* represents a hindrance to the development of a therapeutic nurse-to-patient discussion and should be avoided. Choice *A* displays understanding, Choice *B* encourages deeper dialogue, and Choice *D* shows comprehension of what the patient communicated.

38. A: Regulatory compliance standards required to maintain accreditation include infection control, staff qualifications, and emergency preparedness. Patient satisfaction scores, Choice *A*, are not part of the regulatory compliance review process. However, maintaining accreditation status will greatly increase the trust of patients and provide a positive impact on patient satisfaction.

39. A: When teaching and communicating with patients and families, nurses should strive for an assertive communication style. In this style, nurses communicate and convey their thoughts and beliefs without coming off as antagonistic or unsure of their ideas. Choice *B* is incorrect because aggressive styles of communication do not encourage collaborative communication and may come off as offensive to patients. Choices *C* and *D* are incorrect because passive and submissive communication styles may make it seem as though the nurse lacks confidence and knowledge. Additionally, nurses may not complete their intended educational goals and objectives with this style if they cannot competently present their knowledge or ideas.

40. D: The SBAR technique is a best practice that allows nurses to focus on providing patient care because it decreases the amount of time they spend writing. Also, the design of this process promotes open communication among the nursing team. SBAR can be used face-to-face or by telephone, and it should always be a verbal conversation.

41. B: Sharing, supporting, and explaining the patient's point of view are activities that are consistent with advocacy. The remaining choices contribute to good professional practice but are not specifically related to the concept of advocacy.

42. A: Review of existing policies is completed during the assessment phase. Choice *B* is incorrect, as this is the implementation stage. Choice *C* is incorrect, since conducting a root cause analysis occurs during the identifying issues, problems, or trends stage of the process. Choice *D* is incorrect, as this describes the evaluation phase.

43. C: Digital communications—such as email—and certified electronic healthcare record (EHR) systems are generally secure for accessing and transmitting confidential patient information. However, no system is foolproof, and it is important that the medical assistant educates patients about the risks of data management when using an EHR.

44. C: The Synergy Model shows how client characteristics and nursing competencies work together in a healthcare environment to affect quality outcomes. Resiliency and stability are aspects of client characteristics in the Synergy Model. Other client characteristics include vulnerability, resource availability, participation in care, decision-making ability, predictability, and complexity. Choices *A, B,* and *D* are incorrect because these characteristics are not part of those sections of the Synergy Model.

45. A: A major benefit of an electronic health record is that it can be easily accessed by multiple providers, which increases access to coordinated, interdisciplinary care for patients, improves quality of care, and reduces medical errors. Additionally, patients can access their medical records easily, which can improve patient satisfaction. At this time, types of health records used vary by country, and accessing one's record in a different country will likely require additional steps. Therefore, Choice *B* can be eliminated. Training is extensive, as users need to be trained on data input, data management, security, and other administrative protocols, so Choice *C* can be eliminated. Rural facilities have had a harder time with the implementation and adoption of electronic health record systems due to lower tech literacy in patient populations and limited tech and internet availability; therefore, Choice *D* can be eliminated.

46. C: Immediate action needs to be taken when lapses in established procedures are observed. Posting a notice could be done to reach the greatest number of people without taking up too much time. Retraining the entire staff, Choice *B*, or waiting for more feedback, Choice *D*, are processes that would take too long to organize. Choice *A* would also take too long and cause too much loss of work time for procedures that have already been taught.

47. A: The best general definition of a patient portal is a secure website that gives patients convenient 24-hour access to their personal health information, such as recent doctor visits, discharge summaries, prescribed medications, and lab results. Choices *B, C,* and *D* are incorrect because they all describe specific activities that may be available with some, but not all, patient portals.

48. D: The Occupational Safety and Health Administration (OSHA) was created in 1970 as the main federal government agency that has responsibility for ensuring the health and safety of Americans in their places of employment through the enforcement of federal regulations and laws. OSHA is an agency within the Department of Labor, but the department as a whole has numerous other responsibilities, so Choice *A* is incorrect. The Department of Health and Human Services (HHS) is responsible for enhancing the health and well-being of all Americans—not just workers—by providing various services, so Choice *B* is incorrect. The Centers for Disease Control and Prevention is an agency within HHS that is tasked with protecting public health through the control and prevention of infectious diseases, injuries, and disabilities and through education and research, so Choice *C* is incorrect.

49. B: Competitive benchmarking can help reveal how comparable organizations solved defects similar to what a given healthcare organization is facing. The comparative analysis can also illuminate how the current processes are outpacing the competitors, which encourages the integration of what works with what does not work well enough. This approach will help the leadership team deliver on the promise of providing exceptional care. All hospitals are required to post their quality information on their websites for public view, which can be utilized for competitive benchmarking, as in Choice *B*. Choice A is incorrect since the Joint Commission does not discourage this practice. Choices *C* and *D* are incorrect since they refer to internal benchmarking.

50. D: Risk managers are trained in comprehensive evaluation of the potential for harm, outcomes of events, and patient safety, making Choice *D* correct.

51. C: Understanding the patient concerns validates the patient's viewpoint, which can enhance the patient's self-image. A positive self-image can increase self-efficacy, which is the patient's perception of the ability to succeed. Choice *A* engages the patient with an open-ended question; therefore, Choice *A* is incorrect. Choice *B* asks for clarification, but it will not enhance self-efficacy, so Choice *B* is incorrect. Choice *D* is part of a summary statement that is giving the patient the opportunity to contribute more information, so Choice *D* is incorrect.

52. A: When working with adult learners, it is important for the nurse to relate the teachings to real-world experiences. This acknowledges patients' prior knowledge and experience and helps provide a more robust teaching and understanding that adult learners can utilize. Choice *B* is incorrect because the nurse should not assume the patient has no prior knowledge, as this can come off as belittling and limit the extent to which the nurse can teach. Instead, the nurse should assess the prior knowledge the patient has and tailor the teaching level and material accordingly. Choice *C* is incorrect because by maintaining authority and control, the nurse does not allow the patient to be involved in learning and may invalidate concerns they have. This approach may also come off as disrespectful when trying to educate adult learners. Instead, the nurse should have a professional and collaborative approach. Choice *D* is incorrect because keeping objectives fluid and subjective may make it more difficult for patients to understand the goals they are trying to reach and more difficult for the nurse to assess their learning. Objectives should be clear, measurable, and goal focused.

53. D: Choice *D* includes bringing about the greatest good for the greatest number of people, which is what the nurse does when prioritizing patient care. Choices *A*, *B*, and *C*, while all ethical considerations, do not align with the nurse's actions at this time.

54. A: The Pre-Crisis stage of the CISM model provides tools for nursing staff to relax, mentally prepare any traumatic incidences, and voice any concerns they have for the day. The other stages listed address actions during and after traumatic incidences.

55. A: Patient safety and confidentiality is the most important consideration when it comes to remote monitoring. Data should be transferred to the patient's overseeing provider through secure networks to protect their private health information. Choices *B* and *D* are both important considerations but not the most important, making them incorrect. Choice *C* is also an important consideration, but the data recorded via remote monitoring doesn't necessarily go to the patient's PCP; instead, it goes to the provider that ordered the remote monitoring. However, the PCP can review data to provide continuity of care if needed.

56. A: Organizations that have a more diverse workplace experience higher rates of employee retention, making Choice *A* correct. Additionally, employees are generally more satisfied and perform at a higher level than employees in workplaces that lack diversity, making Choices *B*, *C*, and *D* incorrect.

57. D: Scheduling mandatory in-person training with employee involvement, such as skits, role plays, and mock juries, encourages engagement and focus on real-world implications, making Choice *D* correct. Workplace conduct is a topic that HR should emphasize for all employees with a high level of engagement. HR has made the right first step in deciding to proactively address workplace harassment and misconduct; however, establishing clear guidance and creating a culture of civility comes from true engagement with employees. For this reason, Choice *C* is not the best choice, because employees will be passive learners. Also, while Choice *A* might be a good supplementary resource, employees also need positive modeling and information about how they *should* behave in the workplace, rather than just negative information about how they *should not* behave. Finally, Choice *B* is not the best choice because abstract legal implications may not have a strong connection to employees. Instead, Choice *D* gives employees a chance to explore situations that affect their everyday workplace interactions.

58. C: Facility-specific checklists and resources published on the CDC website include all the information required to plan and conduct an effective audit. Choice *A* is incorrect; although reviewing facility policies and procedures is part of an audit, creating a checklist from existing policies may miss a policy that has not been updated to meet a new regulation or requirement. Choice *B* is incorrect because although past experience has value, audit items specific to an outpatient facility might be missed if relying on previous experience alone. Choice *D* is incorrect because data for gap analysis are not available until the audit is completed.

59. C: An open-door policy specifically encourages openness and transparency with employees. Managers and leadership often implement an open-door policy to ensure that employees know they are welcome to provide insights and feedback without fear of recourse. Choice *A* is incorrect because a communications policy is a broad policy that encompasses all areas of communication, including a social media policy, which is Choice *B.* Choice *D* is incorrect because a code of conduct policy is written to ensure employees are aware of and understand ethical and appropriate behaviors in the workplace.

60. D: Equality of healthcare means that all people are treated equally. For instance, patients should be added to donor lists based only their medical needs. Equitable healthcare refers to the proper management of scarce resources, which can be illustrated by the use of donated organs. The difference can be explained by viewing equality at the level of the individual patient, and equity at the level of the provider. Therefore, Choices *A, B,* and *C* are incorrect.

61. B: Achievement and improvement scores are the two kinds of measurements used to determine a healthcare provider's score for a particular performance domain of the CMS VBP program. Both scores are calculated as a percentile, with achievement scores being compared against other health providers' scores for that particular measurement and improvement scores being compared against the healthcare provider's previously recorded measurements. The number of points a provider ultimately receives is determined by first choosing whichever score is higher and then comparing that score against a threshold and benchmark score, set at the 50th percentile and the mean of the top decile, respectively. If the provider scores at or above the benchmark score, they receive full points for that measurement. Therefore, the correct answer is Choice *B.* As described, the other answer choices cannot be correct in this scenario.

62. A: Value stream mapping is a tool from the Six Sigma approach that shows the value added by each step within a process. HRIS (Choice *B*) refers to information systems. SMART (Choice *C*) is an acronym to guide goal setting. Flow state diagrams (Choice *D*) are not a business tool.

63. B: A patient's social history, which is one aspect of the documentation of care, should include such items as alcohol, smoking, and recreational drug use; living accommodations and arrangements; marital status; occupation; and baseline functioning. Choice *A* is incorrect because the number of friends and relatives and types of social activities are features of social behavior, but they do not accurately represent a medically relevant social history. Choices *C* and *D* are incorrect because chief complaint, review of symptoms, past medical history, family history, occupation history, compliance with treatment, and test and examination results are other aspects of the documentation of care.

64. D: When patients are physically or psychologically unable to provide verbal or written consent to treatment, healthcare providers rely on implied consent, acting on the belief that the patient would like the best treatment to benefit their life.

65. C: Choice *C* indicates a thorough understanding of cultural considerations to care as this behavior represents normal cultural conduct. Choices *A*, *B*, and *D* are inappropriate as this behavior does not insinuate anything more than cultural norms regarding the patient's level of understanding, agreement, or pace of discussion.

66. A: It is not a requirement for the informed consent to list all members of the team involved in the treatment or procedure. However, the patient should still have a general understanding of the care they will be receiving from team members. Choices *B, C,* and *D* are incorrect because these are required components in informed consent. Other required components include risks and benefits of not having the procedure.

67. D: Using a hands-on workshop would be a beneficial teaching style for drawing up and injecting insulin since this is a hands-on, tactile technique to learn. Additionally, hands-on workshops are also conducive for small group settings, such as this one with a patient, spouse, and parent. Choice *A* is incorrect because lecture-style learning would be more beneficial for a large group setting. It may also be more difficult to learn a practical procedure in a lecture setting. Choice *B* is incorrect because, although a discussion group is a good style for a smaller group, it does not have the benefit of being able to teach the practical and technical skills needed for insulin administration. Choice *C* is incorrect because online or computer-based learning would be more beneficial if the learners were remote; however, this group is still in the hospital before being discharged.

68. B: The problem list in the POMR demonstrates the effect of the interventions on the resolution of the individual problems. This chronological record can be used as an outcome measure that is an essential element of the meaningful use standard. The SOMR does not specifically track the resolution of individual problems and therefore is less useful for outcomes assessment than the POMR. Any provider that renders care for the patient documents that care in the SOMR; therefore, Choice *A* is incorrect. There is no evidence that the SOMR generates less paper. In fact, the opposite may be true because each provider maintains a separate entry in the medical record; therefore, Choice *C* is incorrect. The POMR is a chronological compilation of the patient care documentation by all disciplines; therefore, Choice *D* is incorrect.

69. B: The ADKAR model is a change management framework that includes five stages: Awareness, Desire, Knowledge, Ability, and Reinforcement. The model suggests that in order for change to be successful, individuals must progress through each of these stages in order. In this scenario, the nurse is expressing frustration with having to learn a new system, indicating that they may not have a strong desire to change. In order to move forward with the implementation of the new EMR system, the nurse will need to progress through the remaining stages of the ADKAR model, including gaining knowledge about the new system, developing the ability to use it, and receiving reinforcement and support to sustain the change. Choice *A* is incorrect because the nurse is already aware that the organization is implementing a new EMR system. Choice *C* is incorrect because the nurse has not yet completed the training on the new EMR system, indicating that they may not have the necessary knowledge to use the new system. Choice *D* is incorrect because the nurse has not yet gained the ability to use the new EMR system, as they have not yet completed the necessary training.

70. A: The first step to culturally sensitive practice is the assessment and acknowledgment of one's own biases and stereotypes. Without this self-awareness, the nurse's actions can be unduly influenced by these personal beliefs. Cultural awareness is necessary to gain the knowledge and skills needed to implement culturally competent patient care. Therefore, Choices *B, C,* and *D* are incorrect.

71. D: While you should not discriminate for any reason, the EEOC guideline on ageism protects those above the age of forty. Pregnancy status, genetic information, and disability are all protected under the Equal Employment Opportunity Commission, making Choices *A*, *B*, and *C* incorrect.

72. C: There are three levels of responding to diversity in the Synergy Model: levels 1, 3, and 5. According to the Synergy Model of responding to diversity, a nurse who is seeking information about the cultural background of a patient and beginning to incorporate some of this diversity into the patient's care is said to be at a level 3 of diversity response. Choice *A* is incorrect because at level 1, the nurse is just beginning to assess different cultural backgrounds with basic questions and may not be incorporating these findings into diverse care. Choice *B* is incorrect because level 2 is not one of the levels of responding to diversity in the Synergy Model. Choice *D* is incorrect because level 5 is when the nurse is actively incorporating diverse cultural knowledge into the patient's care and can help think of alternative or preferred models for delivery of care that are aligned with the patient's diverse cultural beliefs.

73. B: Electronic syndromic surveillance systems may be used locally, state-wide, or nationwide. The national version receives data from local and state facilities as well as the Center for Disease Control and Prevention (CDC). This type of system can predict an outbreak or threat based on symptoms even before a diagnosis is confirmed. Choice *A* is incorrect; although the CDC does maintain a database of health issues to monitor outbreaks, the CDC database relies on reports from other health professionals and facilities. Choice *C* is incorrect because FEMA directs efforts to prepare for and recover from natural disasters. FEMA does not collect health data. Choice *D* is incorrect because although electronic medical records are great tools to track individual patients, these software programs do not offer an option to track diagnostic data among populations.

74. A: The novice nurse is comparing her own beliefs to the patient's beliefs and lacks the knowledge to understand the patient's point of view. This is the definition of ethnocentrism, which can adversely affect the nurse-patient relationship. The remaining observations could potentially affect the patient's refusal of the therapy; however, the patient's refusal in this example is clearly related to the religious objection.

75. D: There are three levels of caring practice for the nurse: level 1, level 3, and level 5. A nurse who is completely involved in a patient's care and able to anticipate needs to provide safe, dignified, and comfortable care is considered to be at the highest level of caring practice, level 5, Choice *D*. Choice *A* is incorrect because level 1 care provides the most basic care of creating a safe environment for a patient. Choice *B* is incorrect because level 3 care involves kind and compassionate care from a nurse, but the nurse may not be as fully engaged in managing and anticipating a patient's needs. Choice *C* is incorrect because level 4 is not one of the levels of caring practice for the nurse.

76. A: Each state board of nursing has a Nursing Practice Act that sets the standards of care a nurse is expected to maintain in practice. All 50 states do not require nurses to maintain a minimum number of CEUs. Policies and procedures vary from institutions within each state. Nursing Practice Acts are regulated by states, not federally.

77. B: When creating and implementing new evidence-based practice guidelines, the nurse should ask a question of clinical inquiry, gather evidence, appraise this evidence, act and implement new guidelines, and then evaluate the effectiveness of their guidelines. Choices *A, C,* and *D* are incorrect because they do not have the steps of evidence-based practice inquiry in the correct order.

78. A: When implementing remote monitoring in a telehealth program, a priority for the nurse administrator is to ensure that nursing staff are trained on the proper use of remote monitoring equipment and software. Adequate training is vital to ensure accurate data collection, interpretation, and appropriate response to patient data received through remote monitoring. Choice *B* may be a consideration, but training nursing staff is more essential to the successful integration of remote monitoring. Choice *C* is a broader goal that may be pursued after ensuring the successful implementation of remote monitoring. Choice *D* is not the top priority in ensuring the successful integration of remote monitoring, although this option can be valuable for staying informed.

79. A: Postoperative follow-up calls are an opportunity for perioperative staff to assess recovery of the patient, address questions, provide reinforcement education, and identify any discrepancies that could have a negative impact on the patient's postoperative period. Patient satisfaction calls are not typically conducted by the perioperative staff.

80. A: The communication style in which someone sends a message or instruction, someone receives the message, the receiver repeats the message back, and then the initial sender verifies the message is called closed-loop communication. Closed-loop communication is important in the healthcare setting and when delegating tasks to ensure that the instructions are clear and received accurately. Choices *B* and *C* are incorrect because they are each only one step of the closed-loop communication style. Choice *D* is incorrect because in open-loop communication there is no feedback step and the person receiving the instruction does not repeat it back for verification. This communication style is faster but allows more room for error.

81. B: Recognition programs are programs used to promote a positive organizational culture by recognizing individual employees for the work they have done. Recognition programs can be formal or informal and can have a large impact on employees. Special event programs (Choice *A*) are designed to promote a positive culture; they generally do not reward employees for their work. Inclusion programs (Choice *C*) are incorporated into day-to-day operations to ensure that all employees' voices are heard. Incentive programs (Choice *D*) provide financial rewards to those employees who perform at a higher level than others and have a larger impact on the organization.

82. A: The first step of conflict resolution should be for both sides to present their side of the disagreement calmly and professionally. This allows whoever is mediating the conflict to understand the opinions of both sides. Choices *B* and *C* are incorrect because these steps come later in conflict resolution. After presenting the sides of the argument, the disagreement should be discussed in detail, eventually coming to a compromise or some negotiation or re-evaluation. Choice *D* is incorrect because disagreements should not be dismissed. Using conflict resolution can help teams grow and build better communication.

83. C: An online handbook (Choice *C*) is the best option, as it is a paperless method with an immediate notification system that minimizes waste yet keeps all employees informed. Choice *A* and *B* are not as immediate or up-to-date, making them incorrect. Social media, Choice *D,* is not an appropriate place to house policies and practices.

84. C: In this case, the nurse should first check the connections of the PCA device and reposition as needed to ensure proper delivery of medication to the patient. Choices *A, B,* and *D* may be appropriate actions if the issue cannot be resolved through assessment and troubleshooting.

85. D: A literature review does not include test data performed by the researcher. It only reviews work done in the past, and validation of the source is based on the source's credentials and information provided, not on the ability to reproduce its data. It consists of an examination of all the literature compiled for research on a subject, including opinions, Choice *A,* analyses, Choice *B,* and summaries, Choice *C,* of each source.

86. B: According to the AACN Synergy Model, a nurse who is at a level 3 of team collaboration helps initiate collaborative efforts with interdisciplinary team members and actively tries to find activities that continue collaboration. Choice *A* is incorrect because only participating in collaboration with team members is level 1. Choices *C* and *D* are incorrect because teaching and mentoring others to continue to spread and grow collaboration is level 5, the highest collaborative level in the Synergy Model.

87. A: In the AACN Synergy Model, there are three levels: levels 1, 3, and 5. A nurse at a level 1 in facilitation of learning can deliver their planned education to a patient; however, this may be done without fully assessing learning readiness and ability. The ability to competently and expertly facilitate learning requires the nurse to not only create their educational content, but also assess any barriers and adapt these lessons to the individual patient or group. Choice *B* is incorrect because level 2 is not one of the levels in the ability to facilitate learning. Choice *C* is incorrect because level 3 facilitation would exhibit the nurse tailoring some of their teachings to the basic needs or obstacles in a patient's learning. Choice *D* is incorrect because level 5 facilitation of learning would have the nurse able to completely understand the patient's preferred learning styles, teaching methodology, and ability to learn. The nurse would then also be able to fully adapt their teaching and lesson plan to these preferences.

88. B: Choice *B* aligns with the ethical principle to maintain truthful engagements. Choice *A* aligns with ethical fairness. Choice *C* aligns with refraining from harm. Choice *D* promotes doing right by the patient.

89. D: The style of leadership most often associated with motivating team members and improving their work satisfaction is transformational leadership style. Unlike other styles of leadership, transformational leadership style has as its central concept the idea that team members work best and hardest when they feel the internal motivation to do so. Therefore, the correct answer is Choice *D*. The other answer choices refer to styles of leadership that are not known to be particularly effective at motivating team members or helping them find satisfaction in their work.

90. A: The patient described in Choice *A* is the least likely to experience suboptimal care relating to implicit bias. Implicit bias is the unconscious stereotypes, beliefs, and values that influence our decisions and behaviors. Females, people of color, and the elderly are all at risk for receiving substandard patient care relating to negative stereotypes. Therefore, Choice *B* is not correct because this patient is a Hispanic female. Choice *C* is incorrect because this patient is elderly. Lastly, Choice *D* is incorrect because this patient is an African American female. Patients with lower socioeconomic status and non-heterosexual orientation are also more at risk for experiencing the adverse effects of implicit bias. Lastly, individuals with disabilities, mental health disorders, history of drug abuse, and obesity are also at increased risk of receiving substandard care related to caregiver bias.

91. C: All of the answer choices are types of standard precautions, but research has shown that handwashing is the best way to prevent the spread of germs.

92. D: The nurse demonstrates professional competence as a result of a commitment to lifelong learning that is required for all areas of nursing. The other choices each contain only a single element of the five elements of caring: commitment, conscience, competence, compassion, and confidence.

93. B: A checklist can only be useful if all active members work together to use it at the same time; otherwise, it cannot produce standardized results. Aesthetically pleasing checklists can be nice but aren't necessary.

Checklist tasks should always be repeatable and reliable; therefore, diverse tasks would make a poor checklist. A checklist doesn't need a global presence to be a reliable tool; it simply needs to be accepted by the organization and staff where it's being used as a quality tool.

94. C: Quality incentives refer to a form of value-based payment in which a healthcare provider can receive additional reimbursement based on their standard of care. Typically, such an arrangement is made between a private health insurance company and a provider, with the insurance company incentivizing the healthcare provider to hopefully increase the effectiveness and efficiency of care at a facility their clients use. Therefore, the correct answer is Choice *C*. All the other answer choices describe other types of VBP (value-based purchasing) reimbursement methods, none of which have the same reward structure as quality incentives.

95. B: MedWatch is the Food and Drug Administration's system for both healthcare providers and the public to report medical errors, drug reactions, product quality problems, and drug failures, as well as problems with medical devices, dietary supplements, foods, and cosmetics. Choice *A* is incorrect because MedWatch is not only for the public. Choices *C* and *D* are incorrect because MedWatch is not a program of the National Institutes of Health, and the stated purposes of the program are inaccurate.

96. A: Choice *A* indicates an action that aligns with the scope of practice of the unlicensed assistive personnel (UAP) and can safely be delegated by the nurse. Choices *B*, *C*, and *D* indicate actions that should be carried out by the nurse, as they align with the scope of practice of the nurse and not with the scope of the UAP.

97. D: Diversity and inclusion (D&I) should be part of an organization-wide policy that involves all employees in each level of the organization, making Choice *D* correct. Choice *A* is not the best answer because key training messages may get lost in translation as they travel from leadership-level employees to their subordinates. Choice *B* is also not the best answer because it reacts to past problems rather than working to proactively create a workplace culture that avoids such conflict. Choice *C* is incorrect because long-standing employees also need training to adapt to changing workplace conditions.

98. D: Adherence to discharge plans is not one of the eight indicators of nursing competencies; however, it is one of the six indicators of quality outcomes in the healthcare setting. Choices *A, B,* and *C* are incorrect because they are all indicators of nursing competencies. The other nursing competencies are clinical judgement, advocacy, caring practices, collaboration, and diversity response.

99. C: A root cause analysis is a process used to examine all of the factors that contributed to an error, to analyze where changes are most appropriate, and to create a plan for change. Choice *A* is incorrect because it assumes the root cause is human error and takes a punitive approach. Choice *B* is incorrect since this is a risk-management approach to the problem, not a root-cause approach. Choice *D* is incorrect because, while a literature search on ways to prevent the problem in the future may be a final step in a root cause analysis, it does not best describe the overall goal.

100. C: Observational data that has been recorded and validated (Choice *C*) is always more credible than unpublished accounts, such as personal anecdotes, Choice *B*. Student publications, Choice *A*, or surveys, Choice *D*, might also contain fabrications because the information could be falsified by individuals who are participating, and the data collected from their accounts cannot be validated as accurately as hospital data.

101. D: Federally assisted care institutions are held to mandatory compliance with the communication standards of the CLAS criteria, such as the provision of skilled interpreters. The remaining standards are focused on providing culturally sensitive care but do not require mandatory compliance and reporting; therefore, Choices *A*, *B*, and *C* are incorrect.

102. C: "Patient will be able to walk for ten minutes, twice daily, prior to discharge." is the best example of a patient-centered goal statement. Effective goal statements can be formulated using the *SMART* goal criteria: specific, measurable, achievable, relevant, and time-bound. Choice *A* is not the best example of a patient-centered goal statement, as the statement could be more specific and is not measurable or time-bound. Choice *B* is also not the best example of a patient-centered goal because this is not patient-driven and is not specific or measurable. Choice *D* is also not the best choice because this goal does not provide a specific means to achieve the pain level of five out of ten or less.

103. B: The database entries should include the problem, the date of onset, the interventions, and the date of resolution of the problem. The problem list is a chronological record of the patient's progress from the time of the current interventions, which means that details such as the patient's weight and previous medications have already been considered in the development of the problem list. Therefore, Choices *A*, *C*, and *D* are incorrect.

104. A: Although of all these actions may be appropriate at times to address the issue, the first thing Evelyn should do is to provide training to the managers and supervisors, making Choice *A* correct. This training should include information on the process, forms, and timeline, as well as coaching on how to deliver an effective evaluation. Evelyn should respond to questions and provide real-life examples to situations that may arise during the process.

105. D: Change management is the process that seeks to support significant transitions within an organization and could include large-scale changes, resource allocation, operations changes, and an updated business process. Effective change management can help an organization to be successful during transition periods. Choices *A*, *B*, and *C* relate to management of risk, strategy, and evaluation processes, rather than assisting with change.

106. C: The statement provided in the question is the ANA definition of nursing practice: "The protection, promotion, and optimization of health and abilities, prevention of illness and injury, alleviation of suffering through the diagnosis and treatment of human response, and advocacy in the care of individuals, families, communities, and populations."

107. B: Moral agency refers to decision-making that includes accountability for right and wrong decisions by the moral agent. Advocacy is an ethical principle that is not legally enforced. However, many argue that paternalism is contrary to advocacy because of the assumption that the "system" knows what is best for the patient without concern for the patient's wishes. Moral agency is not restricted to a specific population; however, the nurse will assess the ability of all patients to make informed decisions.

108. B: When creating a lesson plan, the nurse should create definite and measurable goals and objectives. Creating open-ended objectives makes it more difficult to create a structured lesson and assess if the learner gained the desired knowledge. Choices *A, C,* and *D* are incorrect because these are all accurate and important components to include in a lesson plan when educating a patient. Additionally, the material in the lesson should encompass both the goals and objectives of the teaching.

109. A: Medical libraries are great sources to find information that was validated and published in the past, especially when looking for older information such as the question suggests. Choice *B*, web browsing, and Choice *D*, recent medical journals may only contain recently acquired data without describing past procedures in detail. Choice *C*, television dramas, can be left out entirely because they most likely contain fictional information that should not be used to further an investigation of disease.

110. B: Choice *B,* a Pareto chart, is a quality improvement tool that uses a bar graph to determine the frequency of causative factors. Choice *A* is not correct because a fishbone diagram focuses on a main problem statement and identifies causative factors in linear form. Choice *C* is not correct because a flow chart produces a step-by-step diagram of a process or workflow. Choice *D* is not correct because a gap analysis identifies the needs or barriers between a desired goal of an implementation strategy and the actual clinical situation.

111. B: Quality standards and guidance can be found at NCQA for professional development nurses to drive quality improvement initiatives. Choice *A* is incorrect, as the CDC provides information on disease prevention, maintenance, and public health matters. Choice *C* is incorrect, as CMS provides information and regulations regarding the joint federal and state insurance programs. Choice *D* is incorrect, as the WHO is an intergovernmental organization focused on improving health on a global scale.

112. B: OSHA, the Occupational Safety and Health Administration, is responsible for creating and enforcing workplace safety standards, making choice *B* correct. OSHA sets minimum standards, provides job training in multiple languages to ensure understanding, and protects employees. The other abbreviations, listed in choices *A, C,* and *D,* are not relevant to workplace safety standards.

113. B: Achievement and improvement scores are both used to assess a healthcare provider's performance in a specific performance domain and their compliance with the guidelines of CMS's VBP program. As the names imply, achievement scores are designed to quantify a hospital's overall quality of care, whereas improvement scores depict how a particular healthcare provider's quality of care has changed compared to previous years. Achievement scores are calculated by comparing an individual healthcare provider's score to other similar healthcare providers' scores, whereas improvement scores are calculated by comparing an individual healthcare provider's score with their previous scores. Therefore, the correct answer is Choice *B.* Choice *A* is incorrect because both achievement and improvement scores are measures determining effectiveness and efficiency of treatment. Choice *C* is incorrect because achievement and improvement scores are assessed for an entire healthcare provider and cannot be used to quantify an individual's performance. Choice *D* is incorrect because achievement and improvement scores are calculated for all healthcare providers, regardless of the percentile of their performance.

114. D: According to the updated Bloom's Taxonomy, the most complex level of cognitive learning listed is the step of evaluating. Bloom's Taxonomy outlines three different domains that are needed for effective learning: cognitive, affective, and psychomotor. The correct order of the steps from least to most complex in cognitive learning are as follows: remembering, understanding, applying, analyzing, evaluating, and creating. Choices *A, B,* and *C* are incorrect because they are not the most complex level of cognitive learning in Bloom's Taxonomy listed in the answer options.

115. D: The HCAHPS survey is a revolutionary survey that attempts to collect, synthetize, and publish consumer experiences when seeking and receiving health care. The HCAHPS survey is used to determine a healthcare provider's performance according to the person and community engagement performance domain of CMS's VBP program. Therefore, the correct answer is Choice *D.* All of the other answer choices refer to other healthcare metrics and do not reflect consumer experience at all.

116. D: When critically reading a new research article, it is not imperative that the nurse sees where funding comes from for the research. While funding can have some influence over research and should be examined when appraising research, it is not necessary when trying to critically read and understand new research information. Choices *A, B,* and *C* are incorrect because the nurse should determine the thesis, process, and outcomes when critically reading research.

117. C: The suggested preparatory schedule for accreditation typically involves a year of planning along with close monitoring. The other choices represent incorrect timelines for planning.

118. C: This patient has recently received the difficult news that she has cancer and has just started chemotherapy, all of which can be very emotionally taxing. Being in a heightened or overly emotional state may make it more difficult for a patient to comprehend new knowledge and decrease their readiness to learn. There is not an indication that this patient has any physical restrictions that may affect learning; therefore, Choice *A* is incorrect. Choice *B* is incorrect because the question stated that the patient is educated and can work in a high-functioning position, so the patient would likely not suffer from a literacy barrier. Choice *D* is incorrect because this patient would most likely suffer from emotional lability. Even if a patient is educated, they can still have barriers to learning. It is important to assess every patient fully for barriers that may not be apparent and adapt one's teaching style accordingly.

119. C: Innovation involves developing a new process, policy, or standard that improves upon the quality outcomes of previous processes. Choice *A* refers to diffusion. Choice *B* refers to patient analytics and medical informatics. Choice *D* refers to internal benchmarking.

120. C: HIPAA protects patient rights around confidentiality, release of medical information, and privacy. A Patient Bill of Rights is a document that communicates the patient's rights and responsibilities when it comes to healthcare. The WHO Surgical Safety Checklist was launched by the WHO in 2004 to examine patient safety in the settings of primary and acute care. TJC's National Patient Safety Goals (NPSGs) are formulated from reviewing best practice guidelines as well as sentinel events.

121. A: Public health is educating and connecting resources to the general public. Topics on healthy foods and chronic disease prevention are applicable to all members of a community. Choice *B* is incorrect, as healthcare law may refer to topics such as health insurance issues, filing grievances, or representation for navigating healthcare matters. Choice *C* is incorrect since home health refers to care needed inside the home for individuals with chronic and debilitating health problems, disabilities, or mental health issues. Patient rights, Choice *D*, is not correct since this type of advocacy assists patients with ensuring that their rights are protected.

122. A: The use of mobile workstations, electronic medical records, integrated clinic and pharmacy systems, and patient portal systems all indicate a medical organization that's fully utilizing healthcare information technology. The online practices illustrated in the case are helping the providers access, document, and maintain patient files more efficiently. The case also illustrates how online systems allow an interdisciplinary team to work together to deliver treatment that the patient needs. Paper-charting systems aren't relevant to this case. The proximity of the pharmacy and the demeanor of the pharmacist is a benefit for the patient, but these aren't recurring themes presented in the case.

123. D: A patient portal generally provides access to the patient's health information and provides the ability to message providers or schedule new appointments. Therefore, Choice *D* is correct. It does not generally provide access to financial or insurance information, so Choice *C* is incorrect. Choice *A* is incorrect because if a new prescription is required, the patient must meet with a provider to receive the prescription. Choice *B* is incorrect because an ROI should be signed in person, not online.

124. A: The Lean Six Sigma format that targets current processes is DMAIC, which stands for define, measure, analyze, improve, and control.

125. D: The federal Family and Medical Leave Act guarantees that some employees have 12 weeks of protected, unpaid leave for family and medical reasons. A number of stipulations to this act include that the organization granting leave must have 50 or more employees, the employee in consideration must have been employed for 12 months before asking for protected leave under the act, and the employee must ask for leave for certain medical conditions. Other rules may also apply based on the organization and employee.

Practice Test #2

1. Which of the following should the nurse prioritize when providing education about breastfeeding to expectant parents?
    a. The use of pre-recorded video demonstration
    b. The use of practice dolls
    c. The use of written step-by-step instructions
    d. The use of verbal discussion

2. A nurse is preparing for an education session with a Spanish-speaking patient. Which of the following is a best practice to provide culturally congruent care?
    a. Asking the patient about their preferred language in which to receive written education
    b. Researching common cultural considerations when caring for Hispanic patients
    c. Requesting that a family member serves as the interpreter to provide familiarity
    d. Speaking loudly and slowly

3. Which action performed by an oncology care site would best evaluate if they are meeting the requirements of their patient education program?
    a. Distribution of patient satisfaction surveys
    b. Staff polling to determine the current process
    c. Review of current standards of practice
    d. Discussion with community stakeholders

4. When meetings have dysfunctions, they impact which of the following?
    a. The quality agenda
    b. The cost and team confidence
    c. The cost, schedule, quality, and project manager's credibility
    d. The schedule and cost

5. A professional development nurse has received committee approval to move forward with a nursing initiative aimed at improving fall rates. What would be the best way to communicate details of the initiative to all nursing staff?
    a. An online forum that is recorded
    b. A memo posted on the unit huddle board
    c. Information provided to nurse managers to be shared with staff
    d. An email with an overview consisting of bullet points

6. Using the Synergy Model, a nurse who is at a level 1 of clinical inquiry would have which of the following characteristics?
    a. Seeks new knowledge
    b. Questions industry standards
    c. Is aware of the problem and asks others for advice
    d. Deviates from industry standards using evidence-based practice

7. Which aspect of employee performance management is defined as identifying when an employee has demonstrated knowledge and ability to do certain work?
    a. Mentoring
    b. Coaching
    c. Teaching
    d. Competency validation

8. A patient experiences a urinary tract infection (UTI) as a result of an improperly inserted catheter. Which of the following performance measures is the professional development nurse most likely to notice a change in as a result?
   a. Clinical outcomes
   b. Person and community engagement
   c. Safety
   d. Efficiency and cost reduction

9. What is the most appropriate nursing intervention for providing education to a patient who speaks a different language?
   a. Use a professional interpreter.
   b. Use a family member to interpret, as they know the patient best.
   c. Speak slowly and loudly to help the patient understand.
   d. Provide the patient with written instructions in their language.

10. An employee must file a complaint charge of discrimination with the Equal Employment Opportunity Commission (EEOC) within how many days of the alleged incident?
   a. 180 days
   b. 90 days
   c. 120 days
   d. There is no time limit associated with filing a complaint charge of discrimination with the EEOC.

11. A professional development nurse is reviewing patient satisfaction data over the last quarter from an acute care unit. The scores have decreased significantly compared to the previous two quarters. What quality metric may be used to evaluate quality and delivery of care?
   a. Bed occupancy rate
   b. Average hospital stay
   c. Insurance reimbursement claims
   d. Hours per patient day

12. Which of the following communication strategies is used to establish a relationship where employees feel comfortable speaking directly with management about problems and suggestions?
   a. Town hall meetings
   b. Management by Walking Around (MBWA)
   c. Open-door policy
   d. Department meetings

13. The professional development nurse is reviewing areas for improvement with an interdisciplinary team that includes nurses, doctors, pharmacists, and other care providers. Which of the following would the nurse understand to be most directly influenced by nursing practice?
   a. Incidence of patient falls
   b. Proper patient consent before procedures
   c. Sterile preparation of blood products
   d. Rate of handwashing among healthcare professionals

14. What is the purpose of the ANA Code of Ethics?
   a. Defines nursing practice and ethical duties
   b. Promotes pay grades for nurses
   c. Defines nurse-to-patient ratios for safe care
   d. Differentiates between the moral compass for nurses versus primary care providers

15. The nurse is providing discharge teaching to a patient on how to de-access a portacath after delivery of a three-day infusion. Which technique will best prepare the patient to perform the de-access successfully and safely?

a. Providing and reviewing detailed written instructions from the hospital's patient education library
b. Explaining the process to the patient and then asking the patient questions to assess whether they have understood
c. Referring the patient to a hospital-approved video on the process
d. Using a model portacath and port needle to teach the patient and then having the patient teach the process back to the nurse

16. Which category of adverse drug reactions (ADRs) is commonly considered to be due to incorrect administration of the drug?

a. Rapid reactions
b. First dose reactions
c. Early reactions
d. Intermediate reactions

17. To obtain as much information as possible, which approach would be best to use when interviewing patients?

a. Focus on closed-ended questions to obtain specific, relevant information.
b. Use mainly open-ended questions to allow patients to express themselves.
c. Emphasize probing questions to clarify responses and resolve contradictions.
d. Use a mix of closed- and open-ended questions to get a range of information.

18. The nursing unit recently discovered a high rate of UTIs amongst post-op patients. As a result, nurses have begun removing indwelling foley catheters within 24 hours after surgery, instead of 48 hours, to try to reduce the rate of UTIs. This nursing unit is at which stage of a problem-solving strategy?

a. Evaluation of solution
b. Development of solutions
c. Identification of the problem
d. Implementation of solution

19. Which of the following statements is consistent with the major premise of the Synergy Model?

a. Family participation in patient care improves outcomes.
b. The model is based on the condition of patients and the function of the nursing staff.
c. The model only relates to critical care environments.
d. Synergy is said to exist when the environment and nursing competencies are consistent with the needs of the patient and the patient's family.

20. When creating education for a community event, which of the following would be subject to organization authorization prior to the publication?

a. Author's name and title
b. Organizational logo
c. Page count
d. Font type

21. Which of the following would be the most appropriate action the nurse could take to help facilitate continuous learning for a patient that has just received a colostomy?
   a. Provide diagrams and written instructions on how to apply the appliance.
   b. Show a video on colostomy care to the patient.
   c. Demonstrate colostomy care to the patient and allow them to practice on a mannequin.
   d. Have the patient participate in a colostomy support group.

22. Which of the following is the most effective way for organizations to secure their electronic health records and access to networks?
   a. Multi-factor authorization
   b. Single-factor authorization
   c. Guest wi-fi access
   d. Use of SSN for passwords

23. Which of the following statements about strategic plans is NOT correct?
   a. Strategic plans involve objectives, analysis, looking at strengths and weaknesses, and implementation.
   b. Strategic plans are executed by employees and HR professionals to ensure these employees have the necessary skills to accomplish the identified goals.
   c. Strategic plans are a one-time activity that should always guide the organization toward the overall goals and objectives.
   d. Strategic plans should maximize the organization's strengths, take advantage of industry opportunities, and regularly be improved.

24. The nurse is caring for a patient who is terminally ill. Which of the following actions can help mitigate ethical dilemmas in this patient population?
   a. Provide thorough explanations of care for decision making.
   b. Promote active treatments to help extend life.
   c. Use nursing expertise to help make decisions for the patient and the family.
   d. Give the patient the highest prescribed dose of analgesic for comfort.

25. The professional development nurse is providing an educational session on asthma triggers and management for individuals with asthma. Which of the following actions by the nurse will help facilitate learning the best?
   a. Present a PowerPoint lecture.
   b. Show a video on asthma management.
   c. Encourage people in the group to share their personal asthma triggers and experiences.
   d. Hand out pamphlets on asthma triggers and management.

26. At which level of the caring practices continuum identified in the Synergy Model is death initially viewed as an acceptable patient outcome?
   a. Level 1
   b. Level 2
   c. Level 3
   d. Death is considered as an acceptable outcome at all levels of caring practice.

27. A nurse is a member of a peer review committee at a hospital. The committee is tasked with reviewing a case in which a nurse has been accused of providing substandard care to a patient who ultimately suffered harm. The reviewing nurse is a longtime friend of the accused nurse, and the two have worked together for many years. The committee has been unable to come to a consensus on the appropriate action to take. What is the best course of action for the reviewing nurse in this scenario?

a. Removing themselves from this case due to their personal relationship with the accused nurse
b. Advocating for the accused nurse and presenting evidence in their favor
c. Making an unbiased decision based on the evidence presented, despite their personal relationship with the accused nurse
d. Abstaining from voting and allowing the other members of the committee to make the decision

28. Recording virtual presentations is an advantageous option because it allows attendees to do which of the following?

a. Eliminate the need for live, virtual meetings.
b. Review content at their own pace.
c. Not be marked absent for attendance.
d. Avoid post-educational surveys.

29. The six key processes in communication are thinking, encoding, transmitting the signal, decoding, understanding, and which of the following?

a. Writing
b. Calculating
c. Listening
d. Perceiving

30. A professional development nurse has created a document containing data on readmitted patients within the last 90 days. When preparing to share the document via email with the executive team, what must the nurse do when emailing this sensitive information?

a. Include visuals to engage leadership interest.
b. Encrypt the email for document security.
c. Nothing, as internal emails do not have to comply with HIPAA
d. Make sure information is attached as a document and not in body of email.

31. Which of the following word pairs identifies the six Cs of caring practices that are most closely associated with caring for acutely ill patients?

a. Compassion and curiosity
b. Confidence and collaboration
c. Conscience and creativity
d. Commitment and competence

32. When should the nursing team monitor for changes to regulatory guidelines and recommendations?

a. Annually
b. Quarterly
c. Only when it contradicts the facility's policies and procedures
d. Constantly

33. A nurse consults with a busy emergency room doctor about the exact dosage of medication to give a patient after noticing that it is more than double the recommended dose. Is she practicing proper resource utilization, and why or why not?

a. No. By interrupting the emergency room doctor, the nurse is preventing the doctor from effectively and efficiently carrying out their duties.
b. No. By restricting the dosage of medication given to a patient, the nurse is attempting to limit the hospital's billable amount.
c. Yes. By attempting to restrict the dosage of medication given to a patient, the nurse is ensuring that minimal resources are expended by each patient.
d. Yes. By consulting with the doctor on the exact dosage, the nurse is ensuring that services provided to a patient are delivered as effectively and efficiently as possible.

34. A nurse is preparing a teaching plan for a patient with the following characteristics: moderately impaired resiliency, stability, and complexity. Which of the following teaching-learning approaches is most appropriate for this patient?

a. Provide a one-hour teaching-learning session twice a day for the next two days.
b. Provide the patient with written information from a nursing journal.
c. Leave the instructions for the outpatient care provider.
d. Meet with the patient for 15–20 minutes to assess their ability to participate.

35. What is the most common initial assessment finding used to diagnose child abuse?

a. Patient report
b. Bruising
c. Onset of bed wetting
d. "Acting out" behavior

36. Doug is an oncology nurse working with a 50-year-old male patient with advanced skin cancer. Besides the cancer, he has no history of any mental, emotional, or physical health issues. As Doug begins to provide education relating to the diagnosis and the next treatment session, the patient begins to look very angry, and his eyes glaze over. As Doug is talking, the patient falls asleep. Doug tries again a few hours later, but the patient ignores him and begins to listen to music on his phone. When Doug asks if the patient would like to know any more about the treatment, the patient rolls away and grumbles under his breath. What should Doug do next?

a. Accept that the patient is not interested in patient education and leave the patient alone.
b. Assume his teaching methods are boring and spend some time figuring out how to make the material more interesting.
c. Double-check the patient's health records to ensure there is no history of cognitive dysfunction.
d. Speak with the patient's next of kin or caregiver to ask if he can share the patient education material with them.

37. Utilitarianism can place a limit on which other ethical principle?

a. Autonomy
b. Beneficence
c. Nonmaleficence
d. Justice

38. Which of the following best describes the first step in Rogers' Five-Stage Change Theory?
   a. Implement change and ensure that staff are adhering to the new practice.
   b. Initiate a trial of the new practices indicated after gathering data.
   c. Announce the change that will be taking place, when it will start, and how it will be measured.
   d. Communicate the reason for the change, what will happen, and who will be most affected.

39. Which of the following best represents the purpose of Six Sigma?
   a. To eliminate ineffective and wasteful techniques that diminish productivity
   b. To organize management and employee councils
   c. To gain valuable feedback from employees to determine the most ineffective use of company resources
   d. To increase productive capacities by recruiting employees with the most experience

40. Which research provides the strongest evidence to support a proposed change in practice?
   a. A single randomized controlled trial (RCT)
   b. A meta-analysis of multiple RCTs
   c. A prospective cohort study
   d. A meta-analysis of multiple retrospective case-control studies

41. What is the advantage of identifying process champions for process and performance improvement projects?
   a. Process champions provide a visual representation of the current processes in an effort to find areas that are redundant and lacking in value.
   b. Process champions consider the importance of adding to, rather than detracting from, the value delivered to customers.
   c. Process champions can identify potential pitfalls during the brainstorming phase of process improvement.
   d. Process champions ensure that the VOC (voice of the client) is heard and confirm that there is a precisely defined focus on the correct processes.

42. Which of the following is a key principle in communication for the professional development nurse?
   a. Active listening
   b. Ambiguity
   c. Speaking quickly
   d. Multitasking

43. Which of the following tools would NOT be used to determine why goals were not achieved or why there was a discrepancy between expected outcomes and actual outcomes?
   a. Six Sigma
   b. Gap analysis
   c. Root cause analysis
   d. Cause-and-effect diagram

44. A leader who discusses ideas with their group but then seldom incorporates the group's suggestions into their presented changes is said to be which kind of leader?
   a. Democratic leader
   b. Consultative leader
   c. Participatory leader
   d. Delegative leader

45. The initial data collected for analysis of a problem is called what?
    a. Aggregate data
    b. Baseline data
    c. Correlative data
    d. Qualitative data

46. The nurse is participating in a shared decision-making model in all of the following examples EXCEPT:
    a. Discussing the side effects a patient is experiencing in treatment with the attending physician
    b. Reinforcing information about different treatment options with the patient after a visit with the physician
    c. Requesting referral to occupational therapy for a patient who is having difficulty managing ADLs after surgery
    d. Performing a chart review to determine if a patient has received the necessary education prior to treatment

47. A significant benefit of utilizing presentation software while delivering nursing education includes:
    a. The ability to grade quizzes in real-time
    b. The use of visual aids
    c. EHR integration
    d. Increased attendance

48. What are the four steps of systems thinking in order?
    a. Anticipate, design, transform, react
    b. React, anticipate, design, transform
    c. Design, anticipate, react, transform
    d. Transform, react, anticipate, design

49. Which of the following hospital wards/centers would most likely have the lowest HPPD value?
    a. Neonatal intensive care unit (NICU)
    b. Burn unit
    c. Psychiatric ward
    d. Hospice care ward

50. Which feature in spreadsheets allows for manipulation of quality improvement project data?
    a. Mail merge
    b. Pivot tables
    c. Charts and graphs
    d. Functional formulas

51. The nursing team is briefed on a patient advocacy concern in which the care that family at the bedside is demanding does not align with the incapacitated patient's stated wishes in their durable power of attorney for healthcare (DPOAH). What is the next best step to protect the patient's rights?
    a. Continue providing care according to the patient's DPOAH.
    b. Call security and have the family removed.
    c. Refer the case to the ethics committee for review and recommendation.
    d. Have the provider explain to the family that they are wrong.

52. The professional development nurse must ensure that the healthcare staff is proficient in responding to a choking incident. Which of the following is the first step in demonstrating this competency?
   a. Ask for the full name and date of birth.
   b. Verify choking and call for help.
   c. Swipe the person's mouth with a bare finger.
   d. Encircle the person's torso with arms and thrust the fist deep into the epigastric area.

53. The Americans with Disabilities Act (ADA) provides for the elimination of discrimination in the workplace and hiring practices. Which of the following is NOT a strategy for the professional development nurse to employ to maintain compliance with the ADA?
   a. Providing a handicapped-accessible environment
   b. Creating reasonable accommodations for the job or work environment
   c. Making broad descriptions of job duties
   d. Determining mandatory job functions

54. The professional development nurse is holding an informational group for parents about childhood immunizations. Which of the following teaching methods would be the most effective to facilitate learning for the parents?
   a. Hand out copies of the childhood immunization schedule.
   b. Have a group discussion on common immunization concerns and misconceptions.
   c. Show an informational video on the importance of childhood immunizations.
   d. Teach parents how to administer the immunizations.

55. According to the Synergy Model, at what level of nursing competence do the nursing competencies of clinical inquiry and clinical reasoning become inseparable in the research process?
   a. The experienced nurse
   b. The novice nurse
   c. The expert nurse
   d. All levels of competency

56. Susan finds that she usually works best when she can go directly to whichever supervisor is responsible for handling the area in which she has a problem. Which type of authoritative structure would best suit Susan's work style?
   a. Line authority
   b. Team authority
   c. Management authority
   d. Staff authority

57. What is NOT a purpose of employee performance appraisals?
   a. Assessment of employee performance
   b. Development of an action plan for advancement
   c. Editing job description and job duties
   d. Encouraging continued development

58. Employee competency validation does NOT provide which of the following?
   a. Risk mitigation
   b. Nursing knowledge and clinical skill
   c. Standardization of care
   d. Critical thinking

59. Two employees who perform well individually have been placed on a project team together. However, in a team setting, they often clash due to very different work styles and attitudes. How can the professional development nurse help resolve this issue?
   a. Separate the two team members and put them on different projects.
   b. Put them on a probationary warning.
   c. Provide coaching to the employees to find common ground.
   d. Allow them to resolve it autonomously, as this is more empowering.

60. When providing trending, tracking, and comparison data related to the CLABSI rates for three different units, which tool is best for analyzing and presenting the information in a meaningful way?
   a. Spreadsheets
   b. Website
   c. Video
   d. Portable document file

61. What is the purpose of a root cause analysis?
   a. To determine the foundation-level reason as to why an overarching issue is occurring
   b. To determine the exact employee that caused an error during a process
   c. To determine the best source of external funding
   d. To determine how to allocate fixed funds within an organization

62. Which of the following is NOT one of the benefits of line authority?
   a. It is a temporary structure that lasts only as long as necessary.
   b. Each employee has only one "boss" to whom they report.
   c. Dealing with problems is a more straightforward process.
   d. There is a clear chain of command, eliminating confusion about who is responsible for what.

63. What is the primary advantage of holding multiple virtual nursing unit-based council committee meetings for participants?
   a. It increases accessibility for attendees.
   b. It facilitates improved conversation.
   c. It decreases employee productivity.
   d. It eliminates the need to keep records.

64. Which of the following steps helps ensure accuracy and clarity before submitting a document?
   a. Using complex terminology
   b. Relying on spellcheck to correct errors
   c. Having a colleague proofread the document
   d. Increasing word count

65. An emergency room calculates that it has an HPPD value for its nursing staff of 0.4. Which of the following statements provides the correct interpretation of that value?
   a. A patient at that emergency room saw an average of 0.4 nurses on a particular day.
   b. A physician at that emergency room saw each patient for 0.4 hours on average for a particular day.
   c. A patient at that emergency room saw nurses for an average of 0.4 hours on a particular day.
   d. A nurse at that emergency room saw an average of 0.4 patients an hour on a particular day.

66. Which strategy assumes individuals are rational and will naturally follow a path that benefits their self-interest?
   a. The power-coercive strategy
   b. The empirical-rational strategy
   c. The technology-innovation strategy
   d. The normative-reductive strategy

67. According to the Synergy Model, which of the following choices is associated with the patient's vulnerability?
   a. The patient is financially stable.
   b. The patient smoked cigarettes for thirty years prior to quitting five years ago.
   c. The patient is married.
   d. The patient actively participates in decisions related to the plan of care.

68. Who would be the best featured speaker(s) for a training on workplace misconduct?
   a. A panel of employees who have made workplace misconduct complaints in the past
   b. Someone from the C-suite (e.g., CEO, CFO, or COO)
   c. A Department of Justice representative
   d. The HR professionals who organized the training

69. Having which of the following characteristics promotes a systems thinking approach?
   a. Independent work dynamic
   b. Organization-wide perspective
   c. Self-focused views
   d. Reliance only on past experiences

70. Performance appraisals and the regular evaluation of performance issues have all of the following in common EXCEPT what?
   a. Employee development
   b. Recognizing accomplishments
   c. Determining training needs
   d. A set time frame

71. The Synergy Model proposes a novel paradigm of nursing. Which of the following statements correctly identifies a characteristic of nursing practice in this model?
   a. Resiliency
   b. Creativity
   c. Collaboration
   d. Complexity

72. Nursing informaticists must ensure that there is widespread knowledge among employees of how to recognize phishing risk. Which of the following best describes this activity?
   a. Clinical simulation skills
   b. Cybersecurity best practice
   c. Improved virtual presentations
   d. Efficacy in holding dial-in meetings

73. A nurse is caring for a patient who is recovering from a prostatectomy earlier in the day. The nurse works with the patient to identify a goal to complete their first ambulation during the nurse's shift. This is an example of which step in the nursing process?

a. Outcome identification
b. Implementation
c. Planning
d. Assessment

74. The nurse is providing education for a patient that has recently had a stroke. The patient is having difficulties with communication. Which of the following actions by the nurse would be an example of caring practice?

a. Use nonverbal communication to show empathy and support.
b. Restrict visitors to prevent excessive stimulation.
c. Speak to the patient in a slow and loud voice.
d. Pretend that the patient is speaking normally.

75. Virtual meetings have many benefits, including cost savings to employees. Which of the following would support this statement?

a. Free continuing education credits
b. Increased access to information
c. Elimination of travel time and expense
d. Reduced usage of company cars

76. Which of the following statements best reflects the similar thinking that underlies both transformational leadership style and transactional leadership style?

a. Leaders are most effective when there is the least oversight.
b. Leaders are most effective when their team members are most satisfied in their work.
c. Leaders are most effective when they listen to feedback.
d. Leaders are most effective when they can adjust how they lead situation to situation.

77. A patient is able to follow the steps in written instructions from a nurse to get their blood glucose level using a new glucometer. According to Bloom's Taxonomy, this patient is at which step of psychomotor learning?

a. Complex overt response
b. Guided response
c. Mechanism
d. Perception

78. To support work-life balance, an organization is allowing applicable nursing staff to work remotely one day per week. In what way can presentations best support remote learning?

a. They do not interrupt patient care.
b. They can be shared virtually.
c. They may be printed and sent to participants.
d. They eliminate the need for in-person meetings.

79. How might an institution best support diversity?

a. By requiring all employees to speak a second language
b. By providing mandatory cultural sensitivity training for all managers
c. By offering alternative food services
d. By providing alternative solutions to all patient requests

80. What are the correct steps to follow when using a fire extinguisher?
   a. Pull the pin, Squeeze the handle, Aim the nozzle, Swirl around the fire
   b. Pull the pin, Aim at the base of the fire, Squeeze the handle, Sweep from side to side
   c. Squeeze the handle, Aim at the base of the fire, Pull the pin, Sweep from side to side
   d. Stand back, Pull the pin, Squeeze the handle, Sweep from side to side

81. An individual believes that being a good leader is an innate trait and cannot be taught to others. This individual most likely subscribes to which of the following theories of leadership?
   a. Autocratic Leadership Theory
   b. Laissez-faire Leadership Theory
   c. The Great Man Theory of Leadership
   d. Democratic Leadership Theory

82. What is the primary purpose of data encryption?
   a. Controlling data duplication
   b. Ensuring timely software updates
   c. Restricting unauthorized access
   d. Decreasing FTE needs for IT staff

83. Which of the following is NOT one of the categories for notifiable diseases?
   a. Outbreak
   b. Infectious
   c. Noninfectious
   d. Reproducible

84. Interdisciplinary communication may be enhanced during virtual meetings through which of the following methods?
   a. Turning off the chat feature to eliminate distractions
   b. Disabling the video of attendees
   c. Limiting cross-department influence
   d. Allowing multiple disciplines to collaborate at their comfort levels

85. Which of the following describes reflective communication?
   a. Actively involving the audience through enthusiasm, imagery, or humor
   b. One person communicates a message, and the recipient confirms with a response
   c. Questioning, listening, and speaking
   d. Actively listening and restating the message in one's own words

86. While creating an evidence-based practice guideline, a nurse is conducting research and wants to use research that has the highest level of evidence, level A. From which of the following studies should the nurse draw information?
   a. Meta-analysis
   b. Randomized-control trial
   c. Integrative interviews
   d. Cohort study

87. Which of the following should be reported to the FDA as an ADR?
   a. Intractable vomiting following oral chemotherapy
   b. Acute cirrhosis secondary to self-induced acetaminophen overdose
   c. Intervention is required to prevent permanent damage following the reported ADR.
   d. Alteration of the pharmacotherapeutic plan is required due to the reported ADR.

88. A professional development nurse believes her team works best when goals and incentives are clearly communicated and quickly rewarded. What style of leadership could she best be described as having?
   a. Situational leadership style
   b. Autocratic leadership style
   c. Transactional leadership style
   d. Transformational leadership style

89. A nurse educator is tasked with tracking the organization's CE content credits. Which of the following technology resources would be appropriate to manage this information?
   a. A word processing document
   b. Spreadsheet tables
   c. Printed logs
   d. A slide deck

90. The professional development nurse works in a community health clinic. Which of the following actions by the nurse aims to improve healthcare services to underserved communities?
   a. Implement a COVID-19 vaccination program for the clinic's staff.
   b. Provide health education sessions for clinic patients.
   c. Hang informational posters in the clinic.
   d. Collaborate with local religious organizations to organize health fairs.

91. A preceptor likes to sit down with her preceptee toward the end of every week, checking in with them about their goals for the work week and their personal ambitions. Which of the following components of transformational leadership could this preceptor be described as exhibiting?
   a. Intellectual stimulation
   b. Individual consideration
   c. Inspirational motivation
   d. Idealized influence

92. Which of the following accurately represents the Fishbone Diagram?
   a. It focuses on the analysis of management and does not consult the entire organization.
   b. It identifies the strengths and weaknesses of an organization.
   c. It investigates the causes of problems.
   d. It provides a visual representation of a distribution of data.

93. What is the rationale for including individual patient identifiers for reportable diseases?
   a. To identify patients with multiple illnesses
   b. To measure the effectiveness of the prescribed medications
   c. To enroll the patient in a mandatory treatment program
   d. To provide immediate disease control and prevention

94. The National Patient Safety Goals are determined and measured by which organization?
   a. The Institute of Medicine (IOM)
   b. The National Institutes of Health (NIH)
   c. The Joint Commission (TJC)
   d. The American Hospital Association (AHA)

95. A patient developed shortness of breath and tachycardia while having a CT diagnostic exam. The time to call for help was delayed due to lack of a clear policy for staff to follow. What intervention would be most effective in improving this staff's knowledge of calling for help during an emergency?
   a. Develop an algorithm to define emergencies and appropriate clinical responses.
   b. Reassign staff to other non-patient areas of the hospital.
   c. Provide additional BLS training to staff in the emergency department.
   d. Quiz staff on the policy to assess their knowledge.

96. When used to implement evidenced-based practice, clinical inquiry can result in which of the following?
   a. Replacing an outdated nursing intervention
   b. The nurse becoming an innovator
   c. Matching patient needs with nursing competencies
   d. All the above

97. A professional development nurse is putting together a presentation and wants to edit visual documents and photos. Which of the following platforms would be best suited for this function?
   a. Microsoft PowerPoint
   b. Google Slides
   c. Prezi
   d. Adobe Photoshop

98. How are diseases designated as reportable?
   a. By the average death rate from a disease in four states
   b. Surveillance case definitions
   c. Consensus as to personal risk for the disease in the community
   d. Published data from the CDC

99. When posting a document with health information and education on a public forum, which of the following should occur?
   a. Archiving to maintain the integrity of original information
   b. Restricting access to contacts only
   c. Regularly updating the information to reflect changes in practice
   d. Utilizing AI to double-check if the information is accurate

100. A pediatric patient is feeling anxious during teaching about their upcoming surgery. Which of the following actions by the nurse indicates caring and compassionate care?
   a. Decrease the child's involvement in their healthcare decision-making to decrease anxiety.
   b. Explain to the child that they do not have anything to worry about and that it will be okay.
   c. Listen to the child's concerns and provide age-appropriate explanations.
   d. Utilize diversion techniques to decrease the child's anxiety.

101. A team has been assembled to complete a root cause analysis and recommend a solution for a safety issue. In reference to goal development, what term is NOT part of a SMART goal?
   a. Standard
   b. Achievable
   c. Measurable
   d. Time-bound

102. Albert is in charge of a committee that is tasked with coming up with better ways to address patients' dietary concerns. His team meets twice weekly, and Albert is responsible for scheduling those meetings and reporting the team's findings to his boss by the end of the month. What type of authority does Albert have?

a. Line authority
b. Team authority
c. Management authority
d. Staff authority

103. The head doctor of a particular ward refrains from checking in frequently with the other doctors of the ward, believing that the best quality of care is provided when each doctor is allowed to work in their own way. What style of leadership might they best be described as having?

a. Transactional leadership style
b. Democratic leadership style
c. Laissez-Faire leadership style
d. Autocratic leadership style

104. When using the empirical-rational strategy to initiate change, what is the best way to accomplish the change successfully?

a. Provide an employee lunch when communicating the change.
b. Educate employees with new information on the change.
c. Incentivize the change to relay the benefit employees will experience.
d. Have the leader of the organization communicate the change.

105. Systems thinking uses which of the following?

a. A centrist approach
b. Cognitive mapping
c. Scorecards
d. Technology to drive ideas

106. Elias has been a registered nurse since he received his Bachelor of Science in Nursing in 2005. He loves his job and has decided he would like to return to school to receive his Master's degree. What is this an example of?

a. A promotion
b. Continuing education
c. Specializing
d. Work-life balance

107. A patient is being discharged with a chest tube following a pneumothorax. They request to have a printed diagram showing steps on how to empty the chest tube. This patient is most likely which type of learner?

a. Auditory learner
b. Reader learner
c. Visual learner
d. Kinesthetic learner

108. Which action is a proven method of reducing risk of healthcare-associated hepatitis B among caregivers in medical facilities?

a. Regular, annual employee screening
b. Declining to offer a job to unimmunized individuals
c. Documenting immunizations for all employees
d. Barring exposed employees from the building for seven days

109. Which phase of the nursing process provokes the nurse to prioritize diagnoses?
    a. Assessment
    b. Analysis
    c. Planning
    d. Implementation

110. What is the most common form of elder abuse in community-dwelling individuals?
    a. Physical
    b. Financial
    c. Psychological
    d. Neglect

111. What is the most common reason for failure to report elder abuse?
    a. The patient asks the provider not to report the abuse.
    b. Psychological abuse is too hard to prove.
    c. The provider is afraid of malpractice lawsuits.
    d. Adult abusers rarely leave visible marks.

112. Which of the following communication types, while making it easy to distribute information to a large group of individuals very quickly, may also lead to "information overload"?
    a. Intranet
    b. Email
    c. Newsletter
    d. Word-of-mouth

113. A patient is being discharged following a drug overdose. Before they leave, the nurse prints out information that has resources for support meetings, local mental health clinics, and crisis hotline numbers. This nurse is at which level of systems thinking in the Synergy Model?
    a. Level 1
    b. Level 3
    c. Level 4
    d. Level 5

114. What is the purpose of the cost-benefit analysis in process improvement?
    a. To determine the true costs of a potential solution compared to the actual benefits
    b. To ensure that the outcome actually solves the problem
    c. To confirm the passive and unplanned spread of new practices
    d. To find solutions before they become necessary

115. What is the goal of the improve phase of the DMAIC model?
    a. To enable the management team to visually analyze the KPIs (key performance indicators) of each individual on the healthcare team
    b. To assimilate all the ideas into a strategic plan that prioritizes opportunities for improvement and amends all processes associated with changes, including any process flows and job aids
    c. To implement strategies to determine the sustainability and benefits of the newly defined processes
    d. To enable team members to implement processes themselves

116. According to the 1961 text, *The Planning of Change*, which of the following is NOT a strategy for managing change?
   a. The normative-reductive strategy
   b. The power-coercive strategy
   c. The technology-innovation strategy
   d. The empirical-rational strategy

117. What are the five rights of delegation the nurse must consider when delegating tasks?
   a. Right task, right person, right direction, right supervision, right dose
   b. Right supervision, right person, right dose, right assessment, right facility
   c. Right circumstance, right assessment, right direction, right task, right facility
   d. Right task, right circumstance, right person, right direction, right supervision

118. Documents containing patient information must comply with which regulation?
   a. OSHA
   b. FERPA
   c. HIPAA
   d. ADA

119. A nurse is developing a plan of care for a patient population that is culturally diverse. Which statement correctly identifies the appropriate nursing actions?
   a. The nurse follows the standard protocol for the predominant culture of the community.
   b. The nurse focuses on the cultural needs of the largest group in the population.
   c. The nurse identifies and acknowledges self-biases and addresses the needs of the patient.
   d. The nurse meets the needs of the group according to personal values and beliefs.

120. Which of the following is NOT one of the components of effective assertive communication?
   a. Look for areas of compromise.
   b. Have a defined and clear message.
   c. Use "you" statements.
   d. Control delivery of information.

121. A medical facility recommended that individuals in their waiting room use proper cough etiquette to contain coughs while waiting for medical attention; however, no reduction in infection transmission was seen despite compliance with this tried-and-true advice. What should they do?
   a. Go online to check the latest guidelines issued by the CDC.
   b. Stop recommending proper cough etiquette because it is a waste of time.
   c. Provide a public supply of hand sanitizer for use after a cough.
   d. Go online to research if any other health facility is facing this problem.

122. At which interval does the Joint Commission conduct its unannounced surveys of nursing units?
   a. 24-48 months
   b. Exactly two years
   c. Every year
   d. 18-36 months

123. Which of the following is NOT a type of managerial communication?
   a. Upward communication
   b. Backward communication
   c. Downward communication
   d. Lateral communication

124. What can the professional development nurse specifically do to alleviate employees' fears and concerns about reporting unethical behavior and possible retaliation?

a. Provide annual training regarding the policies and expectations.
b. Provide confidential and/or anonymous reporting methods.
c. Provide all employees with the handbook to ensure knowledge of the policy.
d. Provide frequent updates to the policies and procedures.

125. A nurse is involved in a research study with 500 participants for a new vaccine that would be recommended for all people 18 years of age and older. 450 of the participants were 50 years old and older. This study would likely suffer from which kind of bias?

a. Reporting bias
b. Recall bias
c. Healthy participant bias
d. Selection bias

Answer Explanations #2

1. B: The most effective method to educate families and facilitate learning is utilizing practice dolls and mannequins. This allows those who are learning to gain hands-on experience so they can be comfortable on their own. Although playing a pre-recorded video demonstration may be helpful, it is not the best choice because it does not allow the expectant parents to have hands-on practice, making Choice *A* incorrect. Providing written step-by-step instructions may be helpful as a reference, but it isn't the most effective way to facilitate learning, making Choice *C* incorrect. This is also true for Choice *D*, making it also incorrect.

2. A: Asking questions regarding patient preference rather than making assumptions is important in providing culturally congruent care. Choice *B* is incorrect because the nurse should ask the patient about their preference instead of researching. Choice *C* is incorrect because, whenever possible, family members should not be interpreting information to the patient. It is unnecessary to speak in a different manner than the nurse would for an English-speaking patient, so Choice *D* is incorrect.

3. C: The best way to evaluate if an oncology practice is meeting the requirements of their current patient education program would be to review the current standards of practice, such as the *Chemotherapy and Immunotherapy Guidelines and Recommendations for Practice*, written by the Oncology Nursing Society in 2018. Choice *A* is not the best choice because patient satisfaction surveys would be best suited for identifying ways to improve patient experience, as opposed to compliance with current requirements. Choice *B* is not the best choice, as staff polling would be better for identifying adherence to the process rather than identifying whether the program is meeting guidelines. Lastly, Choice *D* is not the best choice because discussion with community stakeholders would be better suited for identifying needs and concerns within the community, rather than evaluating adherence to requirements.

4. C: Meeting dysfunctions have significant negative impacts on the progress of the project. Dysfunctional meetings impact the cost, schedule, and quality of the project and reduce the project manager's credibility within the team, making only Choice *C* correct.

5. A: Choice *A,* a recorded online forum, allows staff to view the information when time is available and verify attendance, with minimum disruption to patient care. It offers a format that can go into the depth of the material from the direct source, while reaching individuals that are likely on varying shifts. Choices *B* and *C* are not the best options; not all staff may see the memo, and both choices limit the amount of information, accompanying data, and graphics that can be shared. When initiating an action, it is less likely to have drift or misunderstandings when the same information is distributed from a single source, which is not the case with Choice *C.*

6. C: A nurse at level 1 of clinical inquiry in the Synergy Model, the most basic level, has awareness that a problem exists and may ask others for assistance and guidance. Choices *A* and *B* are incorrect because these are characteristics that reflect level 3 clinical inquiry. Choice *D* is incorrect because using evidence-based practice to change delivery of care, even if it goes against industry standards, is the highest level of clinical inquiry, level 5.

7. D: Competency validation is when the knowledge and skills of a nurse are verified for a particular task.

8. C: Situations such as the one described in the question, in which a patient experiences an infection following medical treatment, can be measured using the metric HAI. Such a metric is used to determine a healthcare provider's performance in the safety performance domain. Therefore, the correct answer is Choice *C.* All of the other answer choices describe the other performance domains, none of which HAI is used to calculate.

9. A: Using a professional interpreter is important to provide safe and effective care for the patient. The professional interpreter is trained in medical terminology to help explain medical conditions. Using a family member to interpret is not the best choice as they can be biased and may withhold information if they do not want the patient to know everything that is happening medically. Not only this, but family members may not fully understand medical terminology. This makes Choice *B* incorrect. Choice *C* is incorrect because this will not help the patient's understanding. Choice *D* is also incorrect as they may not be able to read or write in their own language, and they also may not understand medical terminology.

10. A: An employee must file a complaint charge of discrimination with the EEOC within a period of 180 days of the alleged incident.

11. D: Choice *D* measures the number of hours that clinical staff spend per patient. Increased hours per patient day is directly linked to predicting improved patient satisfaction scores, safer care delivery, and a decrease in quality concerns. Choices *A*, *B*, and *C* are tied to financial gain for an organization, not patient satisfaction.

12. C: An open-door policy is used to establish a relationship where employees feel comfortable speaking directly with management about problems and suggestions. Town hall meetings, Choice *A*, are formal gatherings for the entire company that are commonly referred to as "all-hands meetings" and tend to focus on sharing information "from the top down" concerning the overall organization. These meetings are not usually designed to allow feedback from employees about smaller detail issues. Management by Walking Around (MBWA), Choice *B*, as the name suggests, involves having managers and supervisors physically get out of their offices and interact with employees in person. MBWA allows management to check on employee progress, inquire about potential issues, and gain other feedback without relying on employees to "make the first move." Finally, department meetings, Choice *D*, are formal gatherings of employees and management in a given department that typically take place on a set day and time, allow everyone involved to share ideas, and offer solutions to company challenges.

13. A: The rate of patient falls is considered a nurse-sensitive indicator. Of the options presented, patient falls are most directly affected by nursing practice. Choice *B* is incorrect because, while nurses should check for patient consent before procedures, the full responsibility of ensuring informed consent is obtained prior to medical procedures is not within the nursing scope of practice. Choice *C* is incorrect because preparation of blood products is primarily completed by blood bank staff. Choice *D* is incorrect because the responsibility for handwashing falls equally on all participants in direct patient care.

14. A: The ANA Code of Ethics provides guidance for performing nursing duties in an ethical manner. Choice *B* is not correct because the code does not define pay scales or tables for nursing compensation. Choice *C* is not correct since this is defined in ANA's Principles for Nurse Staffing, not the Code of Ethics. Choice *D* is incorrect since only the ethical considerations of nurses, not primary care providers, are covered.

15. D: The hands-on, teach-back method is the most effective of the four methods for teaching the patient this multi-step process. Choice *A* is incorrect because, while the patient should have written instructions to refer to, giving written instructions alone does not allow the nurse to observe or assess if the teaching was effective. Choice *B* is incorrect because, while a verbal teach-back method is helpful, it is not as good as the hands-on practice in Choice *D*. Choice *C* is incorrect because referring the patient to a video does not allow the nurse to assess whether the education has been effective.

16. A: Rapid reactions are often the result of infusing the fluid too quickly or using small hand veins when a larger vein should be used. These reactions can be avoided by adhering to the recommended administration instructions. First dose reactions occur after the first dose and may or may not occur after subsequent doses. Any patients that exhibit these reactions must be closely monitored for worsening reactions, so Choice *B* is incorrect. Providers are cautioned to initiate drug therapies at the lowest therapeutic dose to avoid early reactions; therefore, Choice *C* is incorrect. Intermediate reactions occur after multiple doses in susceptible individuals; therefore, Choice *D* is incorrect.

17. D: When interviewing patients, the best approach is to use a mix of closed- and open-ended questions to get a range of information; listen carefully to each answer and ask probing questions when necessary to clarify the information. Focusing only on closed-ended questions could prevent patients from sharing certain relevant information, so Choice *A* is incorrect. Using mainly open-ended questions could encourage patients to ramble excessively about irrelevant information, so Choice *B* is incorrect. Probing questions should be used when necessary to narrow down facts, but general questions are also useful to include, so Choice *C* is incorrect.

18. D: This team is now at the implementation stage of problem-solving because their team is actively using their possible solution by removing catheters within 24 hours of surgery. Choice *A* is incorrect because evaluation would be the next step in this process and would include the team seeing if this is an effective strategy in reducing UTIs. In this scenario, the nursing team has already identified a problem, in this case high UTI rates, and developed a possible solution of removing catheters earlier in the post-op period; therefore, Choices *B* and *C* are also incorrect.

19. D: The major premise of the Synergy Model states that synergy—optimum health—can only be achieved when agency resources and nursing competencies are congruent with the patient's needs. Family participation in the patient's care may improve outcomes, however, the synergy is related to the patient–nurse–healthcare agency triad.

20. B: Choice *B* is correct, as adding the company logo indicates that it is an official document endorsed by the organization. Prior to distributing to the public, it would require clearance from the organization's authorizing department, typically Public Affairs. Choice *A* would not specifically require authorization from the organization unless there was indication that the author was connected to the facility. Choices *C* and *D* may follow guidelines and rules set by the organization; however, it would have a lower need for permission to distribute than a company logo.

21. D: Although all options may be useful in helping the patient feel more comfortable with their colostomy, having the patient participate in a colostomy support group will help the patient learn more than just how to apply and remove the colostomy appliance. The patient can learn the struggles of other people with colostomies and how they manage them in their daily lives. Choices *A, B,* and *C* should be implemented to help the patient understand how to care for their ostomy, but having the support group will provide a different level of support and insight for the patient.

22. A: Multi-factorial authorization provides an additional layer of protection when accessing a network and is more secure than the other options. Choice *B* does add some security features; however, it is not as secure as multi-factor authorization. Choice *C* is incorrect since it does not add security to authorized network access. Guest wi-fi access is meant for internet access but should not allow the ability to login to the organization's network. Choice *D* is incorrect since using personally identifiable information within a password is a risk and opens an organization to possible access breaches.

23. C: Strategic plans are an ongoing and continuous process; therefore, Choice *C* is correct. Plans should be evaluated to determine effectiveness and whether new strategies or resources should be considered to accomplish the identified goals. Strategic plans should be regularly reviewed and updated as necessary to ensure the mission and vision of the organization are met.

24. A: Providing thorough explanations of continuing or changing care can help terminally ill patients and family members make the most informed decisions for themselves. Choice *B* is incorrect because although active treatments may help extend life, they may not be curative, and the patient could experience a worsening quality of life due to deteriorating health and side effects of treatment. Choice *C* is incorrect because the nurse and medical team should not make decisions for the patients or family members. The patient and family members should be encouraged to make their own decisions to help gain control and ensure their end-of-life care is within their preferences. Choice *D* is incorrect because giving a higher dose of an analgesic, even if prescribed, should be discussed with the patient and family first. Higher doses of analgesic may decrease a patient's awareness, feelings, and interactions with family, and may even speed up the dying process.

25. C: Having the group participate in a discussion regarding their personal asthma triggers and experiences will help enhance the education based on the group's experiences. Although Choices *A, B,* and *D* may be helpful, discussing personal experiences may be more beneficial overall to understanding how asthma triggers can be managed.

26. B: The nurse at the second level of clinical practice continuum understands that the patient's death may be an acceptable outcome based on the knowledge accumulated through engagement with the patient and family and expert assessment of the patient's progress. The level 1 nurse understands that the patient may possibly die, but the nurse does not comprehend that the death is inevitable or acceptable. According to the Synergy Model, experienced nurses possess skills in managing end-of-life care, which benefits both the patient and the family. This special caring practice not only acknowledges death as an acceptable outcome but consists of a plan of care to achieve that outcome in the best way possible. According to the model, death is initially viewed as an acceptable outcome at the second level of caring practices.

27. A: Peer review committees are responsible for evaluating the quality of care provided by their peers and determining appropriate actions when substandard care is identified. To ensure that the process is fair and unbiased, it is important for committee members to avoid conflicts of interest, including personal relationships with the nurse being reviewed. Choices *B* and *C* would compromise the integrity of the peer review process by creating a conflict of interest. Choice *D* is not the best course of action, as it still allows the nurse to participate in the discussion and influence the outcome of the committee's decision.

28. B: Virtual presentations that are recorded allow a participant to review the content in their own time. Choice *A* is incorrect since relying solely upon recorded virtual meetings prevents audience participation. Choices *C* and *D* are incorrect; virtual meetings may be set up to track attendance and require survey completion after an employee has viewed the content.

29. D. Perceiving is the missing key process in communication. The six key processes are thinking, encoding, transmitting the signal, perceiving, decoding, and understanding.

30. B: When patient-identifying information is shared via email, it must be encrypted. This protects messages and attachments from being accessed or read by an unauthorized party. Choice *A* is incorrect; while this option may increase the likelihood of being noticed and read by the intended party, it does not protect against a data breach or HIPAA violations. Choice *C* is incorrect, as sending emails within an organization does not have transient protection from being accessed. Choice *D* is incorrect, as both the content within the body of an email and any attachments may be compromised if not encrypted.

31. D: Nurses demonstrate professional competence because of a commitment to lifelong learning that is required for expert care of acutely ill patients. The remaining pairs each contain only a single element of the six elements of caring, compassion, confidence, and conscience.

32. D: In order to maintain professional accountability, the nursing staff should constantly monitor for changes to regulatory guidelines and recommendations. Subscribing to journals is a great way to stay informed of these changes. If the changes contradict the facility's policies or procedures, the nurse should have their manager review the impact.

33. D: One of the key principles of proper resource utilization is that each member of a care team, from the doctor in charge to the orderlies responsible for transporting a patient, should understand the treatments prescribed and their roles in that process as thoroughly as possible. For the nurse in this situation, proper resource utilization involves confirming with the doctor when a dosage seems inaccurate. It may be that the doctor incorrectly wrote the dosage or is prescribing that larger dose for a particular reason. By consulting with the doctor, the nurse is ensuring that resources are used properly and that the patient's treatment is as effective and efficient as possible. Therefore, the correct answer is Choice *D.* Although Choice *C* is correct in identifying that the nurse used proper resource utilization techniques, the reasoning is faulty—following proper resource utilization does not entail ensuring that minimal resources are expended on each patient. Instead, proper resource utilization is about ensuring that whatever resources are expended on a patient are effectively and efficiently contributing to the patient's treatment plan. Therefore, Choice *C* is incorrect. Choices *A* and *B* are incorrect because the nurse was practicing proper resource utilization.

34. D: The information indicates that the patient may be relatively stable, yet it is necessary to assess their ability to participate in the lesson for more than 15–20 minutes due to fatigue. Teaching-learning sessions of one hour or more will most likely be unproductive for this patient because of the limitations from fatigue. Teaching-learning sessions of one hour or more will most likely be unproductive for the patient with the identified Synergy Model score due to the limitations imposed by their multiple morbidities and moderately impaired resiliency. Literature from a nursing journal may or may not be appropriate to the patient's learning needs, however, simply providing printed information without additional instruction or discussion does not allow for assessment of the patient's comprehension of the information. The nurse caring for a patient in the acute care environment is responsible for assessing the patient's learning and initiating the necessary instruction. The teaching plan and the patient's progress will be reported to the community provider; however, the process should be started by the inpatient nursing staff.

35. B: Bruising is the most common initial assessment finding in child abuse because physical abuse is the most common form of abuse. Disruptive behavior and bed wetting may not be evident in the initial assessment. In addition, the abused child may or may not verbalize the details of the abuse. The professional development nurse also understands that the results of abuse are not all visible, and the reports of the parent or care provider are not always accurate. Therefore, Choices *A, C,* and *D* are incorrect.

36. D: In this case, the patient is blatantly ignoring Doug's attempts to provide patient education. Often, cancer patients who are overwhelmed with their health situation are not cooperative in discussing their treatment options and what to expect. Some simply do not want to know any more than they have to. In these cases, speaking with a close family member (such as a spouse) or caregiver can ensure that adequate patient education is still disseminated to someone who can benefit the patient with it. However, staff must make sure they are speaking with authorized family members or caregivers to ensure they are not violating any privacy laws.

37. A: Utilitarianism is defined as providing the greatest good for the greatest number, which can limit the autonomy of the individual. Therefore, Choice*s B, C* and *D* are incorrect.

38. D: In Rogers' Five-Stage Change Theory, communicating the reasons, content, and impact of the change to staff is the first step. Choice *A* is incorrect because it describes the last step in this approach. Choice *B* is incorrect because it best describes the third, or middle, step in this approach. Choice *C* is incorrect because it describes a top-down approach to the initiation of change, which is not reflected in Rogers' Five-Stage Change Theory.

39. A: Six Sigma is a method used by organizations to reduce inefficiencies and other cumbersome techniques that diminish profitability. It is a rationally organized process that is enlisted to constantly increase productive capacities by eliminating antiquated or outdated machinery and technology, making Choice *A* correct. Furthermore, Six Sigma may scrutinize opaque bureaucratic structures or wasteful practices that obstruct maximum profitability. Grounded in statistical analysis, this methodology exhibits a scientific and technical approach to solving critical problems facing an organization. Employee councils, feedback, and recruitment, Choices *B*, *C*, and *D*, are therefore not central to the purpose of Six Sigma.

40. B: A meta-analysis of randomized controlled trials is the highest level of evidence to support a practice change. Choice *A* is incorrect because a single trial is weaker evidence than multiple trials of the same subject. Choices *C* and *D* are incorrect because neither a prospective cohort study nor a meta-analysis of retrospective case-control studies is stronger evidence than a meta-analysis of RCTs.

41. C: Process champions can identify potential pitfalls during the brainstorming phase of process improvement. These individuals are team members with the administrative authority to allocate time and resources for a project.

42. A. Active listening is a key principle in communication for professional development nurses. Choices *B*, *C*, and *D* are incorrect. Ambiguity should be avoided in communication, and speaking quickly can cause information to be lost in conversation. Finally, multitasking is not possible when actively listening.

43. A: Six Sigma is a specific technique that works to improve business processes by implementing various tools and concepts to reduce errors and eliminate waste. Gap analysis, root cause analysis, and cause-and-effect diagrams (Choices *B*, *C*, and *D)* are incorrect because they are all tools that would be used to determine why goals were not achieved or if there was a discrepancy between the expected results and actual results.

44. B: Someone who allows their group to present ideas and solutions, but does not use the group's ideas, is said to be a consultative leader. In this leadership style, staff may feel that their input is being heard, even if it is not taken seriously into consideration. Choice *A* is incorrect because a democratic leader collaborates with their staff to hear ideas and solutions and will take those ideas into account when making their decision. Choice *C* is incorrect because participatory leadership is another name for democratic leadership and has the same meaning. Choice *D* is incorrect because in delegative leadership, similar to laissez-faire leadership, the leader is hands-off and assigns tasks and problems to their group to complete without the leader's instruction or input.

45. B: When data is initially collected for analysis, the first set of data points is considered the baseline. Choice *A* is incorrect since this is a compilation of similar data. Choice *C* is incorrect since this is data that is compared with other data to seek a mutual relationship. Choice *D* is incorrect since qualitative data refers to a characteristic, a quality, or an individual's experience.

46. D: A shared decision-making model is the process in which health professionals and patients work together to select tests and treatments and manage side effects based on clinical evidence as well as the patient's preferences. Choice *D* does not consider any discussion with the patient to determine if they feel the education thus far has been sufficient and, therefore, does not represent shared decision making. Choices *A*, *B*, and *C* show examples of shared decision making.

47. B: Presentation software allows the presenter to embed visuals, video, and other features that can add interest and increased understanding of the content being presented. Choice *A* is incorrect, as this benefit may be integrated into a learning management system. Choice *C* is incorrect; EHR integration provides easier access to medical records between different departments or organizations but is not a capability within presentation software. Choice *D* is incorrect; while using presentation software is likely to increase learner engagement, it would not be expected to increase attendance, as that is more often affected by external factors.

48. B: The four steps in systems thinking in order are react (to events), anticipate (patterns, trends, causes), design (identify the underlying structures and patterns of influence), and transform (change the beliefs and mental models).

49. C: A good rule of thumb when considering HPPD as a metric is that the more intensive and continuous care a patient or patient type requires, the higher the HPPD value for that ward will be. A psychiatric ward may have many patients living and existing more or less independently of healthcare professionals' direct intervention. Therefore, the correct answer is Choice *C*. The NICU, burn unit, and hospice care ward are all wards that care for high-risk patients who often require intensive, around-the-clock care.

50. B: Pivot tables are a tool within spreadsheets that allows large datasets, such as quality data, to be analyzed and reorganized to identify trends, spotlight drift or outliers, and compare metrics. Choice *A* is incorrect, as mail merge is a tool used to batch documents with personalized details that are pulled from a spreadsheet. Choice *C* is not the best answer, as there are a variety of charts and graphs available to be used within spreadsheets; however, when analyzing data for quality improvement, pivot tables are the most effective. Choice *D* is incorrect, as this option allows users to calculate values within a cell.

51. C: Referral of the case to the ethics committee, Choice *C*, will provide unbiased guidance on how to uphold the patient and family's wishes from the perspective of the law in that state. Choice *A* is incorrect, as it is best for the ethics committee to review the case and ensure the correct steps are followed. Choices *B* and *D* are unprofessional and will break trust with the family.

52. B: The first responder should verify that the person is choking and immediately call for help. Choice *A* is incorrect, as this could waste valuable time if the person's airway is compromised. Choice *C* is incorrect since this action may push a food bolus further into the airway. Choice *D* is not correct, as this would be completed after verifying choking, calling for help, and assisting the person into a standing position.

53. C. A professional development nurse should not create broad job descriptions, as this could be used to demonstrate that an employer did not hire a person with disabilities based on a job function that is not required. Options *A*, *B*, and *D* are ways that the professional development nurse should maintain compliance with the ADA.

54. B: There are a lot of concerns and misconceptions related to childhood immunizations. Having a group discussion will allow the nurse to answer questions and debunk misconceptions so parents can leave the informational group with better knowledge. Choice *A* would not be helpful as parents do not need to know the immunizations needed for their children; this is something that their primary care provider will monitor. The role of the parents is to bring their children for routine well-child and immunization visits. Choice *C* is also incorrect as this may not answer the parents' concerns. An informational video may be helpful to incorporate within the group, but it shouldn't be the only component. Choice *D* is incorrect since parents are not allowed to administer immunizations.

55. C: The Synergy Model identifies expert nursing practice as the level of nursing competency in which clinical reasoning becomes an integrated element in the process of clinical inquiry. According to the model, prior to that point, nurses are capable of performing at some level of clinical inquiry and may be able to use clinical reasoning in patient care, but the total integration of the two does not occur until the expert level of nursing practice.

56. D: Staff authority is a management system wherein supervisors are responsible for their areas of expertise. Employees would go to whichever supervisor is in charge of the area in which there is a problem. Line authority, Choice *A*, refers to a structure in which employees report to their direct supervisor only, and that supervisor will seek out other supervisors if the need arises. Team authority, Choice *B*, is usually task- or committee-based.

57. C: Editing job descriptions and job duties is not part of the purpose of a performance appraisal. Choices *A*, *B*, and *D* are incorrect. Assessing employee performance, developing an action plan for advancement, and encouraging continued development are all components that should be addressed during a performance appraisal.

58. D: Critical thinking skills are not provided through competency validation. Instead, this often comes from experience and thinking through processes. Choices *A*, *B*, and *C* are all provided by validating the competency of employees.

59. C: Professional development nurses should help non-cooperating employees find common ground to work together toward an end goal, Choice *C*, rather than separating or punishing employees (Choices *A* and *B*). If there are too many failed attempts at resolution, it may be necessary to escalate tactics. Additionally, allowing the employees to solve the issue autonomously, Choice D, is not an effective leadership strategy.

60. A: Spreadsheets provide meaningful options to analyze and present data, enabling the presenter to compare data and compile information in a single chart. Choices *B*, *C*, and *D* are options for displaying and presenting data that has already been compiled, but they do not have specific features to organize and visualize data.

61. A: A root cause analysis is a systematic review of a larger issue that is broken down into smaller issues in order to determine the single "root cause" behind the larger issue, making Choice *A* correct. The aim of the root cause analysis is to resolve the root cause in order to have a positive domino effect on larger issues. Root cause analysis does not involve funding or employee blaming, making Choices *B*, *C*, and *D* incorrect.

62. A: Team authority is a temporary structure lasting only as long as the task or committee is needed. Choices *B*, *C*, and *D* are all benefits of line authority, in which each employee has one immediate supervisor to whom they report.

63. A: Unit-based councils typically consist of nurses on a variety of shifts. Providing multiple virtual meetings allows nurses that work alternative shifts an opportunity to attend. Choice *B* is incorrect since in-person meetings encourage candid conversations better than virtual meetings. Choice *C* is incorrect, as employee productivity is increased when an individual's engagement with their work is high. Therefore, increased access to participation in unit-based councils would be expected to increase productivity. Choice *D* is incorrect since virtual meetings do not eliminate the need for unit-based councils to track participant attendance.

64. C: When preparing documents, it can be helpful to have a colleague or co-worker read and check the content for typos, grammatical errors, and overall readability. Choice *A* is incorrect, as language should be chosen based on the level of the reader to enhance their understanding. While it may be appropriate to use complex terminology in academic or high-level medical writings, word choice should be dependent on the target audience. Choice *B* is incorrect, as spellcheck is not always accurate, especially for medical terminology and acronyms. Additionally, spellcheck will only verify correct spelling rather than correct word choice.

Choice *D* is incorrect; while increasing the word count has the potential to increase clarity, it may also overcomplicate the intended message.

65. C: HPPD is a common metric used to assess effectiveness and efficiency of care provided. By dividing the total number of hours worked by a particular kind of medical professionals (e.g., nurses, physician's assistants, medical technicians) by the total number of patients seen at a particular healthcare center over the same 24-hour period, HPPD provides a healthcare provider with an average of how many hours were spent attending to each patient for that particular day. In other words, HPPD estimates how much time the average patient received medical attention by that group of workers over that 24-hour period. Therefore, the correct answer is Choice *C*. All of the other answer choices do not provide the correct interpretation of an HPPD value of 0.4.

66. B: The empirical-rational strategy assumes that individuals are, in general, rational and will follow a path that benefits them. This strategy to affect change works well when individuals are presented with the benefits that will be experienced by embracing a specific change.

67. B: According to the model, vulnerability refers to the presence of any stressor, actual or potential, that could adversely affect the patient's health. A history of smoking increases the patient's vulnerability to additional health alterations. Socioeconomic status and being married are related to resource availability, which refers to the availability of financial and emotional resources that are necessary to support the patient's recovery. The patient's active participation in the plan of care (Choice *D*) is considered to have a positive effect on care outcomes.

68. B: An organization's culture of civility must be rooted in its leadership. If employees sense that rules about workplace conduct do not apply to an organization's executives, or are applied inconsistently, standards of civil behavior are less likely to take hold throughout the organization. It is important to engage leaders from the C-suite (e.g., CEO, CFO, or COO) to lead by example, making Choice *B* correct. Choice *A* is not the best choice because some employees may prefer to keep their complaints confidential; experience with harassment may be personal and hurtful to share with a large audience. Choice *C* is not the best choice because, while guidance from the Department of Justice could be helpful, it is better to begin with leadership from inside the organization. Finally, while HR should be involved with all levels of this training, it is important to reach outside HR to leaders in other areas of the organization.

69. B: Having an organization-wide perspective can help promote systems thinking because it allows nurses to collaborate with more team members, define problems they see in healthcare, and implement solution strategies. Choices *A, C,* and *D* are incorrect because these characteristics are barriers to systems thinking. Instead, strong group dynamics, prospective thinking, and an organization-wide perspective should be used to encourage systems thinking.

70. D: Performance appraisals are completed on a set time frame (typically on an annual basis), but evaluation of performance issues can occur on an ongoing basis. Employee development, recognition of accomplishments, and determining training needs—Choices *A*, *B*, and *C*—are shared components of performance appraisals and regular evaluations.

71. C: In the Synergy Model, optimum patient care is achieved when the nurse facilitates communication and collaboration with the interdisciplinary team. The nurse possesses the clinical competence to anticipate the needs of the patient and respond appropriately by accessing the required system resources. Resiliency refers to the patient's potential for improved functional status. Creativity is not a characteristic of nursing care identified in the Synergy Model. The complexity of the patient's care needs is assessed according to the number of body systems that are involved.

72. B: Teaching staff the risks and prevention of phishing attempts is a best practice of cybersecurity and should be a fundamental part of any general IT education. Choice *A* is incorrect, as phishing is a form of cyber threat in which clickbait is sent to an email address with the intention of luring the receiver to open the email or click on a link; therefore, it is not part of clinical care. Choices *C* and *D* are incorrect, as phishing does not refer to a practice used during meetings or presentations.

73. A: The creation of goals happens in the outcome identification phase. The nurse recognizes that early ambulation is an expected outcome for a post-operative patient. The planning phase involves prescribing strategies to attain the goals, which have not yet been identified in this scenario; therefore, Choice *C* is incorrect. After the planning phase is completed, the nurse moves into the implementation phase, and the plan is carried out, which makes Choice *B* incorrect. Assessment is the first step in the nursing process, in which the nurse gathers necessary data and information. In this scenario, the assessment phase is not the active phase in place, making Choice *D* incorrect.

74. A: Patients who have difficulties with communication may exhibit frustration. The nurse should show empathy and support through nonverbal communication, which can include therapeutic touch, smile, or nodding for reassurance. Choice *B* is incorrect as restricting visitors reduces the patient's social support and can cause unnecessary distress. Choice *C* is also incorrect because even though the patient has communication difficulties, they do not have hearing difficulties; therefore, the nurse should not change how she speaks to the patient because they still understand what she is saying. Choice *D* is also incorrect since pretending like the patient is speaking normally and failing to acknowledge the difficulty can cause even more distress to the patient.

75. C: Virtual meetings provide attendees with the opportunity to participate regardless of their location, given that they have internet access and the required technology. Choice *A* is incorrect, as virtual meetings are not guaranteed to provide continuing education credits. Choice *B* is incorrect; while access to information is generally improved when it can be obtained from any location, this does not have a direct effect on cost savings to the attendee as the question states. Choice *D* is incorrect since decreased employee use of company cars would only provide cost savings to the organization.

76. B: Transformational leadership style and transactional leadership style are two distinct theories of leadership that share the same central premise: a leader's effectiveness is directly related to their team members' ability to feel satisfied and fulfilled in their work. The distinction between the two leadership styles lies in how they believe team members are most satisfied. With transactional leadership style, the belief is that team members are most satisfied when they can best sense the potential rewards associated with their good performance. On the other hand, transformational leadership style is more concerned with transforming team members' relationship to their work and the leader, with the hope of aligning their personal goals and development with that of the organization. Therefore, the correct answer is Choice *B*. Choice *A* is incorrect because there is nothing about either leadership style that is concerned with oversight for leaders and their decisions. Choice *C* is incorrect because it is an example of democratic leadership style thinking. Choice *D* is incorrect because it is an example of situational leadership style thinking.

77. B: In the psychomotor domain of Bloom's Taxonomy, a person who can follow detailed instructions to complete a practical task is at the guided response level. The complete steps of the psychomotor domain from least to most complex are perception, set, guided response, mechanism, complex overt response, adaptation, and origination. Choice *A* is incorrect because complex overt response is an expert level of proficiency where the learner can perform certain tasks proficiently without hesitation or separate guidance and instruction. Choice *C* is incorrect because mechanism is basic proficiency where the learner has some confidence, and psychomotor response has become habitual. Choice *D* is incorrect because perception is the most basic level where the learner is only aware of certain sensory clues and can guide their motor activity for completion of basic tasks.

78. B: Virtual presentations via Teams, Zoom, or other online applications can provide the opportunity to share information with a hybrid team. Choice *A* is incorrect; virtual meetings do not guarantee that patient care is uninterrupted, as care may also be virtual, such as in cases of telehealth. Choice *C* is incorrect since printing and mailing presentations to remote workers would not be effective or efficient. Choice *D* is incorrect; while virtual meetings are convenient, they are not meant to eliminate face-to-face meetings, which may be beneficial for providing emotional connection, relationship building, and a tangible experience.

79. C: The institution can support diversity by providing resources that satisfy cultural practices, such as dietary rules. Institutions also may provide interpreters, information sessions for employees, and accommodations for religious observances. Under normal circumstances, requiring employees to speak a second language would severely limit the pool of eligible employees and would not be an effective strategy; therefore, Choice *A* is incorrect. Educational programs should be provided for all employees and should not be limited to supervisory staff, so Choice *B* is wrong. Choice *D* is incorrect as offering alternative solutions to all requests for accommodation could be viewed as paternalistic and culturally insensitive. The institution is required to consider ways to satisfy all reasonable patient requests.

80. B: Use the acronym PASS to answer this question. The pin should always be pulled first. Choices *A, C,* and *D* are not listed in the correct order or with the correct wording. The correct directions and order are: Pull the pin, Aim at the base of the fire, Squeeze the handle, and Sweep from side to side.

81. C: Most leadership theories have as a central concept the idea that good leadership can be taught and understood by non-leaders. However, the Great Man Theory of Leadership rejects this notion outright, instead positing that good leadership traits and skills are innate and not transmittable. Therefore, the correct answer is Choice *C.* The other answer choices are all styles of leadership that demonstrate that good leadership is a teachable, transferable skill; therefore, they are all incorrect.

82. C: Encrypting data converts it into an unreadable form called ciphertext. This data is then reverted to the original form once accessed by the approved and authorized party through digital keys. Choices *A* and *B* are incorrect since these are not completed through data encryption; however, other IT tools are available to provide these functions. Choice *D* is incorrect, as data encryption is not a task that would be manually completed by an individual. Instead, it is a built-in feature to many computer programs and applications.

83. D: The three categories of notifiable diseases are outbreak, infectious, and noninfectious; therefore, Choices *A, B,* and *C* are incorrect.

84. D: Virtual meetings have the potential to encourage communication between employees from many different fields and backgrounds, as chat is an option for attendees that would normally not feel comfortable speaking up in a different setting. Choices *A, B,* and *C* provide barriers to communication.

85. D. Reflective communication is described as actively listening and restating the message in one's own words. Choices *A*, *B*, and *C* are incorrect. Engaging communication can be described as actively involving the audience through enthusiasm, imagery, or humor. Two-way communication occurs when one person communicates a message, and the recipient confirms with a response. Interviewing is described as questioning, listening, and speaking.

86. A: Evidence is usually graded on a letter scale, with A being the highest level of evidence. The type of research with the highest level of evidence is a meta-analysis. Choice *B* is incorrect because a randomized-control trial is the second highest level of evidence, level B. Choices *C* and *D* are incorrect because integrative interviews and cohort studies have a moderate level of evidence and are both level C.

87. C: An event that requires intervention to prevent permanent damage is considered to be an adverse drug reaction (ADR) by the FDA. Intractable vomiting following chemotherapy is identified as an expected side effect of the treatment and is not reportable as an ADR; therefore, Choice *A* is incorrect. Harmful self-inflicted behaviors are not identified as ADRs by the FDA; therefore, Choice *B* is incorrect. The American Society of Healthcare Pharmacists has proposed that any unexpected or undesired outcome that requires the alteration of the drug dosage should be defined as an ADR. However, currently, the FDA defines the outcomes more narrowly. Therefore, Choice *D* is incorrect.

88. C: A leader who believes her team members work best with clear-cut incentives and rewards can best be described as having a transactional leadership style. In a transactional leadership style, the main focus is the transactional aspect of the relationship between leader and team member. The belief is that team members are most likely to find satisfaction with their own work when the leader is clear about expectations and incentives. Therefore, the correct answer is Choice *C.* All of the other answer choices describe distinct styles of leadership that are not in line with the scenario described.

89. B: By using a spreadsheet table, the owner can track attendance, calculate CE credits earned, and create formulas that indicate if the mandatory expectations are being met. This information may be filtered based on various criteria, such as name, department, number of credits still required, and deficiencies, so that follow-up can occur to ensure compliance. Choices *A, C,* and *D* are not the best options, as they do not have the capabilities to sort and filter data needed for tracking purposes.

90. D: This option can help with outreach to underserved communities since the fairs will be held outside of the clinic. Choice *A* does not have any benefit to the underserved communities, making this choice incorrect. Choice *B* is also incorrect as this only benefits the clinic's patients and not underserved communities that may not receive regular healthcare. Choice *C* is incorrect as this also does not provide appropriate outreach to individuals outside of the clinic.

91. B: Individual consideration refers to a transformational leader's ability to serve as a direct mentor to their team members. Rather than merely engaging in a transactional relationship, individual consideration asks that leaders take a more involved role in their team members' work lives and goals. By doing so, the hope is that each team member feels listened to and prioritized and is consequently more likely to put their best effort in at work. Therefore, the correct answer is Choice *B.* All of the other answer choices are different components of transformational leadership style with distinct actions and mentalities.

92. C: The Fishbone Diagram is a tool that seeks to analyze the primary causes of a problem. Ultimately, the diagram engages problems and investigates remedial efforts for improvement. In a group formation, a consensus is gathered to identify possible causes, such as employee performance, outdated technology, inefficient methods of production, or environmental implications. By isolating each factor, the diagram details organizational procedure to scientifically diagnose potential inefficiencies.

93. C: Individual patient identifiers are necessary to provide treatment of the patient and avoid progression of the disease. Therefore, Choices *A, B,* and *D* are incorrect.

94. C: The National Patient Safety Goals are an initiative of the Joint Commission.

95. A: An algorithm provides guidance for staff to autonomously respond to an emergent situation. Choice *B* is incorrect since this would not solve the issue. Choice *C* is incorrect; beyond Basic Life Support (BLS) training, development of an algorithm is also needed. Choice *D* is incorrect; although quizzing staff may reveal their base level of knowledge, education on the policy and appropriate response would improve staff knowledge of emergent response.

96. D: When used to implement evidenced based practice, clinical inquiry can result in replacing an outdated, even counter-productive nursing intervention with an intervention that effectively addresses the needs of the patient. Matching patient needs with nursing competencies means that professional nurses are responsible for challenging all nursing interventions to be sure that they represent current best practice standards. As innovators, nurses are in the best position to research, implement, and evaluate alternative care practices.

97. D: Adobe Photoshop is a desktop application that has image- and video-editing capabilities. Choices *A* and *B* are suited for creating slide decks or slideshow presentations where altered images may be added. Choice *C* is incorrect, as this online-based presentation program provides an interactive alternative to slide deck presentations.

98. B: Surveillance case definitions serve as the framework for the designation of reportable diseases. The remaining choices are not associated with this process; therefore, Choices *A, C,* and *D* are incorrect.

99. C: Since health information is dynamic and can change based on research and current best practice, the document should be regularly assessed and updated to ensure the content is accurate. Choice *A* is incorrect, as archiving puts the document in a state that is not easily accessible. This would be appropriate for inactive documents being kept for future reference. Choice *B* is incorrect; if the education is meant to be for the public, the access should not be restricted. Emailing, rather than posting on a public forum, would be more appropriate if the document is only meant to be shared with a specific group. Choice *D* is incorrect, as AI may be inaccurate and should not be relied upon for verifying health information.

100. C: The nurse should acknowledge the child's feelings and address their concerns to provide caring and compassionate care. By explaining things in a way that the child can understand, their anxiety may decrease. Choice *A* is incorrect as this may cause increased anxiety since the child might not have any idea of what is going on. Choice *B* is also incorrect as this doesn't represent compassionate and therapeutic care—it does not address the child's concerns. Choice *D*, utilizing diversion techniques, may be helpful to decrease the child's anxiety temporarily, but it will not address the root cause of their anxiety regarding the surgery.

101. A: The "S" of a SMART goal is *specific*, not *standard*. Choices *B*, *C*, and *D* are all terms used to describe a SMART goal.

102. B: Team authority is a structure used to manage particular tasks or committees. While Albert does report the team's findings to his immediate supervisor, suggesting line authority (Choice *A*), Albert is in charge of his committee. Choice *D* refers to an organizational structure in which employees report to the supervisors of whichever department is having the issue.

103. C: A leader who is not particularly involved in the decision-making process of their teammates may be described as having a laissez-faire leadership style. Under the philosophy of laissez-faire leadership style, team members work best when supervised least because each member knows their own strengths and weaknesses and does not feel hampered by the expectations of the leader. Therefore, the correct answer is Choice *C.* All of the other answer choices describe separate and distinct styles of leadership and do not align with the scenario described.

104. C: In order to effectively manage change with the empirical-rational strategy, it is important to incentivize the change. If employees undergo a change but understand how it can positively impact them, they are more likely to accept it and agree with it. While providing lunch, communication, and education are important (Choices *A*, *B*, and *D*), incentives increase the success rate of change.

105. B: Systems thinking uses cognitive mapping, Choice *B*, to represent physical locations. Reviewing areas where each department connects to others can help identify more points of interaction that contribute to incidents. A centrist approach, scorecards, and technology to drive ideas, Choices *A*, *C*, and *D*, are not central to systems thinking.

106. B: Elias is choosing to further his education, which is a component of lifelong learning. While this may lead to promotion, specializing in a particular field of nursing, or work-life balance, pursuing an advanced degree is directly related to maintaining competence in his field. Nurses should expect to continue their education throughout the course of their careers, as technology, regulations, and other external factors influence the shape of the industry.

107. C: Patients who prefer to use diagrams, visual aids, charts, and videos are likely visual learners. The four types of learning styles are visual, auditory, reader/writer, and kinesthetic. Choice *A* is incorrect because auditory learners prefer to learn through listening and may benefit from lectures, discussion groups, and audiotapes. Choice *B* is incorrect because reader learners, also called reader/writer learners, prefer to learn through handouts, written instruction, and taking their own notes. Choice *D* is incorrect because kinesthetic learners prefer hands-on learning where they can physically hold the equipment or explore the teachings in a tactile manner. Patients may prefer one or a combination of multiple styles of learning. The nurse should be able to assess the styles and tailor the teaching approaches to meet these preferences.

108. C: Since the hepatitis B vaccine became available in 1982, risk of healthcare-associated hepatitis B among caregivers in medical facilities has been significantly reduced. Use of PPE and environmental controls also help reduce risk. Choice *A* is incorrect because screenings are done for TB, not hepatitis B. Choice *B* is incorrect because not every previous work experience requires hepatitis B immunization. A "catch-up" period is advisable to ensure adequate staffing rather than refusing to hire unimmunized individuals. Choice *D* is incorrect. Although seven days is the minimum duration of time that hepatitis B pathogens can survive outside of a host, once exposed, there is no guarantee that this action will prevent the care provider from contracting the disease.

109. C: Choice *C* provokes the nurse to prioritize diagnoses while developing a nursing plan and setting goals. Choice *A* involves a review of subjective and objective data. Choice *B* involves interpreting signs and symptoms to identify the patient's needs. Choice *D* involves providing patient education and carrying out procedures.

110. C: The most commonly reported form of elder abuse in community-dwelling individuals is psychological abuse. The remaining forms of abuse are less likely in this population.

111. C: The most common reason for providers to not report elder abuse is concern about malpractice claims by the patient's family. The remaining choices are not identified as reasons for non-reporting of abuse. Therefore, Choices *A, B*, and *D* are incorrect.

112. B: Email makes it easy to get information to a lot of people very quickly. However, this communication method can result in employees suffering from "information overload" from too many emails. The intranet, Choice *A*, has the benefit of no risk of important information being accessed by someone outside the organization. Intranets can be effective at communicating important ongoing information about the company, such as policies and procedures. Newsletters, Choice *C*, can provide a variety of information and have the potential to do so in an engaging and welcoming manner. However, newsletters can be labor-intensive. Finally, word-of-mouth, Choice *D*, can quickly spread information throughout a group of people.

However, information can become muddled, misinterpreted, and unrecognizable as it is passed from person to person.

113. D: For systems thinking according to the AACN Synergy Model, a nurse who has a deep understanding of community resources outside of themselves and can actively promote these to assist in a patient's care and recovery is at the highest level of systems thinking, level 5. Choice A is incorrect because a nurse at level 1 systems thinking is only able to offer themself as a resource and does not know or offer outside resources. Choice *B* is incorrect because a nurse at level 3 systems thinking can look for external resources and help for a patient, but may not have an expert understanding. Choice *C* is incorrect because level 4 is not one of the levels of systems thinking.

114. A: A cost-benefit analysis is used in the Lean Six Sigma methodology to determine the true costs of a potential solution, as compared to the actual benefits. Choices *B*, *C*, and *D* are not goals of a cost-benefit analysis.

115. B: The goal is to assimilate all the ideas into a strategic plan that prioritizes opportunities for improvement and amends all processes associated with changes, including any process flows and job aids. Choice *A*, visually analyzing team members' performance, may come before this, while Choice *C*, implementing strategies, would come after.

116. C: The technology-innovation strategy is not a strategy for managing change, making Choice *C* incorrect. The text *The Planning of Change* outlines three strategies for managing change: normative-reductive, power-coercive, and empirical-rational, Choices *A*, *B*, and *D* respectively.

117. D: The five rights of delegation are right task, right circumstance, right person, right direction, and right supervision. If the nurse is unsure if a task falls within these guidelines, they should not delegate that task and should check their facility policy for future delegation. When the nurse is delegating a task to unlicensed assistive personnel, they must make sure they include the five rights of delegation for the safety of the patient as well as coverage for their own license. Choices *A, B,* and *C* are incorrect because they do not correctly outline the five rights of delegation.

118. C: The Health Information Portability and Accountability Act was enacted in 1996 to protect the privacy and security of patient health information. Choice *A* is the federal agency that oversees safe working conditions. Choice *B* protects the type of access that is allowed for educational records and information. Choice *D* was established in 1990 to protect discrimination against individuals based on disability.

119. C: Nurses must acknowledge their own biases and recognize that those biases will affect their ability to provide culturally sensitive care. Standard protocols related to cultural beliefs and practices are an imperfect solution to the problem of culturally sensitive care because they are not individualized to the specific patient. Meeting the needs of the largest group in a population generally means that the cultural needs of the minority groups within the population are not met. As previously stated, culturally competent care results when caregivers first consider their own biases and the possible effect of those beliefs on patient care. If nurses base their care only on their own beliefs, the patient's beliefs and practices will be ignored.

120. C: Using "you" statements may place needless blame and pressure on the patient or learner. In the case of disagreement and communication, it is better for the nurse to use "I" statements to help them take responsibility for both ideas and feelings to help move a conversation forward. Choices *A, B,* and *D* are incorrect because these are encouraged communication tactics in successful assertive communication.

121. A: The CDC and the World Health Organization constantly review and update recommendations of risk reduction measures based on the latest scientific data; therefore, conducting research for a better answer is the best approach. Choice *B* is incorrect because entirely stopping any previous CDC recommendation is not the best answer. Choice *C* is incorrect because hand sanitizer will not remove the airborne infectious particles launched by the cough into the air that others are breathing. Choice *D* is incorrect because although researching other facilities may reveal shared challenges, this type of research will not always provide a solution for improvement in risk reduction measures.

122. D: According to the Joint Commission, "An organization can have an unannounced survey between 18 and 36 months after its previous full survey."

123. B. Backward communication is not a type of managerial communication. Choices *A, C,* and *D* represent different types of managerial communication.

124. B: The professional development nurse can specifically alleviate employees' fears and concerns about reporting unethical behavior and possible retaliation by providing them with a confidential and/or anonymous reporting method. This will protect their identity while still allowing for a proper and thorough investigation to occur. Although Choices *A, C,* and *D* are all appropriate actions to ensure a robust policy that is compliant with the law and understood by employees, these actions may not specifically address employees' concerns about making a report.

125. D: Since most of the participants are over 50 years old and the treatment is for all adults over 18 years old, these participants do not accurately reflect the population for which the vaccine is intended. This can lead to skewed results due to a selection bias, a bias that comes from study participants not being reflective of the true population. Choice *A* is incorrect because reporting bias comes from under-reporting or over-reporting certain characteristics or variables to skew results. Choice *B* is incorrect because recall bias is when participants are not able to accurately or completely remember information that is asked in a study. Choice *C* is incorrect because healthy participant bias is when someone is more likely to participate in a medical study if they are already careful and considerate about their health.

Practice Test #3

To keep the size of this book manageable, save paper, and provide a digital test-taking experience, the 3rd practice test can be found online. Scan the QR code or go to this link to access it:

testprepbooks.com/online387/npd

SCAN ME

The first time you access the test, you will need to register as a "new user" and verify your email address.

If you have any issues, please email support@testprepbooks.com

Dear Nursing Professional Development Test Taker,

Thank you for purchasing this study guide for your Nursing exam. We hope that we exceeded your expectations.

Our goal in creating this study guide was to cover all of the topics that you will see on the test. We also strove to make our practice questions as similar as possible to what you will encounter on test day. With that being said, if you found something that you feel was not up to your standards, please send us an email and let us know.

We would also like to let you know about other books in our catalog that may interest you.

CNOR

amazon.com/dp/1637753004

Medical Surgical Nurse

amazon.com/dp/1637754647

We have study guides and flashcards in a wide variety of fields. If the one you are looking for isn't listed above, then try searching for it on Amazon or send us an email.

Thanks Again and Happy Testing!
Product Development Team
support@testprepbooks.com

Online Resources & Audiobook

Included with your purchase are multiple online resources. This includes the practice tests in an interactive format and this book in audiobook format. There is also a convenient study timer to help you manage your time.

Scan the QR code or go to this link to access this content:

testprepbooks.com/online387/npd

SCAN ME

The first time you access the page, you will need to register as a "new user" and verify your email address.

If you have any issues, please email support@testprepbooks.com.

Thank you for letting us be a part of your studying journey!